AF397649

Access Surgery

Access Surgery

*Proceedings of the International Congress on Access Surgery,
held at The University of Limburg, Maastricht,
on 22–24 April 1982*

**A review of current techniques for vascular access for
Haemodialysis,
Chemotherapy and
Total parenteral nutrition**

Edited by

Gauke Kootstra, MD, PhD,

*Professor of Surgery,
University of Limburg, Hospital St. Annadal,
Maastricht, The Netherlands*

and

Paul J. G. Jörning, MD, PhD,

*Surgeon,
University of Limburg, Hospital St. Annadal,
Maastricht, The Netherlands*

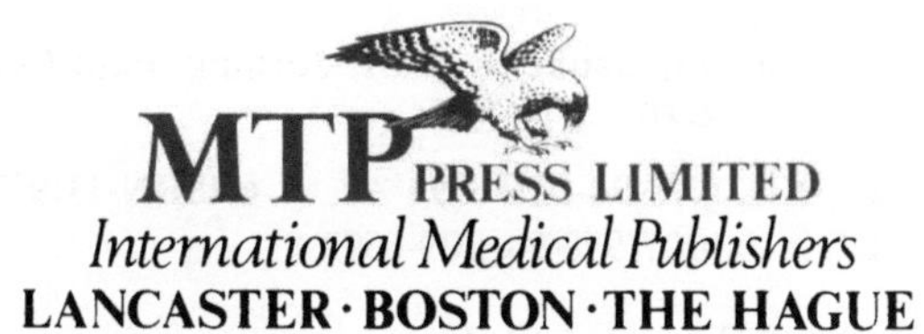

MTP PRESS LIMITED
International Medical Publishers
LANCASTER · BOSTON · THE HAGUE

Published by
MTP Press Limited
Falcon House
Lancaster, England

British Library Cataloguing in Publication Data

Access surgery.
   1. Surgery—Congresses
   I. Kootstra, Gauke   II. Jörning, Paul J.G.
   617   RD1

   ISBN-13:978-94-009-6594-2   e-ISBN-13:978-94-009-6592-8
   DOI: 10.1007/978-94-009-6592-8

Butler & Tanner Ltd, Frome and London

Contents

CONTENTS

List of Contributors

D. ABET
C.H.U.
Hôpital Nord
Service de Néphrologie
80000 Amiens
France

G. F. ADAMI
Università di Genova
Patologia Chirurgica I
Ospedale S. Martino
16132 Genova
Italy

T. AGISHI
Tokyo Women's Medical College
Kidney Centre
10 Kawada-cha Shinjuku-ku
162 Tokyo
Japan

J. AGOSTI
Clinica Nefrológica Bilbaina
Gordóniz 9
Bilbao
Spain

LINDA C. AMAN
Henry Ford Hospital
2799 W. Grand Blvd
48202 Detroit
USA

M. AMMATUNA
Anesthesiology
Istituto Nazionale Tumori
Via Venezian
20133 Milano
Italy

K. AMPLATZ
University of Minnesota Hospitals
Dept. of Surgery and Radiology
Box 263 Mayo
55455 Minneapolis
USA

R. ANDERSEN
Surgery
Hennepin County Medical Center
701 Park Avenue
55415 Minneapolis
USA

T. ANDERSSON
Central County Hospital
S-701 85 Örebro
Sweden

R. ARA
Tokyo Women's Medical College
Kidney Centre
10 Kawada-cha Shinjuku-ku
162 Tokyo
Japan

J. M. VAN BAALEN
Catharina Hospital
Dept. of Surgery
Michelangelolaan 2
5623 EJ Eindhoven
The Netherlands

U. BACIGALUPO
Università di Genova
Patologia Chirurgica I
Viale Benedetto XV
16132 Genova
Italy

R. BAMBAUER
Med. Universitätsklinik
Dept. of Nephrology
D-6650 Homburg
Germany

J. BANCEWICZ
Hope Hospital
Eccles Old Road
M6 8HD Salford
UK

ACCESS SURGERY

H. W. M. BARENBRUG
University Hospital
Dept. of Surgery
Rijnsburgerweg 10
2333 AA Leiden
The Netherlands

A. D. BARNES
Queen Elizabeth Hospital
Renal Unit
Birmingham
UK

N. M. A. BAX
Wilhelmina Children's Hospital
Dept. of Surgery
Nieuwe Gracht 137
3512 LK Utrecht
The Netherlands

J. BECART
97 Ave. Albert 1er
92500 Rueil Malmaison
France

B. K. BEGEMAN
University Hospital
Oostersingel 59
9713 EZ Groningen
The Netherlands

P. R. F. BELL
Dept. of Surgery
University of Leicester
Leicester Royal Infirmary
Leicester
UK

V. BELWE
J.W. Goethe Universität
St. Markus Krankenhaus
W. Epsteinstrasse 2
D-6000 Frankfurt/Main
Germany

F. O. BELZER
University of Wisconsin
Dept. of Surgery
600 Highland Avenue
53792 Madison
USA

Ø. BENTDAL
The National Hospital
Dept. of Surgery
Pilestredet 32
Oslo 1
Norway

L. BERARDINELLI
Ospedale Policlinico
Dept. of Vascular Surgery and Kidney
Transplantation
Via F. Sforza 35
20122 Milano
Italy

C. BERETTA
Ospedale Policlinico
Dept. of Vascular Surgery and Kidney
Transplantation
Via F. Sforza 35
20122 Milano
Italy

J. H. BERGMEIJER
Sophia Children's Hospital
Dept. of Surgery
Gordelweg 160
3038 GE Rotterdam
The Netherlands

J. F. BERNARD
Hôpital Beaujon
Service d'Hématologie
92210 Clichy
France

J. R. BEUKHOF
University Hospital
Oostersingel 59
9713 EZ Groningen
The Netherlands

N. BILGIN
Hacettepe University Hospital
Transplantation Unit
Ankara
Turkey

M. BITKER
Hôpital de la Pitié
Dept. of Nephrology and Urology
Bd de l'hôpital
75013 Paris
France

D. BLANCHARD
Broussais Hospital
Dept. of Cardiovascular Radiology
96 Rue Didot
75014 Paris
France

LIST OF CONTRIBUTORS

E. BLOOM
C.H.R. Purpan
Chirurgie Sud
31059 Toulouse Cedex
France

J. H. van BOCKEL
Academisch Ziekenhuis Leiden
Heelkundige Kliniek
Rijnsburgerweg 10
2333 AA Leiden
The Netherlands

J. BOMMER
University of Heidelberg
Bergheimerstrasse 58
D-6900 Heidelberg
Germany

U. BONALUMI
Università di Genova
Patologia Chirurgica I
Ospedale S. Martino
16132 Genova
Italy

H. BONDEVIK
The National Hospital
Dept. of Surgery
Pilestredet 32
Oslo 1
Norway

G. BONFANTI
Clincial Oncology
Istituto Nazionale Tumori
Via Venezian
20133 Milano
Italy

PH. BONNAUD
Hôpital Necker
Clinique Urologique
161 Rue de Sèvres
75015 Paris
France

F. BORCHARD
University of Düsseldorf
Dept. of Pathology
Moorenstrasse
D-4000 Dusseldorf
Germany

D. BOUGLÉ
Hôpital des Enfants Malades
149 Rue de Sèvres
75 730 Paris Cedex 15
France

P. BOURQUELOT
Deptartment of Urology
Hôpital St. Joseph
7 rue Pierre Larousse
75674 Paris Cedex 14
France

J. M. BOUTON
Brugmann Univ. Hospital
Dept. of Pediatric Surgery
van Gehuchtenplein 4
B-1020 Brussels
Belgium

F. BOZZETTI
Clinical Oncology G
Istituto Nazionale Tumori
Via Venezian
20133 Milano
Italy

M. BRODIN
Central County Hospital
S-701 85 Örebro
Sweden

M. E. DE BROE
University of Antwerp
Dept. of Nephrol.-Hypertension
B-2520 Antwerp
Belgium

C. M. A. BRUYNINCKX
St. Joseph Hospital
Dept. of Surgery
Aalsterweg 259
5600 RC Eindhoven
The Netherlands

P. BUCHMANN
University Hospital
Surgical Clinic A
Ramistrasse 100
8091 Zürich
Switzerland

J. A. C. BUCKELS
Queen Elizabeth Hospital
Renal Unit
Birmingham
UK

J. BURNAY
C.H.U.
Hôpital Nord
Service de Néphrologie
80000 Amiens
France

F. G. M. BUSKENS
University of Nijmegen
Dept. of Thoracic/Cardiovascular Surgery
Geert Grooteplein 10
6500 HB Nijmegen
The Netherlands

KOCO CAKALAROSKI
Medical Faculty
Clinic of Nephrology
Vodnjanska 17
91000 Skopje
Yugoslavia

R. CANAL
Ospedale Policlinico
Dept. of Vascular Surgery and Kidney
Transplantation
Via F. Sforza 35
20122 Milano
Italy

W. R. CASTENADA-ZUNIGA
University of Minnesota Hospitals
Dept. of Surgery and Radiology
Box 263 Mayo
55455 Minneapolis
USA

F. CASTRO
Hospital N. S. Esperanza
Mariano Cubi 155
21 Barcelona
Spain

L. CATIZONE
M. Malpighi Hospital
Dept. of Nephrology and Dialysis
P. Palagi 9
40138 Bologna
Italy

C. CAVICCHIONI
Catholic University
Inst. of Surgical Pathology
Largo A. Gemelli
00168 Roma
Italy

F. CERIATI
Catholic University
Inst. of Surgical Pathology
Largo A. Gemelli
00168 Roma
Italy

J. A. CHACON
Clinical Nefrologica
S. Cirurgia Vascular
Gordoniz 9
Bilbao
Spain

D. CIVALLERI
Università di Genova
Patologia Chirurgica I
Ospedale S. Martino
16132 Genova
Italy

M. de CLIPPELE
University Hospital
Renal Division
De Pintelaan 185
B-9000 Gent
Belgium

B. COEVOET
C.H.U.
Hôpital Nord
Service de Néphrologie
80000 Amiens
France

G. A. COLES
Cardiff Royal Infirmary
Institute of Renal Disease
Newport Road
Cardiff, S. Wales
UK

A. J. COLLINS
Medicine
Regional Kidney Disease Program
701 Park Avenue
55415 Minneapolis
USA

L. COSENTINO
Renal Systems Inc.
14905 28th Avenue
Plymouth MN55441
USA

J. L. COY
97 Ave. Albert 1er
92500 Rueil Malmaison
France

A. De CUBBER
Department of Medicine
Service of Nephrology
Akademisch Ziekenhuis
De Pintelaan 185
B-9000 Gent
Belgium

LIST OF CONTRIBUTORS

A. DANA
Hôpital Necker
161 Rue de Sèvres
75 730 Paris Cedex 15
France

A. E. DAUL
Department of Renal and Hypertensive
Diseases
Medical Clinic and Policlinic
Universitätsklinikum
D43 Essen
West Germany

F. DAVIES
Cardiff Royal Infirmary
Institute of Renal Disease
Newport Road
Cardiff, S. Wales
UK

E. DECHELETTE
C.H.U.R.
Dept. of Nephrology
and Vascular Surgery
Grenoble
France

P. DECONINCK
Brugmann Univ. Hospital
Dept. of Pediatric Surgery
van Gehuchtenplein 4
B-1020 Brussels
Belgium

M. DECURTINS
University Hospital
Surgical Clinic A
Rämistrasse 100
8091 Zürich
Switzerland

R. DEREERE
Brugmann Univ. Hospital
Dept. of Pediatric Surgery
van Gehuchtenplein 4
B-1020 Brussels
Belgium

R. J. van DET
Surgery
Hospital Leyenburg
2504 LN The Hague
The Netherlands

F. DIDERICH
St. Franciscus Hospital
Dept. of Surgery
Kleiweg 500
3045 PM Rotterdam
The Netherlands

R. A. DONALDSON
Belfast City Hospital
Renal Unit
Lisburn Road
BT9 7AB Belfast
N. Ireland

G. DONGRADI
97 Ave. Albert 1er
92500 Rueil Malmaison
France

J. F. DOUGLAS
Belfast City Hospital
Renal Unit
Lisburn Road
BT9 7AB Belfast
N. Ireland

J. DRINOVEC
University Medical Centre
Dialysis Centre
Zaloska 7
61000 Ljubljana
Yugoslavia

T. DRUËKE
Hôpital Saint Joseph
7 Rue Pierre Larousse
75 730 Paris Cedex 15
France

M. ELSENER
C.H.U.R.
Dept. of Nephrology and Vascular Surgery
Grenoble
France

M. M. ELSEVIERS
University of Antwerp
Dept. of Nephrol.-Hypertension
B-2520 Antwerp
Belgium

F. VAN ELST
Stuivenberg Hospital
Lge Beeldekensstraat
Antwerp
Belgium

ACCESS SURGERY

L. G. J. ENGELS
University Hospital
Dept. of Internal Medicine
Geert Grooteplein 8
6500 HB Nijmegen
The Netherlands

H. ERASMI
Deptartment of Surgery
Kreislauflabor
Altbau, Haus 6
University Hospital of Cologne
Josef-Stelzmann Strasse 9
5000 Köln 41
West Germany

B. ESKUBI
Clinica Nefrologica
S. Cirurgia Vascular
Gordoniz 9
Bilbao
Spain

E. degli ESPOSTI
M. Malpighi Hospital
Dept. of Nephrology and Dialysis
P. Palagi 9
40138 Bologna
Italy

J. EVERS
Medizin. Klinik I
Ostmerheimstrasse 200
D-5000 Köln-Merheim
Germany

M. Y. EZZIBDEH
Queen Elizabeth Hospital
Renal Unit
Birmingham
UK

A. FARINELLI
Renal Unit
Arcispedale
S. Anna U.S.L. 31
44100 Ferrara
Italy

P. FAUCHALD
The National Hospital
Dept. of Surgery
Pilestredet 32
Oslo 1
Norway

Z. FEDJELLI
Hôpital Necker
161 Rue de Sèvres
75 730 Paris Cedex 15
France

D. FERLUGA
University Medical Centre
Dialysis Centre
Zaloska 7
61000 Ljubljana
Yugoslavia

A. FLATMARK
The National Hospital
Dept. of Surgery
Pilestredet 32
Oslo 1
Norway

J. A. FLENDRIG
Catharina Hospital
Dept. of Internal Medicine
Michelangelolaan 2
5623 EJ Eindhoven
The Netherlands

S. FLOREZ
Clinica Nefrológica Bilbaina
Gordóniz 9
Bilbao
Spain

T. C. FLYNN
Department of Surgery
The University of Texas Health Science
Center—Houston
6431 Fannin Suite MSMB 4.284
Houston, Texas 77030
USA

M. FORET
C.H.U.R.
Dept. of Nephrology and Vascular Surgery
Grenoble
France

B. FORSBERG
University Hospital
Dept. of Nephrology
221 85 Lund
Sweden

L. FORSBERG
University Hospital
Dept. of Diagnostic Radiology
221 85 Lund
Sweden

LIST OF CONTRIBUTORS

A. FOURNIER
Hôpital Saint Joseph
7 Rue Pierre Larousse
75674 Paris Cedex 14
France

D. M. A. FRANCIS
Royal Victoria Infirmary
Dept. of Surgery
NE1 4LP Newcastle upon Tyne
UK

P. FRANTZ
Hôpital de la Pitié
Dept. of Nephrology and Urology
Bd de l'hôpital
75013 Paris
France

J. F. DE FREMONT
C.H.U.
Hôpital Nord
Service de Néphrologie
80000 Amiens
France

J. L. GALLEGO
Hôpital de la Pitie
Dept. of Urology and Nephrology
83 Bd de l'hôpital
75013 Paris
France

J. GARCIA-ALONSO
Clinica Nefrológica
S. Cirurgia Vascular
Gordoniz 9
Bilbao
Spain

A. GARCIA-ALFAGEME
Clinica Nefrológica
S. Cirurgia Vascular
Gordoniz 9
Bilbao
Spain

J. C. GAUX
Broussais Hospital
Dept. of Cardiovascular Radiology
96 Rue Didot
75014 Paris
France

M. J. C. VAN GEMERT
St. Joseph Hospital
Dept. of Medical Technology
Aalsterweg 259
5600 RC Eindhoven
The Netherlands

M. GEORGIEFF
Inst. Anästhesiologie/Reanimation
Chirurgische Klinik
Theoder Kutzer Ufer
D-6800 Mannheim
Germany

P. G. G. GERLAG
St. Joseph Hospital
Dept. of Internal Medicine
Aalsterweg 259
5600 ML Eindhoven
The Netherlands

S. GEROULANDS
Surgical Clinic
University Hospital
Rämistrasse 100
CH-8091 Zürich
Switzerland

J. GERSTOFT
Hvidovre Hospital
Dept. of Nephrology
2650 Hvidovre
Denmark

J. A. VAN GERWEN
St. Joseph Hospital
Dept. of Medical Technology
Aalsterweg 259
5600 RC Eindhoven
The Netherlands

E. GIANETTA
Università di Genova
Patologia Chirurgica I
Ospedale S. Martino
16132 Genova
Italy

J. F. GILLETTE
Centre René Huguenin
de Lutte contre le Cancer
5 Rue Gaston Latouche
92211 Saint-Cloud
France

G. GO
University Hospital
Oostersingel 59
9713 EZ Groningen
The Netherlands

E. VAN GOGH
University Hospital
Oostersingel 59
9713 EZ Groningen
The Netherlands

ACCESS SURGERY

R. GOKAL
Manchester Royal Infirmary
Oxford Road
MI3 9WL Manchester
UK

A. L. GOLDING
University Clinics
Los Angeles
California
USA

E. M. GORDON
Charing Cross Hospital
Medical School
Fulham Palace
W6 8RF London
UK

J. L. GOUZI
C.H.U. Purpan
Chirurgie Sud
31059 Toulouse Cedex
France

N. GRABEN
Department of Renal and Hypertensive
Diseases
Medical Clinic and Policlinic
Universitätsklinikum
D.43 Essen
West Germany

F. GRIFFANTI-BARTOLI
Università di Genova
Patologia Chirurgica I
Ospedale S. Martino
16132 Genova
Italy

P. J. A. GRIFFIN
Cardiff Royal Infirmary
Institute of Renal Disease
Newport Road
Cardiff, S. Wales
UK

A. GUČEK
University Medical Centre
Dialysis Centre
Zaloska 7
61000 Ljubljana
Yugoslavia

B. GUIDET
Broussais Hospital
Dept. of Cardiovascular Radiology
96 Rue Didot
75014 Paris
France

M. C. GUIMOT
Hôpital de la Pitié
Dept. of Nephrology and Urology
Bd de l'hôpital
75013 Paris
France

H. GÜLAY
Hacettepe University Hospital
Transplantation Unit
Ankara
Turkey

T. HAAS
97 Ave. Albert 1er
92500 Rueil Malmaison
France

M. HABERAL
Hacettepe University Hospital
Transplantation Unit
Ankara
Turkey

M. HAIMOV
The Mount Sinai School of Medicine
1 Gustave Levy Plaza
10028 New York
USA

F. HARDER
University Hospital
Dept. of Surgery
Ch-4031 Basel
Switzerland

F. W. J. HAZEBROEK
Sophia Children's Hospital
Dept. of Surgery
Gordelweg 160
3038 GE Rotterdam
The Netherlands

R. VAN HEE
University of Antwerp
Dept. of Surgery
B-2520 Antwerp
Belgium

G. K. VAN DER HEM
University Hospital
Oostersingel 59
9713 EZ Groningen
The Netherlands

L. HENDRICKX
Stuivenberg Hospital
Lge Beeldekensstraat
Antwerp
Belgium

J. M. M. P. H. HERMAN
Catharina Hospital
Dept. of Surgery
Michelangelolaan 2
5623 EJ Eindhoven
The Netherlands

D. J. HOELZER
Division of Pediatric Surgery
The University of Texas Health Science
Center – Houston
6431 Fannin
Suite MSMB 6.264
Houston, Texas 77030
USA

T. HOLMIN
University Hospital
Dept. of Surgery
221 85 Lund
Sweden

S. HORSCH
Department of Surgery
Kreislauflaber
Altbau Haus 6
University Hospital of Cologne
Josef-Stelzmann Strasse 9
5000 Köln 41
West Germany

A. HUBENS
Stuivenberg Hospital
Nutrition Team
Lge Beeldekensstraat
Antwerp
Belgium

B. HUSBERG
Malmö General Hospital
Dept. of Surgery
S-214 01 Malmö
Sweden

A. HVALA
University Medical Centre
Dialysis Centre
Zaloska 7
61000 Ljubljana
Yugoslavia

K. ILSTRUP
Nephrology
Regional Kidney Disease Program
701 Park Avenue
55415 Minneapolis
USA

J. J. JAKIMOWICZ
Catharina Hospital
Dept. of Surgery
Michelangelolaan 2
5623 EJ Eindhoven
The Netherlands

A. JAKOBSEN
The National Hospital
Dept. of Surgery
Pilestredet 32
Oslo 1
Norway

H. D. JAKUBOWSKI
University of Essen
Dept. of General Surgery
Hufelandstrasse 55
D-4300 Essen
Germany

R. W. G. JOHNSON
Royal Infirmary
Dept. of Surgery
Manchester
UK

M. C. J. DE JONG
University of Nijmegen
Dept. of Thoracic/Cardiovascular Surgery
Geert Grooteplein
6500 HB Nijmegen
The Netherlands

P. C. M. DE JONG
St. Annadal Hospital
Dept. of Surgery
P.O. Box 1918
6201 BX Maastricht
The Netherlands

C. A. De JONGH
Program of Oncology,
University of Maryland Cancer Center
University of Maryland School of Medicine
22 S. Greene Street
21201 Baltimore
USA

C. JUANENA
Clinica Nefrológica Bilbaina
Gordóniz 9
Bilbao
Spain

H. M. KARNAHL
Strahleninstitut AOK
D-5000 Köln
Germany

ACCESS SURGERY

B. M. KEMKES
University of Munich
Dept. of Cardiac Surgery
Marchioninistrasse 15
D-8000 Munich 70
Germany

P. KESHAVIAH
Medicine
Regional Kidney Disease Program
701 Park Avenue
55415 Minneapolis
USA

F. KHAZINE
97 Ave. Albert 1er
92500 Rueil Malmaison
France

V. KINDHÄUSER
University of Essen
Dept. of General Surgery
Hufelandstrasse 55
D-4300 Essen
Germany

P. KINNAERT
Université Libre de Bruxelles
Hôpital Erasme
808 Route de Lennik
B-1070 Brussels
Belgium

L. J. KOEP
Phoenix Transplant Center
1010 E McDowell Road
201 Phoenix
85006 Arizona
USA

K. KONNER
Medizin. Klinik I
Ostmerheimerstrasse 200
Köln-Merheim
D-5000
Germany

G. KOOTSTRA
University Hospital
Dept. of Surgery
St. Annadal 1
6214 PA Maastricht
The Netherlands

B. J. L. KOTHUIS
University Hospital
Dept. of Surgery
Rijnsburgerweg 10
2333 AA Leiden
The Netherlands

G. KRÖNUNG
Chir. Universitätsklinik
Sigmund Freud Strasse
Bonn
Germany

F. KUENTZ
C.H.U.R.
Dept. of Nephrology and Vascular Surgery
Grenoble
France

R. KVEDER
University Medical Centre
Dialysis Centre
Zaloska 7
61000 Ljubljana
Yugoslavia

T. S. KWAN
St. Franciscus Hospital
Dept. of Surgery
Kleiweg 500
3045 PM Rotterdam
The Netherlands

L. LAMY
Hôpital Saint Joseph
7 Rue Pierre Larousse
75674 Paris Cedex 14
France

J. LANDMANN
University Hospital
Dept. of Surgery
Ch-4031 Basel
Switzerland

B. LANE
Ninewells Hospital and Medical School
Ninewells
DD1 9 SY Dundee
Scotland

F. LARGIADÈR
University Hospital
Surgical Clinic A
Rämistrasse 100
8091 Zürich
Switzerland

I. De LEEUW
University Hospital
Antwerp
Belgium

LIST OF CONTRIBUTORS

E. LEGARRETA
Clinical Nefrologica
S. Cirurgia Vascular
Gordoniz 9
Bilbao
Spain

R. LERMA
Hospital N.S. Esperanza
Mariano Cubi 155
21 Barcelona
Spain

N. W. LEVIN
Henry Ford Hospital
2799 W. Grand Blvd
48202 Detroit
USA

B. I. LEVY
Inserm U141
41 Bd. de la Chapelle
75475 Paris Cedex 10
France

D. H. E. LICHTENDAHL
Department of Surgery
Academisch Ziekenhuis
Oostersingel 59
9713 EZ Groningen
The Netherlands

P. D. LIGHT
University of Maryland
22 S Greene Street
21201 Baltimore
USA

M. R. LILIEN
Academisch Ziekenhuis Leiden
Heelkundige Kliniek
Rijnsburgerweg 10
2333 AA Leiden
The Netherlands

E. LINDBERG
Central County Hospital
Dept. of Gastro-enterology
S-701 85 Örebro
Sweden

M. J. LINDOP
Addenbrooke's Hospital
Hills Road
Cambridge
UK

E. LINDSTEDT
University Hospital
Dept. of Urology
221 85 Lund
Sweden

R. LINS
University of Antwerp
Dept. of Nephrol.-Hypertension
B-2520 Antwerp
Belgium

C. LISBONA
Hospital N.S. Esperanza
Mariano Cubi 155
21 Barcelona
Spain

H. LUTZ
Inst. Anästhesiologie/Reanimation
Chirurgische Klinik
Theodor Kutzer Ufer
D-6800 Mannheim
Germany

N. P. MALLICK
Manchester Royal Infirmary
Oxford Road
MI3 9WL Manchester
UK

M. MALOVRH
University Medical Centre
Dialysis Centre
Zaloska 7
61000 Ljubljana
Yugoslavia

N. K. MAN
Hôpital Necker
Clinique Urologique
161 Rue de Sèvres
75015 Paris
France

E. MANZO
Chir. Spermentale e
Trapianti d'Organo
Via S. Pansini 5
80131 Napoli
Italy

R. MARGREITER
I. Univ. Klinik für Chirurgie
Anichstrasse 35
A-6020 Innsbrück
Austria

I. R. MARINO
Catholic University
Inst. of Surgical Pathology
Largo A. Gemelli
00168 Roma
Italy

J. P. MARTINEAUD
Hôpital Saint Joséph
7 Rue Pierre Larousse
75674 Paris Cedex 14
France

P. MARTÍNEZ
Clinica Nefrológica Bilbaina
Gordóniz 9
Bilbao
Spain

R. MARTINEZ CERCOS
Hospital N.S. Esperanza
Mariano Cubi 155
21 Barcelona
Spain

MARY G. McGEOWN
Belfast City Hospital
Renal Unit
Lisburn Road
BT9 7AB Belfast
N. Ireland

P. Y. MEAULLE
C.H.U.R.
Dept. of Nephrology and Vascular Surgery
Grenoble
France

H. MEFTAHI
C.H.U.R.
Dept. of Nephrology and Vascular Surgery
Grenoble
France

G. MEIDER
Medizin. Klinik I
Ostmerheimerstrasse 200
D-5000 Köln-Merheim
Germany

M. F. von MEYENFELDT
St. Annadal Hospital
Dept. of Surgery
P.O. Box 1918
6201 BX Maastricht
The Netherlands

P. MICHIELSEN
University Hospital St. Rafaël
Dept. of Internal Medicine
Kapucijnenvoer 33
B-3000 Leuven
Belgium

L. MILITANO
Ospedale Policlinico
Dept. of Vascular Surgery and
Kidney Transplantation
Via F. Sforza 35
20122 Milano
Italy

C. D. MISTRY
Manchester Royal Infirmary
Oxford Road
M13 9WL Manchester
UK

N. B. MOGENSEN
Hvidovre Hospital
Dept. of Nephrology
2650 Hvidovre
Denmark

K. MÖHRING
University of Heidelberg
Berliner Strasse
D-6900 Heidelberg
Germany

J. C. MOLENAAR
Sophia Children's Hospital
Dept. of Surgery
Gordelweg 160
3038 GE Rotterdam
The Netherlands

Ph. MORINIÈRE
C.H.U.
Hôpital Nord
Service de Néphrologie
80000 Amiens
France

C. MORRIS
Université Libre de Bruxelles
Hôpital Erasme
808 Route de Lennik
B-1070 Brussels
Belgium

J. MORTENSEN
Hvidovre Hospital
Dept. of Nephrology
2650 Hvidovre
Denmark

R. MOSIMANN
Centre Hospitalier Universitaire
Service de Chirurgie B
1011 Lausanne
Switzerland

A. MOUTON
Hôpital Saint Joseph
7 Rue Pierre Larousse
75674 Paris Cedex 14
France

N. H. MULDER
University Hospital
Oostersingel 59
9700 RB Groningen
The Netherlands

J. M. MÜLLER
Chir. Universitätsklinik
Jos. Stelzmannstrasse
Köln–Lindenthal
Germany

G. NAPPI
Chir. Sperimentale e
Trapianti D'Organo
Via S. Pansini 5
80131 Napoli
Italy

R. A. F. v.d. NESTE
St. Clara Hospital
Olympiaweg 350
3078 HT Rotterdam
The Netherlands

K. A. NEWMAN
Program of Oncology
University of Maryland Cancer Center
University of Maryland School of Medicine
11 S. Greene Street
21201 Baltimore
USA

R. NEWTON
Ninewells Hospital and Medical School
Ninewells
DD1 9SY Dundee
Scotland

H. NISHI
Shinseikai Hospital
1-3-2 Tamamizu-cho
467 Mizuho-ku
Japan

T. O'BRIEN
Surgery
Hennepin County Medical Center
701 Park Avenue
55415 Minneapolis
USA

H. K. OH
Henry Ford Hospital
2799 W. Grand Blvd
48202 Detroit
USA

A. ONCEVSKI
Medical Faculty
Clinic of Nephrology
Vodnjanska 17
91000 Skopje
Yugoslavia

Z. ÖNER
Hacettepe University Hospital
Transplantation Unit
Ankara
Turkey

K. H. ONG
St. Clara Hospital
Olympiaweg 350
3078 HT Rotterdam
The Netherlands

K. ONO
Ono Geka Clinic
Hakataekihigashi
812 Fukuoka
Japan

K. OTA
Tokyo Women's Medical College
Kidney Centre
10 Kawada-cha Shinjuku-ku
162 Tokyo
Japan

A. ÖZENC
Hacettepe University Hospital
Transplantation Unit
Ankara
Turkey

E. de PAOLI VITALI
Renal Unit
Arcispedale
S. Anna U.S.L. 31
44100 Ferrara
Italy

V. PARENT
C.H.R. Purpan
Chirurgie Sud
31059 Toulouse Cedex
France

H. J. PEARSON
The General Hospital
Dept. of Surgery
Gwendolen Road
LE5 4PW Leicester
UK

R. PEETERS
Stuivenberg Hospital
Dept. of Surgery
Lge Beeldekensstraat
Antwerp
Belgium

H. PICHLMAIER
Department of Surgery
University Hospital of Cologne
Josef-Stelzmann Strasse 9
5000 Köln 41
West Germany

J. PIETRI
C.H.U.
Hôpital Nord
Service de Néphrologie
80000 Amiens
France

K. PISTOR
Department of Nephrology
Pediatric Clinic
Universitätsklinikum
D43 Essen
West Germany

J. L. POIGNET
Hôpital de la Pitié
Dept. of Nephrology and Urology
83 Bd de l'hôpital
75013 Paris
France

R. PONIKVAR
University Medical Centre
Dialysis Centre
Zaloska 7
61000 Ljubljana
Yugoslavia

J. C. PONSIN
Hôpital Lariboisiére
41 Bd de la Chapelle
75010 Paris
France

E. POZZOLI
Ospedale Policlinico
Dept. of Vascular Surgery and
Kidney Transplantation
Via F. Sforza 35
20122 Milano
Italy

B. PRADERE
C.H.R. Purpan
Chirurgie Sud
31059 Toulouse Cedex
France

K. PRENNER
Landeskrankenanstalten Salzburg
Dept. of Vascular Surgery
Müllnerhaupstrasse
Salzburg
Austria

G. PROUD
Royal Victoria Infirmary
Dept. of Surgery
NE1 4LP Newcastle upon Tyne
UK

J. PUNCERNAU
Hospital N.S. Esperanza
Mariano Cubi 155
21 Barcelona
Spain

A. PUPA
Anesthesiology
Istituto Nazionale Tumori
Via Venezian
20133 Milano
Italy

C. QUESADA
C.H.U.R.
Dept. of Nephrology and Vascular Surgery
Grenoble
France

F. QUINTANA RIERA
Hospital N.S. Esperanza
Mariano Cubi 155
21 Barcelona
Spain

A. RAYNAUD
Broussais Hospital
Dept. of Cardiovascular Surgery
96 Rue Didot
75014 Paris
France

LIST OF CONTRIBUTORS

W. P. REED
The Oncology Program
Department of Surgery
University of Maryland School of Medicine
22 S. Greene Street
21201 Baltimore
USA

D. T. REILLY
Dept. of Cardiovascular Surgery
St. Mary's Hospital
Praed Street
London W2
UK

J. J. REILLY Jr
University of Pittsburgh
1087 Scaife Hall
Pittsburgh 15261 PA
USA

H. H. M. REINAERTS
University of Nijmegen
Dept. of Thoracic/Cardiovascular Surgery
Geert Grooteplein
6500 HB Nijmegen
The Netherlands

K. RENDL
Landeskrankenanstalten Salzburg
Dept. of Vascular Surgery
Müllnerhaupstrasse
Salzburg
Austria

Y. RÉVILLON
Hôpital des Enfants Malades
149 Rue de Sèvres
75 730 Paris Cedex 15
France

C. RICOUR
Hôpital des Enfants Malades
149 Rue de Sèvres
75 730 Paris Cedex 15
France

S. RINGOIR
University Hospital
Renal Division
De Pintelaan 185
B-9000 Gent
Belgium

P. RINGOT
C.H.U.
Hôpital Nord
Service de Néphrologie
80000 Amiens
France

P. S. RITTER
University of Pittsburgh
1087 Scaife Hall
Pittsburgh 15261 PA
USA

E. RITZ
University of Heidelberg
Bergheimerstrasse 58
D-6900 Heidelberg
Germany

L. RODRIQUEZ
Clinica Nefrologica
S. Cirurgia Vascular
Gordoniz 9
Bilbao
Spain

P. ROJAS
Hôpital de Pitié
Dept. of Nephrology and Urology
Bd de l'hôpital
75013 Paris
France

G. ROMANO
Chir. Sperimentale e
Trapianti D'Organo
Via S. Pansini 5
80131 Napoli
Italy

P. DE ROSA
Chir. Sperimentale e
Trapianti d'Organo
Via S. Pansini 5
80131 Napoli
Italy

J. ROTTEMBOURG
Hôpital de la Pitié
Dept. of Nephrology and Urology
Bd de l'hôpital
75013 Paris
France

B. ROWLANDS
Health Science Center of Houston
Dept. of Surgery
6431 Fannin Suite MSMB 4.162
Houston
USA

C. H. RUEGSEGGER
Centre Hospitalier Universitaire
Service de Chirurgie B
1011 Lausanne
Switzerland

U. RUSCHEWSKI
University of Essen
Dept. of General Surgery
Hufelandstrasse 55
D-4300 Essen
Germany

J. A. SADLER
University of Maryland
22 S. Greene Street
21201 Baltimore
USA

E. DI SALVO
Chir. Sperimentale e
Trapianti d'Organo
Via S. Pansini 5
80131 Napoli
Italy

F. SALZANO DE LUNA
Chir. Sperimentale e
Trapianti d'Organo
Via S. Pansini 5
80131 Napoli
Italy

M. L. SANTAGELO
Chir. Sperimentale e
Trapianti d'Organo
Via S. Pansini 5
80131 Napoli
Italy

A. SANTORO
M. Malpighi Hospital
Dept. Nephrology and Dialysis
P. Palagi 9
40138 Bologna
Italy

C. SASSAROLI
Chir. Sperimentale e
Trapianti D'Organo
Via S. Pansini 5
80131 Napoli
Italy

D. SCARPA
Anesthesiology
Istituto Nazionale Tumori
Via Venezian
20133 Milano
Italy

A. M. de SCHEPPER
University of Antwerp
Dept. of Nephrol.-Hypertension
B-2520 Antwerp
Belgium

I. SCHICHT
Academisch Ziekenhuis Leiden
Department of Medicine
Rijnsburgerweg 10
2333 AA Leiden
The Netherlands

R. van SCHILFGAARDE
Academisch Ziekenhuis Leiden
Department of Surgery
Rijnsburgerweg 10
2333 AA Leiden
The Netherlands

S. C. SCHIMPFF
Program of Oncology
University of Maryland Cancer Center
University of Maryland School of Medicine
22 S. Greene Street
21201 Baltimore
USA

R. SCHMIDT
Department of Surgery
Kreislauflaber
Altbau Haus 6
University Hospital of Cologne
Josef-Stelzmann Strasse 9
5000 Köln 41
West Germany

W. SCHOEPPE
J. W. Goethe Universität
St. Markus Krankenhaus
W. Epsteinstrasse 2
D-6000 Frankfurt/Main
Germany

B. H. SCRIBNER
University of Washington
School of Medicine
Division of Nephrology
Box RM–11
Seattle, Washington 98195
USA

C. SERVADIO
Beilinson Medical Center
Transplant Unit
Dept. of Urology
49 100 Petah Tiqva
Israel

M. SEUROT
Broussais Hospital
Dept. of Cardiovascular Radiology
96 Rue Didot
75014 Paris
France

Z. SHAPIRA
Beilinson Medical Center
Transplant Unit
Dept. of Urology
49 100 Petah Tiqva
Israel

F. SHAPIRO
Medicine
Regional Kidney Disease Program
701 Park Avenue
55415 Minneapolis
USA

D. SHMUELI
Beilinson Medical Center
Transplant Unit
Dept. of Urology
49 100 Petah Tiqva
Israel

O. SIMONS
97 Ave. Albert 1er
92500 Rueil Malmaison
France

S. H. SKOTNICKI
University of Nijmegen
Dept. of Thoracic/Cardiovascular Surgery
Geert Grooteplein 10
6500 HB Nijmegen
The Netherlands

D. Th. SLEYFER
University Hospital
Oostersingel 59
9700 RB Groningen
The Netherlands

R. SLIFKIN
The Mount Sinai School of Medicine
1 Gustave Levy Plaza
10028 New York
USA

M. J. H. SLOOFF
University Hospital
Dept. of Surgery
Oostersingel 59
9700 RB Groningen
The Netherlands

D. W. SMITH
Statistical Research Laboratory
University of Michigan
106 Rackham
Ann Arbor, MI 48109
USA

M. F. SMITH
Addenbrooke's Hospital
Hills Road
Cambridge
UK

P. J. H. SMITS
University Hospital
Oostersingel 59
9713 EZ Groningen
The Netherlands

S. K. S. SO
University of Minnesota Hospitals
Dept. of Surgery and Radiology
Box 263 Mayo
55455 Minneapolis
USA

G. SØDAL
The National Hospital
Dept. of Surgery
Pilestredet 32
Oslo 1
Norway

P. B. SOETERS
St. Annadal Hospital
Dept. of Surgery
P.O. Box 1918
6201 BX Maastricht
The Netherlands

R. SQUERZANTI
Renal Unit
Arcispedale
S. Anna U.S.L. 31
44100 Ferrara
Italy

J. W. J. L. STAPERT
St. Annadal Hospital
Dept. of Surgery
P.O. Box 1918
6201 BX Maastricht
The Netherlands

D. L. STEED
University of Pittsburgh
1087 Scaife Hall
Pittsburgh 15261 PA
USA

G. STORELLI
Ospedale Policlinico
Dept. of Vascular Surgery and
Kidney Transplantation
Via F. Sforza 35
20122 Milano
Italy

L. W. STORZ
Inst. Anästhesiologie/Reanimation
Chirurgische Klinik
Theodor Kutzer Ufer
D-6800 Mannheim
Germany

J. SUSINI
Centre René Huguenin
de Lutte Contre
le Cancer
5 Rue Gaston Latouche
92211 Saint-Cloud
France

D. E. R. SUTHERLAND
University of Minnesota Hospitals
Dept. of Surgery and Radiology
Box 263 Mayo
55455 Minneapolis
USA

K. TAKAHASHI
Tokyo Women's Medical College
Kidney Centre
10 Kawada-cha Shinjuku-ku
162 Tokyo
Japan

R. M. R. TAYLOR
Royal Victoria Infirmary
Dept. of Surgery
NE1 4LP Newcastle upon Tyne
UK

A. M. TEGZESS
University Hospital
Oostersingel 59
9713 EZ Groningen
The Netherlands

G. TERNO
Anesthesiology
Istituto Nazionale Tumori
Via Venezian
20133 Milano
Italy

M. B. THOMSEN
University Hospital
Dept. of Surgery
S-581 85 Linköping
Sweden

P. TONDELLI
University Hospital
Dept. of Surgery
Ch-4031 Basel
Switzerland

J. H. M. van TONGEREN
University Hospital
Dept. of Internal Medicine
Geert Grooteplein 8
6500 HB Nijmegen
The Netherlands

J. H. M. TORDOIR
Catharina Hospital
Dept. of Surgery
Michelangelolaan 2
5623 EJ Eindhoven
The Netherlands

G. K. UHLSCHMID
University Hospital
Surgical Clinic A
Rämistrasse 100
8091 Zürich
Switzerland

A. UHRENHOLDT
Hvidovre Hospital
Dept. of Nephrology
2650 Hvidovre
Denmark

G. VALLANCIEN
Hôpital de la Pitié
Dept. of Nephrology and Urology
Bd de l'hôpital
75013 Paris
France

B. A. VANDERWERF
Good Samaritan Hospital
Phoenix Renal Transplant Center
1010 East McDowell Road
85006 Phoenix
USA

R. VANHOLDER
University Hospital
Renal Division
De Pintelaan 185
B-9000 Gent
Belgium

J. VARL
University Medical Centre
Dialysis Centre
Zaloska 7
61000 Ljubljana
Yugoslavia

LIST OF CONTRIBUTORS

A. VEGETO
Ospedale Policlinico
Dept. of Vascular Surgery and
Kidney Transplantation
Via F. Sforza 35
20122 Milano
Italy

C. J. H. van de VELDE
University Hospital
Dept. of Surgery
Rijnsburgerweg 10
2333 AA Leiden
The Netherlands

H. A. VEREYCKEN
University of Antwerp
Dept. of Nephrol.-Hypertension
B-2520 Antwerp
Belgium

J. P. VERMYNCK
C.H.U.
Hôpital Nord
Service de Néphrologie
80000 Amiens
France

G. A. VERPOOTEN
University of Antwerp
Dept. of Nephrol.-Hypertension
B-2520 Antwerp
Belgium

F. VIDAL-BARRAQUER
Hospital N.S. Esperanza
Mariano Cubi 155
21 Barcelona
Spain

J. VILLEBOEUF
97 Ave. Albert 1er
92500 Rueil Malmaison
France

A. VIZJAK
University Medical Centre
Dialysis Centre
Zaloska 7
61000 Ljubljana
Yugoslavia

J. VLACHOYANNIS
J. W. Goethe Universität
St. Markus Krankenhaus
W. Epsteinstrasse 2
D-6000 Frankfurt/Main
Germany

J. P. VAN WAELEGHEM
University of Antwerp
Dept. Nephrology-Hypertension
B-2520 Antwerp
Belgium

N. WALDSTEIN
Landeskrankenanstalten Salzburg
Dept. of Vascular Surgery
Müllnerhaupstrasse
Salzburg
Austria

M. G. WALKER
Ninewells Hospital and Medical School
Ninewells
DD1 9 SY Dundee
UK

M. K. WARD
Royal Victoria Infirmary
Dept. of Surgery
NE1 4LP Newcastle upon Tyne
UK

E. M. WATKIN
The General Hospital
Dept. of Surgery
Gwendolen Road
LE5 4PW Leicester
UK

J. P. WAUTERS
Centre Hospitalier Universitaire
Service de Chirurgie B
1011 Lausanne
Switzerland

R. I. C. WESDORP
St. Annadal Hospital
Dept. of Surgery
P.O. Box 1918
6201 BX Maastricht
The Netherlands

H. WESTLING
University Hospital
221 85 Lund
Sweden

T. WHITE
University Hospital
221 85 Lund
Sweden

G. WICKBOM
Central County Hospital
Dept. of Surgery
S-701 85 Örebro
Sweden

P. WIERNIK
Program of Oncology
University of Maryland Cancer Center
University of Maryland School of Medicine
22 S. Greene Street
21201 Baltimore
U.S.A.

T. WILLIAMS
909 E. Brill Street
Phoenix
85006 Arizona
USA

Th. WOBBES
Radboud Hospital
Geert Grooteplein 14
6500 HB Nijmegen
The Netherlands

R. F. M. WOOD
Nuffield Department of Surgery
John Radcliffe Hospital
Headington
Oxford OX3 9DU
UK

R. YALIN
Hacettepe University Hospital
Transplantation Unit
Ankara
Turkey

A. YAÑEZ
Clinica Nefrologica
S. Cirurgia Vascular
Gordoniz 9
Bilbao
Spain

T. I. YO
St. Clara Hospital
Olympiaweg 350
3078 HT Rotterdam
The Netherlands

A. YUSSIM
Beilinson Medical Center
Transplant Unit
Dept. of Urology
49 100 Petah Tiqva
Israel

J. ZINGRAFF
Hôpital Necker
161 Rue de Sèvres
75 730 Paris Cedex 15
France

P. ZUCCHELLI
M. Malpighi Hospital
Dept. of Nephrology and Dialysis
P. Palagi 9
40138 Bologna
Italy

A. ZWAVELING
University Hospital
Dept. of Surgery
Rijnsburgerweg 10
2333 AA Leiden
The Netherlands

INTRODUCTORY ADDRESS

Permanent circulatory access – past, present and future

J. J. COLE, R. O. HICKMAN, M. B. DENNIS, JR., W. JENSEN AND
B. H. SCRIBNER, Guest Lecturer

In this chapter the term 'permanent' is used to indicate life-long circulatory access as distinguished from various forms of temporary circulatory access, such as the placement of a needle in a vein to provide a route for intravenous infusion. Furthermore, the term 'circulatory access' as we use it here can be either direct or indirect. Examples of the latter are the use of the peritoneum for long-term dialysis or the subcutaneous route for the continuous infusion of insulin. In the following pages we will describe some of the important evolutionary steps in the history of permanent circulatory access and the interesting interplay among some of the modes of access that have evolved during the last 20 years. We will also discuss possible future developments.

The history of permanent circulatory access began on 9 March 1960, with the placement of an all-Teflon arteriovenous (A-V) shunt in the left arm of the world's first maintenance haemodialysis patient[1]. Although this device represented a very poor solution to the need for permanent circulatory access, it got the job done during the first 2 years of maintenance haemodialysis and the patient survived 11 years without any renal function of his own. He died, not from loss of circulatory access, but from a myocardial infarction.

It is noteworthy that Teflon was selected for use in the first cannula design. The right substance was selected for the wrong reason. A surgical colleague had told us that Teflon should be tried because of its low tissue reactivity. Much later we realized that the 'non-stick' ultrasmooth surface of Teflon was what prevented the early shunts from clotting. Had we chosen any other plastic, the original shunts undoubtedly would not have remained patent. Instead, it was chosen because a roll of Teflon tubing of the correct size, as

1

judged by the intuition of the engineers and physicians involved, happened to be on the shelves in the Central Supply division of University Hospital. Had this material, intended for use as insulation for electrical wiring, not been available and another chosen instead, results of the initial cannulation might have ended quite differently.

Another significant evolutionary step occurred when silicone 'rubber' was introduced into the cannula system. Whereas the development of the all-Teflon A-V cannulas represented the first step in achieving successful long-term blood access, use of these cannulas usually was limited to a few weeks or months, with flows progressively slowing as the vessels immediately proximal to the cannula tips closed. Believing this problem to be due to recurring trauma at the junction of the cannula tip and vessel caused by cannula rigidity, we sought a material which would serve as a 'shock buffer', preventing movement of the vessel tips as the arm was rotated. Silicone rubber, a newly available biologically compatible polymer from the Dow Corning Company, eventually was selected for use in this application[2] and remains a major contributor to successful circulatory access to the present time. Incorporation of a tubular silicone rubber segment as part of the blood conduit immediately produced a two- to threefold improvement in cannula longevity.

In 1966 the course of haemodialysis blood access was abruptly and dramatically altered by the Cimino group's announcement of the successful use of the A-V fistula, thereby making possible permanent blood access for many dialysis patients[3]. It is ironic that the means for a surgically created vascular fistula had existed long before 1960, but the idea simply had been overlooked by the many investigators seeking a better means of circulatory access for dialysis. The originators are to be commended for their innovation and perception.

Although the A-V fistula greatly extends the longevity of blood access for most dialysis patients, it is subject to failure by thrombosis, stenosis, infection, and haematoma at the venipuncture site. These occasional complications, plus the fistula's principal disadvantage, i.e. the need to perform painful venipuncture, have fostered research for a permanent percutaneous blood access method which continues to the present. Notwithstanding these drawbacks, the A-V fistula presently is the most widely used method for dialysis blood access in the world.

Our story now shifts to peritoneal dialysis. In 1963 Dr Fred Boen, while working in Seattle, addressed the serious problem of peritonitis in patients maintained on this therapy. Boen resorted to what he called the 'single-stick method' of peritoneal access, which simply meant that a new intraperitoneal catheter had to be inserted for each dialysis. Using this approach, Boen demonstrated for the first time that long-term peritoneal dialysis could be administered with an acceptably low infection risk for the patient and that it was a serious therapeutic alternative to haemodialysis for the treatment of end-stage renal disease[4]. A new treatment option for the patient with chronic renal disease had been established.

A year or so later, Palmer, Quinton *et al.* developed a new 'intramural' cannula for peritoneal dialysis[5]. Quinton, who had worked with our group in the development of the all-Teflon and later the Teflon–silicone cannulas, chose silicone as the material for the Palmer–Quinton peritoneal catheter. This appliance was an extruded tube with perforations through the wall of the terminal segment for fluid flow, and with sufficient compliance to be atraumatic to the abdominal viscera. Although this catheter had numerous other desirable features, it, like its predecessors, produced unacceptably high rates of infection.

The final step in the evolution of the bacteriologically safe peritoneal catheter occurred when Tenckhoff and Schechter modified the design of the Palmer–Quinton catheter and applied Dacron felt cuffs to its exterior[6]. Tissue ingrowth into these cuffs effectively produced sinus closure and resulted in a dramatic drop in the incidence of infectious complications. With this final development, home peritoneal dialysis became a realistic possibility which soon was realized when the necessary home peritoneal equipment was devised.

In 1969 we developed the concept of 'the artificial gut'[7] to provide life support for patients with chronic bowel disease. Compared to home haemodialysis, which at that time had a history of 5 successful years behind it, this idea was indeed simple. We put a side-arm on an A-V shunt and used it to infuse parenteral nutrients, which recently had been shown both to sustain life and to support normal growth and development[8]. The side-arm worked perfectly when we tried infusing 50% dextrose into dialysis patients. However, when the technique was tried on patients with bowel disease the shunts clotted. What we had not foreseen was that patients with bowel disease usually have poor peripheral veins that thrombose readily and, unlike uraemic patients, they also have a normal clotting mechanism.

As the realization began to sink in that the concept was on the verge of failure, a severely malnourished patient with Crohn's disease arrived for treatment. In a desperate effort to save this patient's life, we decided to try infusion into a major vessel. After preliminary tests in sheep, the catheter was implanted in the superior vena cava of the patient and used over the ensuing weeks to bring him back to near normal weight. This early hyperalimentation catheter consisted of a Teflon intravascular segment coupled to a flexible, percutaneous silicone catheter segment to which the fluid administration system was connected. Based on the experience with the Tenckhoff peritoneal catheter, a subcutaneous Dacron cuff was employed with this catheter to serve as an infection barrier and to anchor it.

Subsequently a revised catheter was prepared constructed wholly of silicone rubber and equipped with an extravascular Dacron cuff. The intravascular length of this new catheter was increased to place the tip in the right atrium where more rapid dilution of the concentrated glucose solutions, required to maintain caloric balance, would take place. This basic catheter design has since become the safest form of indwelling vascular access yet devised and is now employed for purposes not envisaged at the time of its original creation.

One such application began in 1972 with patients at the Fred Hutchinson Cancer Research Center in Seattle undergoing bone marrow transplants for leukaemia[9]. It was obvious that long-term circulatory access in these patients was required for a multitude of reasons and that in many this was impractical because of poor peripheral vessels due to previous therapy. Initially the hyperalimentation catheter was employed for the administration of blood and blood products, and for the withdrawal of blood specimens. However, the internal diameter of the catheter was too small and often clotted when used in this manner, even though it terminated in the atrium.

This experience led to the development of a catheter similar in design and placement to the original hyperalimentation catheter but with a larger internal diameter, 1.6 mm instead of 1.0 mm. Since its redesign this catheter has been placed in over 2000 patients in the city of Seattle, most of whom were under treatment for oncology conditions. This catheter and the hyperalimentation and peritoneal dialysis catheters are available from Evergreen Medical Products, PO Box 296, Medina, Washington, 98039 USA. Catheters have been in place from 7 days to 4 years. The youngest patient was 2 months old. In addition to blood administration and withdrawal the catheter is used for the administration of electrolytes, antibiotics and chemotherapeutic agents to these patients. The major catheter problem in the oncology patient is infection. The infection rate in this high-risk group has been reported at between 1 infection per 490 and 1 per 850 days[10,11].

Recently, another variant of the basic hyperalimentation catheter has come into increasing use. This is the double-lumen catheter used to facilitate oncology treatment by permitting uninterrupted administration of nutrient solutions through one channel while the second lumen is used to deliver all other solutions and for blood sampling. This approach simplifies care and also improves overall nutritional balance since one channel is dedicated to hyperalimentation.

Looking back to 9 March 1960, it is remarkable indeed how widespread the use of the several forms of circulatory access has become. In a little over two decades, therapies that are access-dependent have reached a point where well over 100 000 patients are on long-term haemodialysis and peritoneal dialysis. Additional thousands are on long-term parenteral nutrition and also anticancer therapy.

With this brief span of time for perspective it seems useful to review the present limitations of circulatory access and also to speculate on where this emerging field may evolve in the future.

Two trends in medicine suggest an expanding future need for circulatory access. The first of these is the abolition of infectious disease as the principal cause of death in the western world[12], and a corresponding change in the focus of medicine to the treatment of chronic illness. Implicit in this emerging trend is the need to provide more specialized and focused therapies, some of which must be repeated at intervals and which require blood access. Haemodialysis and peritoneal dialysis are established examples of this trend. Others which are presently evolving include plasmapheresis, haemodetoxification and bone marrow transplantation and cancer chemotherapy. Soon, new procedures such as enzyme haemoperfusion and immune complex removal also may be routinely employed and will be heavily dependent on long-term access.

The second influence which may affect the future expansion in need for circulatory access is economic rather than technological. As the cost of overall health care rises, counter-pressures are exerted to reduce cost wherever possible in order to extend limited health care resources. The existence of percutaneous access may be of increasing importance in this trend since it is convenient to use and may permit various therapies to be administered on an outpatient basis, and even in the home. This potential is exemplified by both haemodialysis and peritoneal dialysis. An emerging example which also reflects this trend is the continuous, variable administration of insulin via intravenous or subcutaneous catheters to achieve euglycaemia in the diabetic.

Despite the numerous advances in circulatory access that have occurred during the last 20 years, the same fundamental problems which caused failure of the earliest crude dialysis cannulas affect performance of all access methods at the present time. None of the methods, direct or indirect, functions without the constant risk of infection. Further, those methods which directly involve the bloodstream and vessels also may be compromised by the threat of vessel stenosis.

Infection should now be considered the most important threat to the longevity of percutaneous prostheses since it is potentially life-threatening when it develops. Standard treatment for infected catheters consists of administering antibiotics once infection is detected. Often, however, this proves insufficient, with infection persisting despite drug therapy or recurring once therapy has been discontinued. We have noted on several occasions that when infected peritoneal dialysis catheters which failed to respond to antibiotics were replaced by sterile catheters in the same tract, infection cleared. These observations point to the need to examine the role of the implant in the infectious process, to determine how organisms remain viable even when antibiotics fill the lumen and surround the intraperitoneal portion of the prosthesis. The implication of these findings is that organisms are somehow being harboured on the catheter, perhaps in minute irregularities on the catheter wall, and that alteration in the physical or chemical nature of the catheter material might greatly increase the ease of dealing with this problem when it occurs.

Historically the build-up of intimal smooth muscle cells with resultant stenosis of the vascular channel has been repeatedly described as a cause of failure at the tip–vessel junction of silicone–Teflon cannulas. It is unfortunate that the common terminology used to describe the end result of this process, 'clotted cannulas', has had the effect of shifting research for a means of prevention from the true cause, tissue hyperplasia, to the cannula materials themselves in the hope that the development of materials more biocompatible would prevent cannula failure.

This same problem of cellular proliferation continues to plague fistulas and vascular grafts, the build-up occurring both at venipuncture sites and at the graft–vein junction. We have observed smooth muscle cell proliferation also causing stenosis of catheterized peripheral vessels[13]. If a means of preventing or delaying this process can be found, it will greatly enhance the longevity of a variety of access methods. In the arm we have noted that the process of stenosis of catheterized vessels does not occur when there are no collateral veins available for the shunting of blood. This observation is further supported by the long-term success of the hyperalimentation catheter which passes through the superior vena cava into the atrium. Whether or not this 'single-channel' principle is valid and can be applied to vascular implants elsewhere in the body is presently unclear, but controlled experimentation to explore the idea seems warranted.

Long-term circulatory access via the larger vessels began with the Thomas femoral shunt[14] and later the right atrial hyperalimentation catheter. More recently the necessities of cancer chemotherapy have expanded use of the central vessels. This trend seems likely to continue, as higher blood flow rates are sought for faster treatment, and because these higher flows more rapidly dilute medications which are potentially thrombogenic or sclerosing. As the more peripheral sites are used up or found to be unsatisfactory we will turn increasingly to the upper arm, the thigh and the central vessels. Conceivably use of the renal vessels for access in haemodialysis patients will eventually be common. The idea was discussed in 1960 but to our knowledge has never been employed.

Catheters with multiple conduits and puncturable surfaces are now being introduced, signalling a trend towards greater convenience and specialization. Perhaps soon we will use exteriorized vascular grafts composed solely of living tissue. It seems clear that the trend is at present towards increased use of percutaneous access prostheses due to convenience and freedom from discomfort. Nevertheless, it should be noted at this time, when access methods and their uses are proliferating, that the limiting factors remain the same as in the early 1960s – infection and stenosis.

References

1 Quinton, W. E., Dillard, D. H. and Scribner, B. H. (1960). Cannulation of blood vessels for prolonged hemodialysis. *Trans. Am. Soc. Artif. Intern. Organs*, **6**, 104

2 Quinton, W. E., Dillard, D. H., Cole, J. J. and Scribner, B. H. (1962). Eight months' experience with Silastic–Teflon cannulas. *Trans. Am. Soc. Artif. Intern. Organs*, **8**, 236

3 Brescia, M. J., Cimino, J. E., Appel, K. and Hurwich, B. J. (1966). Chronic hemodialysis using venipuncture and a surgically created arteriovenous fistula. *N. Engl. J. Med.*, **275**, 1089

4 Boen, S. T., Mion, C. M., Curtis, F. K. and Shilipetar, G. (1964). Periodic peritoneal dialysis using the repeated puncture technique and an automatic cycling machine. *Trans. Am. Soc. Artif. Intern. Organs*, **10**, 409

5 Palmer, R. A., Newell, J. E., Gray, E. J. and Quinton, W. E. (1966). Treatment of chronic renal failure by prolonged peritoneal dialysis. *N. Engl. J. Med.*, **274**, 248

6 Tenckhoff, H. and Schechter, H. (1966). A bacteriologically safe peritoneal access device. *Trans. Am. Soc. Artif. Intern. Organs*, **14**, 181

7 Scribner, B. H., Cole, J. J., Christopher, T. G., Vizzo, J. E., Atkins, R. C. and Blagg, C. R. (1970). Long term total parenteral nutrition. The concept of an artificial gut. *J. Am. Med. Assoc.*, **212**, 457

8 Dudrick, S. J., Wilmore, D. W., Vars, H. M. and Rhoads, J. E. (1969). Can intravenous feeding as the sole means of nutrition support growth in the child and restore weight loss in an infant? An affirmative answer. *Ann. Surg.*, **169**, 974

9 Hickman, R. O., Buckner, C. D., Clift, R. A., Sanders, J. E., Stewart, P. and Thomas, E. D. (1979). A modified right atrial catheter for access to the venous system in marrow transplant recipients. *Surg. Gynecol. Obstet.*, **148**, 871

10 Larsen, E. B., Wooding, M. and Hickman, R. O. (1981). Infectious complications of right atrial catheters used for venous access in patients receiving chemotherapy. *Surg. Gynecol. Obstet.*, **153**, 369

11 Abrahm, J. L. and Mullen, J. L. (1982). A prospective study of prolonged central venous access in leukemia. A three year experience. (In press)

12 Fries, J. F. (1980). Aging, natural death, and the compression of morbidity. *N. Engl. J. Med.*, **303**, 130

13 Dennis, M. B., Cole, J. J., Hickman, R. O., Hall, D. G., Jensen, W. M. and Scribner, B. H. (1979). Secondary blood access by fistula catheter in pediatric and problem dialysis patients. *Int. J. Artif. Organs*, **2**, 410

14 Thomas, G. I. (1969). A large-vessel applique A-V shunt for hemodialysis. *Trans. Am. Soc. Artif. Intern. Organs*, **15**, 288

Section I
Surgical technique and microsurgery

1

Microsurgery for distal A-V fistula in children

P. BOURQUELOT

INTRODUCTION

In 1966 Brescia and Cimino described the distal A-V fistula at the wrist. At the present time it is the best angioaccess for haemodialysis, but due to the small diameter (1 mm) of the vessels, difficulties are observed in small children with conventional techniques.

In the 1960s microsurgery[1] developed and successful small vessel sutures of about 1 mm diameter were successively reported by Jacobson (1960, 1.5 mm), Buncke (1966, 1 mm) and Acland (1969, 0.5 mm).

Microvascular surgery is now used on a routine basis by surgeons. Since 1977, in our Department of Urology, microsurgery is used for all distal A-V fistulas in children and adults. The technique, the instruments and the results will be described in this chapter.

MICROSURGERY

Microinstruments are characterized by small precision tips, light weight, balanced proportions, and dull, non-reflective surfaces. In microsurgery, virtually all surgical movements have been reduced to a pinch mechanism between thumb and index finger, guided by vision through the operating microscope. As forceps we prefer the type as initially proposed by the Swiss Dumont factory. They are classified according to the width of the bit: no. 5 forceps is our preferred one. The needle-holder and scissors are derived from the Gastroviejo type. One of the scissors must be very small for the incision of the vessels. The ideal microvascular clamp has to be atraumatic and to possess a sufficient closing pressure to prevent bleeding and accidental disruption. Acland has perfected a series of clamps of varying widths and closing tension. The smallest one (A1, VI) is used. The diamond knife provides an extremely sharp cutting surface, most useful to initiate the opening of the artery. Its principal disadvantage is high cost.

Frequent irrigation of the wound is necessary to prevent desiccation, to improve visualization, to irrigate the clots out of the vessels and to float the vessel edges apart. Background material is placed behind structures to improve visualization. We prefer the colour to be yellow. Bipolar coagulation is most helpful in coagulating the branches of small vessels during dissection. The alternative is to divide them between two sutures. Standard coagulation should not be used for microvascular surgery, as the current will extend into the main vessel and destroy it. We use 10-0 Ethilon® microsutures with B.V.8 needle with a diameter of 50 μm. The microscope that provides excellent help is the Zeiss® O.P.M.I. 6D. It has two binoculars allowing two surgeons to work together face to face. The focus is 200 mm. A foot control panel changes zoom magnification, translation and focus. One can operate it without touching, and sterilization is not necessary. Magnification ranges from 4 to 40×. Illumination is provided by fibre-optic light source. It is a very efficient instrument, rather expensive, but it is very strongly built and it can be used by surgeons of different specialties.

Skill in microsurgical techniques has to be acquired on the animal. The best way to initiate this is to spend a week in master class, to overcome initial difficulties. Thereafter it will take several months in the research laboratory to perfect microsurgical skills. The rat is the most widely used experimental animal for surgical training and research: housing is easy, short-term experiments can be done, costs are low. Sutures of the aorta (2 mm), femoral artery (1 mm) and epigastric artery (0.5 mm) are ideal models. Any organ transplantation can be done in the rat, including kidney transplantation. Fetal microsurgery in rabbits can be the next step.

MICROSURGICAL ANGIOACCESS

Preoperative evaluation of the radial and the ulnar artery at the wrist is easy to perform with the help of a Doppler apparatus. Evaluation of the cephalic and basilic vein is much more difficult because of the thickness of the subcutaneous tissue in very young children. A venogram is necessary to assess the vein from wrist to elbow and the adequacy of the run-off proximally. The vein may have been damaged mainly at the elbow by repeated punctures or by some previous vascular access procedures which may sometimes preclude the creation of a distal arteriovenous fistula on both forearms.

The operation is performed under general anaesthesia. The operative microscope is used immediately after incision of the skin. A relatively extensive mobilization of the vein is necessary to bring it to the artery without tension or kinking. All the branches are ligated. The vein is divided distally. A long incision is made to spatulate the vein. The dissection of the artery has to be very gentle to avoid spasm, for which papaverine may help. Branches are severed after ligation or bipolar coagulation. External arterial diameter varies from 0.8 to 1.2 mm; vein diameter varies from 1.0 to 1.6 mm. Dilatation of both vessels is prohibited, not only with the Fogarty® catheter but also with saline. The intima should never be grasped. The anastomosis is side (artery) to end (vein). The length of the anastomosis is made equal to three times the diameter of the vein. Vessels are heparinized only between the clamps. Four running stitches are used. After release of the clamps a sterile Doppler probe is placed on the vein to check the permeability of the fistula. In small children a continuous murmur may be absent during the first post-operative hours and patency has to be checked by transcutaneous Doppler examination later on.

Secondary surgical procedure may be necessary some weeks later. This may involve a second anastomosis for stenosis, or superficialization of a vein which is situated too deeply.

CLINICAL EXPERIENCE

Between January 1977 and March 1982, 31 distal arteriovenous fistulas have been created in 24 children with microsurgical techniques. In 26 cases the radial artery, and in five cases the ulnar artery at the wrist, were used. In six children chronic haemodialysis had already been started through a more proximal A-V fistula when the distal fistula was created. Secondary surgical procedures were necessary nine times: three for re-anastomosis, six for super-ficializations of the vein. Mean weight of the children was 7600 g (4500–10 000 g) and the mean age was 20 months (8–36 months).

There were 12 failures: two thrombosed immediately after surgical procedure, four thrombosed later before maturation, six never developed. In addition, one child died before the beginning of dialysis, and one patient was lost for follow-up. In the 17 successful fistulas the vein expanded sufficiently to be used for haemodialysis. Seven of them have not yet come into use while 10 are being or have been used. The mean delay between operation and the first needle puncture was 4 months (1–10 months). At the present time 15 fistulas are patent with a mean patency rate of 20 months. During the follow-up four children died and five children had a successful kidney transplant-ation.

DISCUSSION

Microsurgery is particularly applicable for the distal A-V fistula in small children. The smallest child having successful creation of a distal A-V fistula is the case reported by Sicard[2] in 1978; the child weighed 14 kg. In the same year Gagnadoux[3] reported immediate thrombosis in 50% of distal fistulas in children under 20 kg. The benefit of microsurgery is obvious in our series: 31 distal fistulas were performed in 24 children under 10 kg. The immediate thrombosis rate is 6%, and the definitive success rate (i.e. usable for haemodialysis) is 54%. This brings us to the conclusion that microvascular surgery is a must for vascular access in small children, where it provides in skilled hands a usable access in most of the children.

References

1 Daniel, R. and Terkis, J. (1977). *Reconstructive Microsurgery*. 1st Edn. (Boston: Little, Brown)
2 Sigard, G. and Merrel, R. (1978). Subcutaneous arteriovenous dialysis fistulas in pediatric patients. *Trans. Am. Soc. Artif. Intern. Organs*, **24**, 695
3 Gagnadoux, M. F. and Degoulet, P. (1978). L'Abord vasculaire chez l'enfant traité par hemodialyse périodique (resultats d'une enquête cooperative). *J. Urol. Nephrol.*, **84**, 935

2

Utilization of the 'anatomical snuffbox' for vascular access in haemodialysis

U. BONALUMI, D. CIVALLERI, G. ADAMI, E. GIANETTA AND
F. GRIFFANTI-BARTOLI

It is widely accepted that the arteriovenous fistula is the method of choice in achieving vascular access for maintenance haemodialysis. Since the first report by Brescia and co-workers[1], numerous modifications have been made concerning both site of the procedure[2-5] and type of anastomosis[6,7].

The 'anatomical snuffbox' (AS), at the base of the thumb between the tendons of the extensor pollicis muscles, can be a desirable site for starting vascular surgery for haemodialysis. The following advantages favour this procedure:

(1) very simple operation with easy access to the vessels;
(2) extensive vascular segment for venipuncture:
(3) possibility of performing a new A-V fistula at the distal forearm in case of failure.

The reports on utilization of AS for vascular access are few[2,3,8] and, to our knowledge, no attention has been given to the end-to-end anastomosis at this location.

MATERIAL AND METHODS

From 1 January 1972 to 31 December 1981, 213 patients were submitted to end-to-end A-V fistula at the AS for haemodialysis. There were 85 females and 128 males ranging in age from 15 to 72 years. Mean age was 47 years. Patient follow-up ranged from a minimum of 1 month to a maximum of 120 months.

Under local anaesthesia a 3 cm longitudinal incision is made at the AS

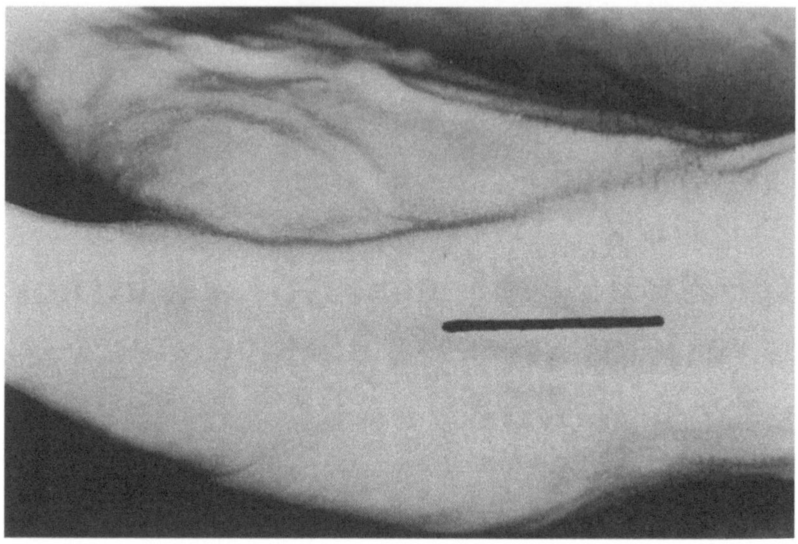

Figure 2.1 Site of incision for performing arteriovenous fistula at the 'anatomical snuffbox'

(Figure 2.1). The cephalic vein is mobilized for a distance of 2–3 cm. Caution must be exercised in order to avoid lesions of a superficial radial nerve branch. The fascia between the tendons is incised and the subfascial layers are gently dissected. After ligation and interruption of two main small branches,

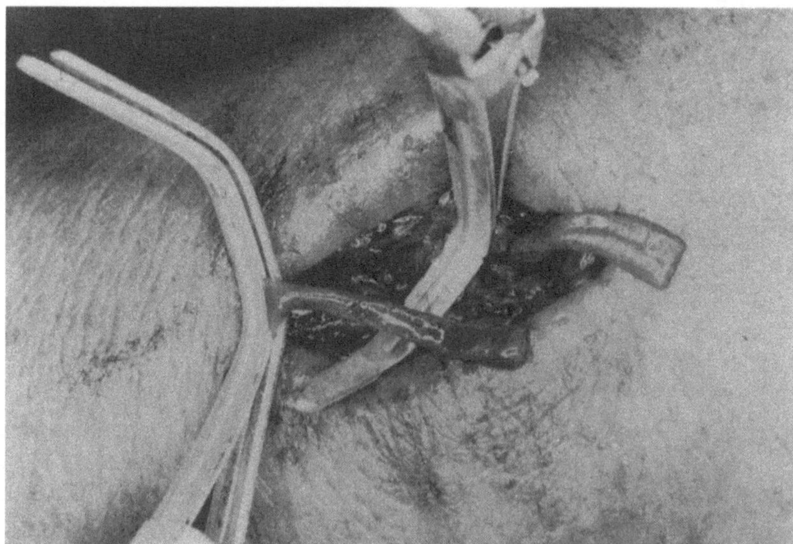

Figure 2.2 The vessels have been prepared for anastomosis. Woman's hair clips are utilized as atraumatic clamps

the artery is mobilized for about 3 cm. Atraumatic clamps are applied to occlude the vessels which are then ligated and sectioned as distal as possible (Figure 2.2). The vessel lumens are gently dilated and then washed out with heparinized saline by means of a small catheter which is introduced into the vein and pushed up along the forearm to be sure of vein patency. It is mandatory to have the artery making the loop and the vein to be in a straight line in order to avoid angulation of the vein. A double semicircle anastomosis is performed in a continuous fashion with 7/O monofilament or woven suture (Figure 2.3). Magnification loupe or other ocular devices are not used. On release of the clamps there must be an immediate thrill and bruit before one can consider the operation a success. The fistula is usually not used before a period of 10–15 days in order to allow the arterialized vein to distend. If the fistula could not be used for regular haemodialysis it was considered a failure. A-V fistulas that stopped functioning within the first 48 h were considered to be an immediate failure. The survival curve for all the A-V fistulas was calculated by the life-table method[9].

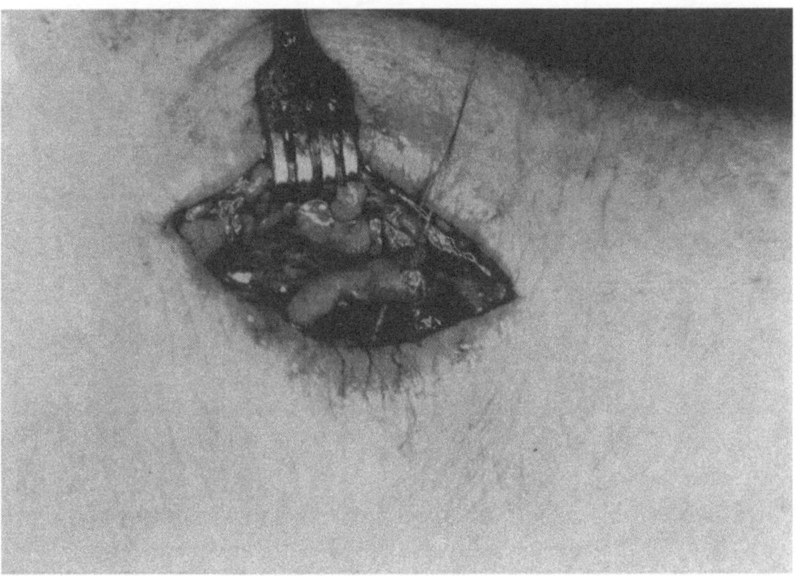

Figure 2.3   The end-to-end anastomosis is completed. Note that the artery makes the loop and the vein is in a straight line

RESULTS

The operation was tolerated quite well. Bleeding from vascular suture line developed 3 h after surgery in one patient, requiring a revision with closure of a small anastomotic leak. Infection was never observed. Figure 2.4 shows the

A-V fistula survival curve for all the patients. Survival rate was 83% at 12 months and 49% at 72 months.

Twenty-four fistulas (11%) stopped functioning within the first 48 h. Thrombosis, responsible for 100% of these immediate failures, was due to technical errors at operation and/or hypotension and/or small size of the vessels.

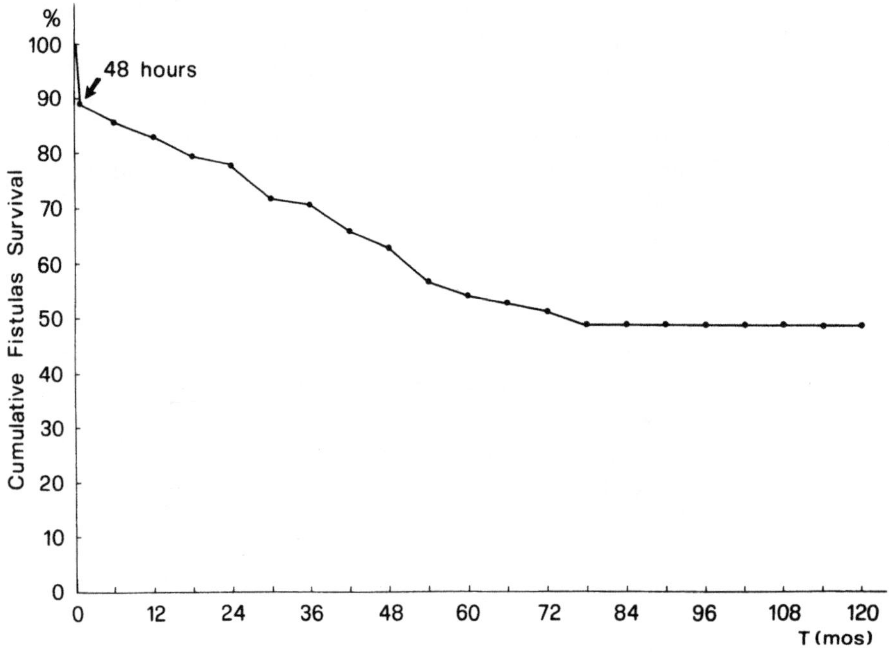

Figure 2.4 Survival curve of 213 arteriovenous fistulas at the 'anatomical snuffbox'

Forty-two fistulas ceased functioning 10 days to 72 months after surgery. Twenty-one of these late failures were due to aneurysm formation and subsequent thrombosis as a result of repeated punctures of the arterialized vein at the same site. Ten fistulas thrombosed because of prolonged hypotensive episodes. Two fistulas failed because of a haematoma constricting the vein which developed after needle puncture. One fistula thrombosed after an abdominal operation. Another failed because the cephalic vein did not dilate in spite of the presence of a thrill, due to the blood flow diversion towards a deep vein. Seven fistulas failed for unknown reasons from 10 to 60 days after surgery.

Ischaemic complications, distal venous hypertension or cardiac failure never occurred.

DISCUSSION

The great improvement in dialysis techniques and improved knowledge of the management of maintenance haemodialysis patients have considerably prolonged the life of these patients. Therefore one of the most important problems regarding the future of these patients could be the progressive reduction in angioaccess for venipuncture. For this reason there is general agreement that surgery for haemodialysis should be performed as distal as possible in order to spare vessels.

The 'anatomical snuffbox' can be considered the most distal location available for vascular access for haemodialysis.

In our opinion the end-to-end anastomosis is preferable to the side-to-side and end-to-side technique for the following reasons:

(1)   easier anastomosis technique;
(2)   no local venous hypertension as compared to the side-to-side technique[10,11];
(3)   no possibility of a steal syndrome[10-12];
(4)   lower risk of cardiac failure[13,14].

Before operation it is important to verify the presence of a suitable vein and a normal pulsating artery at the AS. The vein is confirmed suitable when measuring 3–4 mm after instrumental dilatation. A highly calcified artery

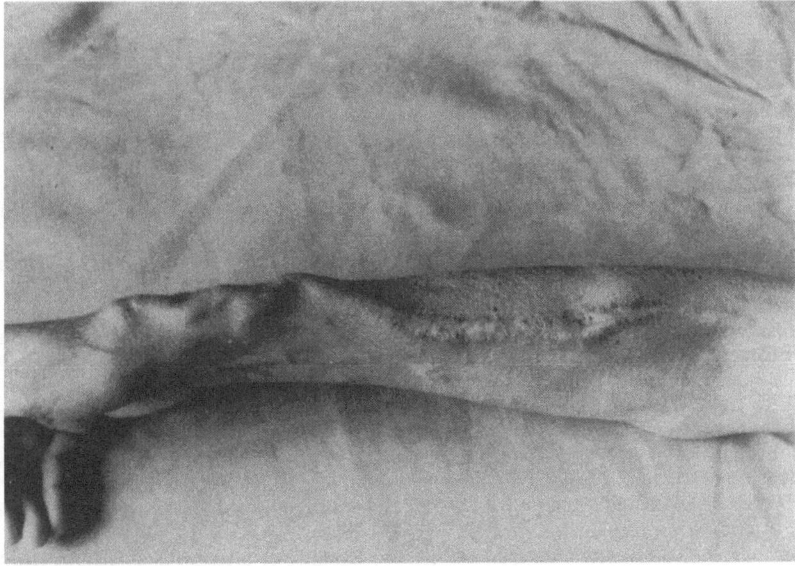

Figure 2.5 A 10-year-old arteriovenous fistula. Note the regular distension of the whole arterialized venous tract

must be discarded for anastomosis if the blood flow from the sectioned vessel is considered inadequate or the suture is impracticable because of the wall stiffness. Vein patency must be ascertained along the forearm as far as the antecubital fossa. It is mandatory to create an arterial loop and to have the vein in a straight line because of the more elastic and consistent wall of the artery.

Fifty per cent of the late failures were due to aneurysm formation for repeated needle venipuncture at the same site and subsequent obliteration of the segment. Two factors seem to lead to this complication: preference for inserting needles in dilated areas by dialysis personnel, and the pressing desire of the patient to be punctured always at the same site because of skin insensibility. The correct fistula management should consist in changing the site of venipuncture at the time of every dialysis, thus allowing a regular distension of the whole venous tract (Figure 2.5).

In case of failure, reoperation at the AS is inadvisable because of the lack of material for a new anastomosis. The creation of an A-V fistula at the wrist is facilitated by the enlarged diameter of both artery and vein by the previous fistula in the AS.

References

1 Brescia, M. J., Cimino, J. E., Appel, K. and Hurvich, B. J. (1966). Chronic hemodialysis using venipuncture and a surgically created arteriovenous fistula. *N. Engl. J. Med.*, **275**, 1089

2 Harder, F., Tondelli, P. and Haenel (1977). Hämodialyse-die arterio-venöse fistel distal des handgelenkes. *Chirurg*, **48**, 719

3 Rassat, J. P. and Moskovchenko, J. P. (1971). 60 fistules artério-veineuses pour épuration extra-rénale. *Ann. Chir. Thorac. Cardiovasc.*, **10**, 79

4 Kinnaert, P., Vereerstraeten, P., Geens, M. and Toussaint, C. (1971). Ulnar arteriovenous fistula for maintenance hemodialysis *Br. J. Surg.*, **58**, 641

5 May, J., Tiller, D., Johnson, J., Stewart, J. and Ross Sheil, A. G. (1969). Saphenous-vein arteriovenous fistula in regular dialysis treatment. *N. Engl. J. Med.*, **280**, 770

6 Sperling, M., Kleinschmidt, W., Wilhelm, A., Heidland, A. and Klutsch, K. (1967). Die subkutane arteriovenöse fistel zur intermittierenden hämodialyse-behandlung. *Dtsch. Med. Wochenschr.*, **10**, 425

7 Thompson, B. W., Barbour, G. and Bisset, J. (1972). Internal arteriovenous fistula for hemodialysis. *Am. J. Surg.*, **124**, 785

8 Mehigan, J. T. and McAlexander, R. A. (1982). Snuffbox arteriovenous fistula for hemodialysis. *Am. J. Surg.*, **143**, 252

9 Armitage, P. (1971). *Statistical Methods in Medical Research*. (Oxford: Blackwell)

10 Lawton, R. L. and Freeman, R. M. (1972). Complications of arteriovenous fistulae. In Cameron, G. S., Fries, D. and Ogg, C. S. (eds.) *Proc. Eur. Dial. Transplant. Assoc.*, **9**, 588 (London: Pitman Medical)

11 Haimov, M., Baez, A., Neff, M. and Slifkin, R. (1975). Complications of arteriovenous fistulas for hemodialysis. *Arch. Surg.*, **110**, 708

12 Bussell, J. A., Abbott, J. A. and Lim, R. C. (1971). A radial steal syndrome with arteriovenous fistula for hemodialysis. *Ann. Intern. Med.*, **75**, 387

13 Ahearn, D. J. and Maher, J. F. (1972). Heart failure as a complication of hemodialysis arteriovenous fistula. *Ann. Intern. Med.*, **77**, 201

14 Anderson, C. B. and Groce, M. A. (1975). Banding of arteriovenous dialysis fistulas to correct high-output cardiac failure. *Surgery*, **78**, 552

3

Side-to-side, side-to-end or end-to-end anastomosis for Cimino–Brescia fistula? Preliminary report of a randomized study

B. FORSBERG, L. FORSBERG, E. LINDSTEDT, H. WESTLING AND T. WHITE

Arteriovenous fistula in the forearm has been the established technique for vascular access in haemodialysis treatment for the last 15 years. The fistula is usually constructed between the radial artery and the cephalic vein if these vessels are available. The anastomosis may be performed side-to-side as was originally described by Cimino, Brescia and others in 1966. It can also be performed side-to-end or end-to-end, and each anastomosis technique has its advantages and disadvantages. To compare the usefulness of various anastomosis techniques we started a randomized study in 27 uremic patients who were prepared for haemodialysis treatment.

PATIENTS AND METHODS

None of the patients had previously been operated upon, and healthy vessels were found at operation. If the anatomical conditions allowed optional anastomosis technique to be used the patient entered the study. In the first group of 10 patients the standard side-to-side anastomosis was performed 5 mm in length. In the second group of eight patients the cephalic vein was cut distally and connected to the side of the artery making a smooth loop. The third group of nine was operated exactly as the second group but a ligature was tied around the artery just distal to the anastomosis, making it functionally an end-to-end anastomosis.

One primary failure occurred in the side-to-end group. In this group another fistula ceased to function after the patient received a kidney

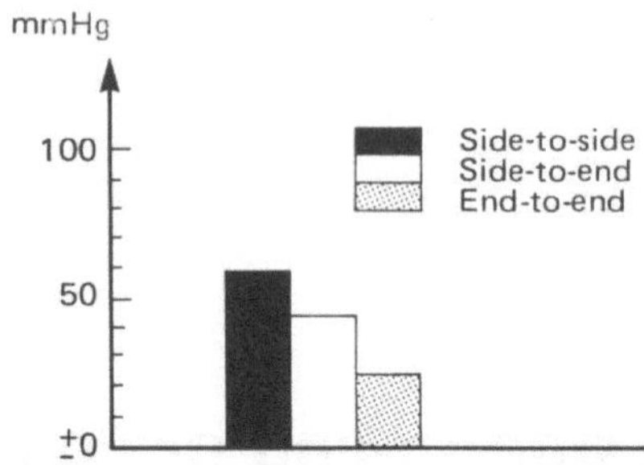

Figure 3.1 Difference in blood pressure in thumb before and after compression of fistula

transplant 6 months later. Apart from this, 16 renal transplantations were performed among the patients without interfering with the function of the fistula. No other secondary failure has occurred after 3 years of use.

The systemic blood pressure of the arm was measured using a mercury sphygmomanometer. The blood pressure of both thumbs was measured by a strain gauge device. Differences in blood pressure between arm and thumb were noted before operation and 3 months thereafter. The systolic blood pressure of the arm was higher than that of the thumb before operation. This blood pressure gradient was found to be equal on both sides. After operation the gradient was more pronounced on the fistula side. Comparisons were made between the three groups of fistulas concerning the changes of the blood pressure gradient of the operated arm. The non-operated arm was used as reference (Figure 3.1). The pressure gradient increased with a mean of 64 mmHg in the group of the side-to-side fistulas, with a mean of 39 mmHg in the side-to-end group and of 18 mmHg only in the end-to-end group. The patient with the most pronounced gradient in the side-to-side group had a fall in systolic blood pressure in the operated arm of 125 mmHg, from 170 in the upper arm to 45 in the thumb.

These variations were found to be statistically significant when comparing the side-to-side group with the end-to-end group; using Wilcoxon's test of

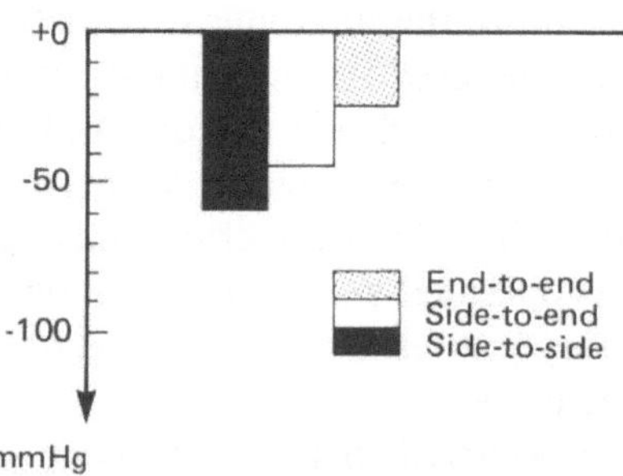

Figure 3.2 Difference in blood pressure fall between thumbs, 3 months after A-V fistula operation

unpaired samples the p value was less than 0.05. We also tried to estimate the function of the fistula, studying the thumb blood pressure on the operated side before and during compression of the fistula (Figure 3.2). The increase in thumb blood pressure after this procedure was more pronounced in the side-to-side group than in the other groups. The mean increase in thumb blood pressure was 59 mmHg in the side-to-side group, 43 mmHg in the side-to-end group and 22 mmHg in the end-to-end group. This difference was significant using Wilcoxon's test.

The blood flow through the brachial artery was measured with Doppler technique in eleven patients (Figure 3.3). There was a wide range of variation of flow from 350 ml/min to 910 ml/min. The arteries and veins of the patients were at operation found to be of almost the same size, the radial artery between 2.5 and 3 mm and the cephalic vein between 3 and 4 mm.

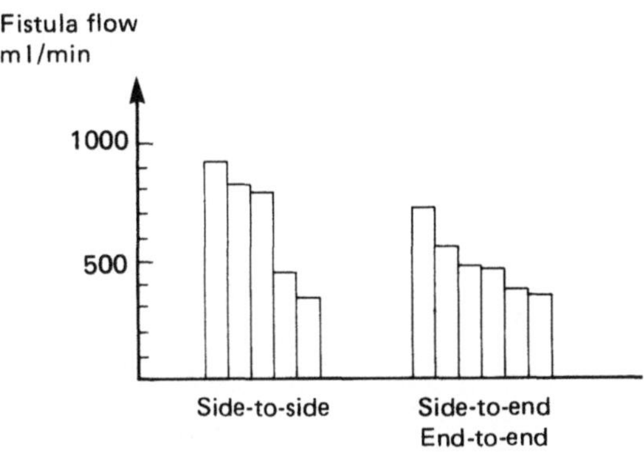

Figure 3.3   Blood flow (Doppler) through the A-V fistula in 11 patients

Some of the patients with highest blood flow were found in the side-to-side group, but this material is small and any significant differences between the groups could not be found.

DISCUSSION

Thus these findings indicate a steal of blood pressure from the arterial collaterals to the fistula. None of the patients had clinical symptoms of arterial steal.

This study shows that side-to-side anastomosis might be the best choice in patients when a high blood flow is needed. Today the fistula function of all patients in this study is quite sufficient when used in ordinary haemodialysis treatment. When considering the increasing treatment with haemofiltration where a minimal flow of 300 ml/min is necessary, some of the fistulas in this study might not have been acceptable. Also in patients with small veins at operation side-to-side anastomosis might be the best choice, obtaining the highest blood flow.

4

Arteriovenous fistula at the elbow for maintenance haemodialysis

C. MORIS AND P. KINNAERT

Over the past years, in an attempt to maintain good vascular access for chronic haemodialysis in uremic patients, an increasing number of arteriovenous (A-V) fistulas in the antecubital fossa have been performed in our department.

This type of A-V fistula was chosen when a more distal fistula had failed, or when the forearm veins were unsuitable for the standard A-V fistula. The purpose of this presentation is to report our experience with four different types of elbow A-V fistulas and to provide actuarial data on the survival of this type of vascular access as well as on its complications.

MATERIAL AND METHODS

Between January 1976 and December 1981 a total of 119 A-V fistulas at the elbow were realized in 103 patients. Over half of the patients had at least one A-V fistula operation before. The age of the patients ranged from 19 to 81 years. Two-thirds of the patients were women. Half of the patients were over 50 years of age.

Follow-up ranged from 6 months to 6 years. Twenty-six patients were in poor condition and died during follow-up. Five patients were lost for follow-up. When either the cephalic or basilic vein in the forearm was still patent and of sufficient calibre, it was dissected free, placed in a U-shaped subcutaneous tunnel created at the volar aspect of the forearm, and:

(a)   sutured end-to-side to the brachial artery in the antecubital fossa (Figure 4.1a). If the veins in the forearm were inadequate, there was still the choice out of three possibilities:

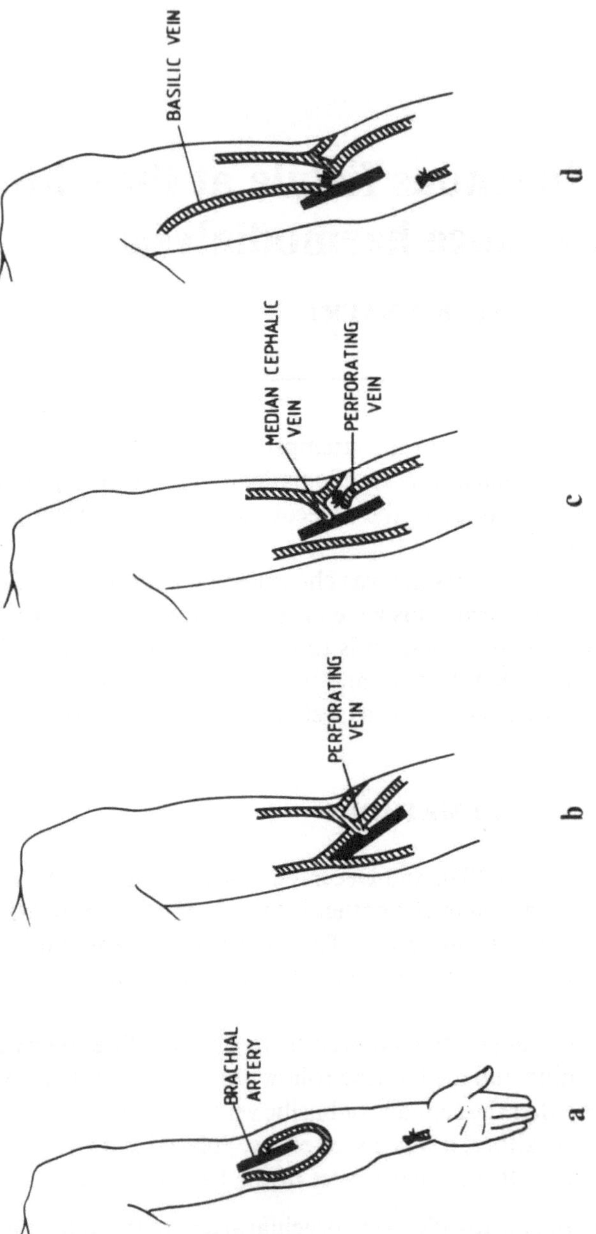

Figure 4.1 Four different types of elbow A-V fistulas

(b)   if a perforating vein at the elbow is present and of good calibre, it is sutured end-to-side to the brachial artery (Figure 4.1b);

(c)   the median cephalic vein can be anastomosed to the brachial artery (Figure 4.1c); or,

(d)   if the basilic vein in the upper arm is of good calibre, it is dissected free to the axillary vein and positioned in a subcutaneous tunnel at the volar aspect of the upper arm and sutured end-to-side to the brachial artery in the antecubital fossa. The subcutaneous positioning of the vein makes it accessible for puncture (Figure 4.1d)[1,2].

Of the 119 A-V fistulas at the elbow, 31 were realized with a vein of the forearm (type a), 27 with an elbow perforating vein (type b), 25 with the median cephalic vein (type c) and 36 with the proximal basilic vein (type d).

The operations were performed either under general or local anaesthesia.

RESULTS

The overall immediate failure rate was 9.2%. It was slightly higher for women (10.3%) than for men (7.1%). There was no significant difference in the immediate failure rate of the four types of fistula (Figure 4.2). Thrombosis was responsible for 85% of these failures. Other causes were infection, false aneurysm or cardiac failure.

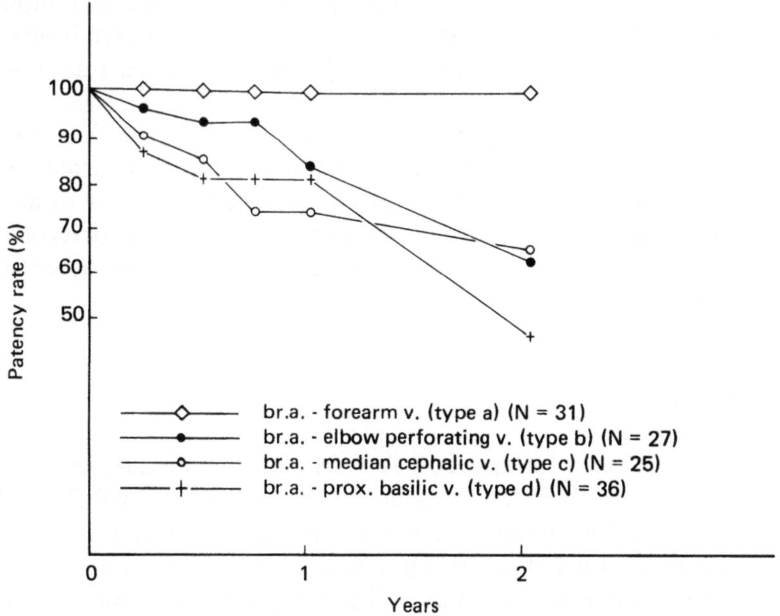

Figure 4.2   Life-table curves for the four different types of elbow A-V fistulas

We had 103 elbow A-V fistulas available for life-table calculations. The overall patency rate was 82% at 1 year and 68% at 2 years. The fistula survival rate was lower in women (respectively 81% and 62% at 1 and 2 years) than in men (82% at both 1 and 2 years). The fistula survival rate between the four types of elbow A-V fistulas is shown in Figure 4.2. There were no late failures among the elbow perforating vein A-V fistula (type b). This 100% survival rate differs significantly from the rates calculated for the other types of fistulas. At 2 years, survival rate was 64% for the forearm vein A-V fistula (type a), only 48% for the median cephalic vein A-V fistula (type c) and 63% for type (d) fistulas. The difference of survival between these latter three fistulas is not statistically significant.

Various complications were observed: a long-lasting oedema was present in eight patients. It eventually disappeared. Two patients presented with a false aneurysm which was responsible for haemorrhage; one of the fistulas had to be ligated for that reason.

Infection at a puncture site occurred five times. Adequate antibiotic treatment was successful in all but one case, where the infected segment had to be excised to avoid septicaemia. All but one patient had good flow-rates, allowing adequate dialysis. One patient developed cardiac failure, but it is doubtful whether the fistula was responsible: its ligation did not improve clinical status.

Ischaemia seems to be by far the most frequent side-effect of this type of fistula: out of 50 patients, carefully interviewed and examined, 23 complained of some degree of ischaemia. In most cases, however, symptoms were very mild, like a cold, pale hand or sometimes Raynaud's syndrome-like phenomena when exposed to cold. Simple precautions, such as wearing gloves outdoors and avoiding contact with cold water, diminished or even abolished symptoms. Six patients complained of typical intermittent claudication of the hand (defined as a cramping pain that occurred during exercise and disappeared quickly at rest) but again, this was not disabling. Two patients presented with very mild trophic lesions of the nails (irregularity, small holes). Symptoms of ischaemia were more frequently observed in women (28%) than in men (18%).

DISCUSSION

Patients were selected for an elbow A-V fistula either because of the poor quality of their vessels in the forearm or because a more distal fistula had failed. With smaller-calibre arteries and veins and a greater tendency to vasoconstriction, it is not surprising to find a higher proportion of women selected for this type of fistula as well as a higher failure rate, and more frequent ischaemia. The reason for the high incidence of 'steal syndrome' with the elbow A-V fistula, could be its haemodynamic similarity with a side-to-side A-V anastomosis. It has been reported that the incidence of ischaemic symptoms was higher with a side-to-side anastomosis at the wrist than with an end-to-side or end-to-end technique[3]. Compared to wrist A-V fistula survival rates at 1 year are not different (respectively 85% for wrist A-V fistula, and 82% for elbow A-V fistula), but a little lower at 2 years (83 and 68% respectively)[4]. Mild ischaemic symptoms are a little more frequent in elbow A-V fistula, respectively 42% in wrist A-V fistula and 46% in elbow A-V fistula[3]. Compared to saphenous vein graft fistulas, complications were less frequent and patency rates were higher. For saphenous vein graft fistulas patency rates are 75% and 48% at 1 and 2 years respectively[5].

In our hands elbow A-V fistulas offer a good alternative when a radial cephalic fistula has failed or cannot be realized due to unsuitable veins. It has the advantage of avoiding the use of prosthetic material or bovine heterografts. It is technically simple and requires only one vascular suture. It results in a good functioning fistula with high flow-rates and few complications.

References

1 Dagher, F. J., Gelber, R. L., Ramos, E. J. and Sadler, J. H. (1976). Basilic vein to brachial artery fistula: a new access for chronic hemodialysis. *South. Med. J.*, **69**, 1438
2 Dagher, F. J., Gelber, R. L., Ramos, E. J. and Sadler, J. H. (1976). The use of basilic vein and brachial artery as an AV fistula for long term hemodialysis. *J. Surg. Res.*, **20**, 373
3 Kinnaert, P., Struyven, J., Mathieu, J., Vereerstraeten, P., Toussaint, C. and Van Geertruyden, J. (1980). Intermittent claudication of the hand after creation of an arteriovenous fistula in the forearm. *Am. J. Surg.*, **139**, 838
4 Kinnaert, P., Vereerstraeten, P., Toussaint, C. and Van Geertruyden, J. (1977). Nine years experience with internal arteriovenous fistulas for hemodialysis: a study of some factors influencing the results. *Br. J. Surg.*, **64**, 242
5 Kinnaert, P., Vereerstraeten, P., Toussaint, C. and Van Geertruyden, J. (1979). Saphenous vein loop fistula in the thigh for maintenance hemodialysis. *World J. Surg.*, **3**, 95

5

Abstracts of posters in Surgical technique and microsurgery

The arteriovenous fistula in the tabatière
J. LANDMANN, F. HARDER and P. TONDELLI

The A-V fistula in the snuffbox (tabatière) distal to the wrist extends accessible vessel length distally leaving the proximal segments intact for further use. Eighty-eight A-V fistulas in the tabatière have been done from 1972 to 1981. Four patients have been lost to follow-up. The remaining 84 patients have been on haemodialysis until renal transplantation or death on an average of 2.6 years. Of these 84 fistulas 59 functioned well, five showed poor function and twenty failed at some time. The outcome of these 25 insufficient fistulas is presented in Table 5.1. Eighty-eight per cent of all patients were finally on haemodialysis with a tabatière or Cimino fistula. Major vascular changes as the cause of renal failure have been found to unfavourably influence the outcome of these A-V fistulas: in four of six patients with vascular pathology the fistula failed. Comparing the different surgeons having done such fistulas shows the correlation between experience and success. Due to the proximity of suitable arterial and venous branches in the tabatière the A-V fistula at this site represents an access that can be created easily and rapidly without jeopardizing the construction of any one of the more proximal fistulas if it fails.

Table 5.1 Initial result and eventual modification of 84 tabatière fistulas

Initial result	Good	Poor	Occlusion	
Final access				
Tabatière	59	1	4	64
Cimino		2	8	10
Other		2	8	10
Total	59	5	20	84

Forming of arteriovenous fistula and arteriovenous shunt by one operation
A. ONCEVSKI and K. CAKALAROSKI

We present an original approach in utilization of the distal segment of A. radialis and V. cephalica to form an A-V shunt made simultaneously with the formation of the Cimino A-V fistula between the A. radialis and V. cephalica.

This is applied in order to reduce the traumatization of the patient, rationalization of vascular access and facilitation of haemodialysis while the Cimino fistula matures.

Our first experiences (nine cases), where we always respected the anatomical and functional features of blood vessels, are encouraging. The objective of our paper is to present this method as a viable vascular approach.

Preoperative regional block with guanethidine may improve patency rates of arteriovenous fistulas
M. B. THOMSEN

Regional intravenous sympathetic block with guanethidine (RGB) was given to patients before construction of A-V fistulas and the effect on early failure rate is investigated in a prospective randomized trial.

Direct type lower forearm fistulas were constructed in 34 patients with renal failure. Seventeen patients were pretreated with RGB and 17 served as controls. RGB was performed essentially as an intravenous regional neural block for local analgesia only the anaesthetic was substituted by guanethidine (0.25 mg/kg body weight). Patency of less than 2 weeks was classified as early failure. Resting arterial flow (RAF) was determined by occlusion plethysmography on two occasions, before and 20 h after block or at equivalent interval in controls. Blood flow through the fistula was measured electromagnetically during operation and venous and arterial diameters as well as arterial BP were recorded. Fistula blood flow resistance was calculated as $BP \times flow^{-1}$.

Blood flow before blockade was 3.8 ± 1.3 ml $\times$ 100 ml tissue^{-1} $\times$ min^{-1} (mean $\pm$ SD) and rose to 9.7 ± 3.2 after block ($p<0.001$). The mean intra-individual increase in RAF in blocked arm was 5.8 ± 3.4 ($p<0.001$). In patients treated with hydralazine as an antihypertensive drug there was only a small increase in blood flow (2.6 ± 2.6; $p>0.05$). In patients not so treated the mean intraindividual increase was 7.8 ± 1.9 ($p<0.001$). At operation there was as significantly lower mean flow resistance (1.7 ± 0.6) in blocked arms than in non-blocked (3.8 ± 2.6; $p<0.05$). Among 21 non-hydralazine patients there was one early failure in 10 RGB-treated individuals and three early failures in 11 controls.

The conclusion is that RGB lowers flow resistance in AVF and may be of value in reducing early failure rates.

Conversion of the external 'short shunt' to an internal arteriovenous fistula
A. GARCIA-ALFAGEME, J. A. CHACON, A. YAÑEZ, L. RODRIGUEZ, E. LEGARRETA, N. ESKUBI and J. GARCIA-ALONSO

In this paper we are analysing the results obtained in 120 patients in which we have used our 'short shunt', placed in the forearm in order to begin the haemodialysis programme with urgency. After obtaining a good 'maturation' of the veins, the device is removed and an internal A-V fistula is performed on the same vessels. The haemodialysis is continued by venipuncture of the new fistula.

The follow-up has been a minimum of 6 months. In 77% of the patients this was the definitive vascular access. We have had complications in 23% of them; in 15% the A-V fistula is well functioning after a short rest, in the other 8% the fistula failed, of these, 4% was due to bad handling of the external shunt previous to its transformation. The other 4% had very bad superficial veins which failed with most access techniques, so we had to use a vascular graft.

The results with this 'short shunt' conversion technique are comparable with the conventional A-V internal fistula. It is of immediate and permanent use, and thus contributes to save the 'vascular access-reserve' of these patients, which is a guarantee of their survival.

Transformation of Buselmeier shunts into arteriovenous fistulas for haemodialysis
J. ROTTEMBOURG, P. ROJAS, M. C. GUIMONT, G. VALLANCIEN, P. FRANTZ and M. BITKER

When the creation of an arteriovenous (A-V) fistula is not immediately possible, temporary upper limb implantation of a Buselmeier shunt (BS) offers adequate blood flow maintenance haemodialysis and allows further transformation into the A-V fistula using the same vessels. Between October 1976 and December 1981 a BS was implanted in 58 adults with end-stage renal failure (30 males, 28 females, mean age 54.8 ± 12.6 years). Implantation was made near the wrist close to the radial (53 cases) or ulnar (5 cases) side. Implantation of a shunt was decided in 14 cases after immediate failure of an A-V fistula construction and in 44 cases as a first-choice procedure because either emergency dialysis was required (12 cases) or small size of blood vessels made the creation and rapid use of an A-V fistula (32 cases) difficult. Very small vessel tips (size 18–20, outside diameter 1.8–1.3 mm) were used in 30 cases on the arterial site and in 18 cases on the venous site. In all cases haemodialysis was easily performed immediately after the implantation of the BS. Transformation of the shunt into A-V fistula was successful within a delay of 46 ± 22 days in 48 cases (82%); two surgical procedures were required in four cases. Transformation was avoided because of local complications in six cases. Haemodialysis using the single-needle procedure was performed within 24–50 h following the transformation. Blood flow rates measured in 10 patients using the Doppler technique increased from 60 ± 12 ml/min on the radial artery before BS to 180 ± 46 ml/min on the BS, and to 226 ± 48 ml/min on the A-V fistula. The technique proposed offers an efficient and safe temporary vascular access for haemodialysis and represents a challenge to other procedures including the use of a subclavian catheter.

Is vessel size a limiting factor in determining success of dialysis fistula?
D. T. REILLY, R. F. M. WOOD and P. R. F. BELL

The longest-lasting procedure for vascular access is the wrist fistula; it would be advantageous to increase the number of primary wrist fistulas in patients who are now undergoing other access procedures because of small veins. To determine whether fistulas adequate for dialysis could be constructed despite small veins and low flow at operation, 33 consecutive fistula operations were studied. At operation vessel dimensions and blood pressure were measured and flow was determined with an electromagnetic flowmeter. Over a mean follow-up time of 7 months, 19 fistulas had been used for dialysis and seven not yet used. Nine patients developed thrombotic or stenotic complications: mean flow for this group was 221 ± 189 ml/min compared with 222 ± 171 ml/min for the whole group. Blood flow correlated with arm blood pressure but there was no greater incidence of problems in patients with low flow, low blood pressure and smaller veins. It is concluded that development of fistulas is independent of the absolute flow rate achieved at operation and other factors such as a relative thrombotic tendency should be investigated.

Bilateral radiocephalic arteriovenous fistulas for prolonged vascular access
K. ONO

In order to prolong the useful life of A-V fistulas for haemodialysis, we have adopted the following policy. Whenever possible, bilateral radiocephalic wrist A-V fistulas are created in patients under the age of 50 who showed no evidence of cardiac failure. Autogenous vein was used only if revision procedures were necessary. Fistulas were always needled by the surgeon who operated on the patient, and when two fistulas were available, these were used alternately. Fifty-two cases were divided into two groups, depending on the number of available access sites. Those with single sites had a fistula at the wrist, elbow or upper arm, depending on the availability of vessels. The results are shown in Table 5.2. Access was significantly prolonged in patients with bilateral fistulas. The haematocrit (Hct) was also higher in this group.

There was no clinical evidence that bilateral fistulas had any adverse effect on the cardiovascular system. In addition, the cardiothoracic ratio (CTR) was not different in the two groups. In conclusion, bilateral fistulas allow alternate needling, which helps to significantly prolong fistula life and allow for unexpected failure of one of them. Careful use of each site with one person inserting the needle may also be important. This approach prolongs fistula life and may avoid the necessity of using more complicated procedures or synthetic graft materials.

Table 5.2

No. of A-V fistulas	No. of patients	Age	Duration of haemodialysis	Longevity of access	CTR	Hct
1	26	48	53 months	32 months	47.9%	26.0%
2	26	47	57 months	48 months	46.8%	29.0%

Arteriovenous shunts transformation into arteriovenous fistulas

M. ELSENER, P. Y. MEAULLE, C. QUESADA, M. FORET, H. MEFTAHI, F. KUENTZ, and E. DECHELETTE

For the past 3 years all our A-V shunts have been placed near the wrist, in view of future A-V fistula transformation of the employed blood vessels. This was performed on 34 patients at a mean 41 days after A-V shunt placing (extremes at 18 and 98 days). Efferent A-V shunt vein arterialization is clinically checked in order to determine earliest possible two needle puncture, and use as a fistula; the A-V shunt is still functioning during this type of dialysis. If blood flow is sufficient and allows for efficient dialysis, the A-V shunt is transformed into an A-V fistula during the following days.

All our patients were dialysed on the newly created A-V fistula from A-V shunt blood vessels, at latest 48 h after surgery. The only problem sometimes encountered was postoperative oedema which required temporary single-needle puncture. This type of A-V fistula was studied from 1 to 40 months (a mean of 12 months). In three cases, initial, non-functional A-V fistula (previous thrombosis, or small blood vessels in a child) was replaced by an A-V shunt. This allowed for a subsequent functional A-V fistula transformation of the same blood vessels developed by the A-V shunt.

At present A-V shunt placing in the upper limb is always performed for its future A-V fistula transformation, or in order to arterialize or preserve blood vessels that are too small for an immediate A-V fistula creation.

6

Invited comment on papers and posters in Surgical technique and microsurgery

B. HUSBERG

Standing here as the first in a row of invited commenters I feel disadvantaged in one way and privileged in another. On the one hand I have to make comments based on very short abstracts of presentations and posters that I have heard or seen as complete presentations only within the last 2 h. Even more important, I think that you ladies and gentlemen have not had the time to study the posters yet. On the other hand, being first I can extend my comments outside the limits of this session, thereby stealing the planned remarks by my successors and knowing there is nothing they can do about it.

A dependable vascular access is literally a question of life and death for many of our patients. It is therefore not surprising that this small but rather specialized field of surgery has now become mature enough to merit its own international congress and the organizers deserve great credit for realizing this. Access surgery should not be looked upon as a specialty on its own, but every surgeon who works within it should have training and knowledge in order to avoid beginners' mistakes and to contribute to a high-quality care for this sensitive group of patients. We are all aware of the strong correlation between experience and success in this field.

The two major groups of patients in need of access surgery today are uraemic patients and patients in need of vessel-irritating cytostatic or nutritive treatment. Naturally the 'access surgeon' also meets occasional patients with other problems, as for instance in my own experience a 1-year-old child with haemophilia in need of regular dependable access for anti-haemophilic globulin administration or a markedly obese asthmatic woman. It is important to realize that vascular access surgery is not a single intervention, but requires the handling of patients over a long period of time, even decades. This handling involves not only surgical procedures, but also care of the patient before the first surgical procedure and between the procedures.

Before the first surgical procedure it is important to protect the vessels of the extremities as much as possible. The surgeon interested in vascular access surgery should be consulted as soon as there is a suspicion that such surgery may be required, and he should give instructions and advice about the management of the veins used for injections, infusions and blood sampling. Great care should be taken to save as many veins as possible for future vascular access surgery. Postoperatively the access surgeon might be consulted regarding, for instance, aneurysm formation, infections, steal phenomena and needling accidents.

The surgeon who performs the first surgical procedure has the golden opportunity to get a good fistula which can last for a long time. I think that most of us agree that this first operation should preferably be done without the use of transplanted material as a simple direct arteriovenous (A-V) fistula side-to-side or end-to-side. If a graft has to be used I think it should preferably be placed straight, with the arterial anastomosis distally rather than in a U-shaped fashion in order to diminish the risk of kinking, to make it easier to needle, and probably give less risk for cardiac strain and steal. The patient's own autogenous vein should always be the first choice as graft material. However, when there is an urgency to give dialysis treatment we seem to have a slight difference of opinion. We all agree that we should try to preserve the vascular tree as much as possible and a separate Scribner shunt should not be inserted for temporary use until the A-V fistula is developed. Today in posters by A. Garcia-Alfageme *et al.*, J. Rottembourg *et al.*, M. Elsener *et al.* and A. Oncevski *et al.* we can learn about ingenious methods to use the same site for a temporary shunt and an A-V fistula. The shunt is then at a later stage transformed into a fistula or the shunt is inserted into the distal stump of the transected artery; right after that an end-to-end A-V anastomosis is constructed. Personally I think that such a shunt must jeopardize the fistula by creating an infectious risk. A counter-argument put forward by Dr Rottembourg in his poster is that a shunt to a small vein has a greater chance to remain open than a fistula to a small vein. Personally I do not believe this, provided that microsurgical technique is used. This review is supported in a poster belonging to this session by Dr Reilly from Leicester, Great Britain. He can find no correlation between flow-rate or vein diameter during the operation and the later development of the fistula. So what is my proposal to save vessels and allow immediate treatment of the patient?

During the last 3 years we have always been able to gain time enough for a fistula to develop by peritoneal dialysis treatment or haemodialysis through a femoral vein catheter repeatedly inserted in the groin by the Seldinger technique. We have patients that have received twice-weekly maintenance dialysis for more than 4 months through such repeated groin vein punctures.

In spite of the fact that the main title for this first section of our congress includes the word 'microsurgery', only Dr Bourquelot in an invited presentation has really been talking about this and microsurgery is not mentioned in the poster presentations. One would hope that this is due to the fact that everybody accepts that delicate microsurgical technique with the use of optical magnification should be used in all patients. I think it is clear that even though it is technically possible to perform A-V fistulas in adults with standard surgical management it is a great advantage to use microsurgical technique and magnification. This gives a higher quality of all the surgical details, and decreases the risk for occlusion. Whatever success rate one has with standard technique it will improve further with a microsurgical one. In other words: 'if you are good, you will be super-good; if you are bad, you will be less bad'.

I would then like to turn my attention to the individual presentations. In the past there has been much discussion about end-to-side, end-to-end or side-to-side fistulas. Today we have heard from the group in Lund that there is really no great difference between these three types, and this seems to be supported by other oral and poster presentations. The risk for occlusion seems to be about the same with all three types and the life-span also apparently is about the same. The one disadvantage of the side-to-side anastomosis could be a tendency to widening and thus a too high shunt-flow.

The reason why there is a difference in thumb blood pressure after side-to-side and side-to-end anastomosis must be that the distal venous branch in the side-to-side fistula will soon have an incompetent valve. Otherwise you would in both instances from a physiological standpoint have a side-to-end situation. Also in the presentation by Dr Forsberg it is claimed that the steal of blood from the thumb is greater with a side-to-side than with an end-to-end fistula. 'Steal' is then defined as blood-pressure difference in the thumb before and after compression of the fistula. Personally I do not quite see that point. One should not expect a difference of thumb pressure at all before and after compression of an end-to-end fistula, unless of course a lot of arterial collaterals have developed bridging the gap down to the distal arterial stump. In my opinion, and from a technical standpoint, one of the great advantages with a side-to-side fistula is that the distal vein branch offers such a nice site for introduction of an embolectomy catheter or diluted contrast medium in case of trouble after completion of the anastomosis or at a reoperation.

Some other points of technique regarding the first operation for vascular access have been stressed in presentations belonging to this section. In one poster and one oral presentation by J. Landmann *et al.* and U. Bonalumi *et al.* respectively the use of the 'tabatière anatomique' or 'anatomical snuffbox' for vascular access is recommended, and large series of patients are presented. It is obviously a comparatively simple technique of anastomosing the cephalic vein and radical artery end-to-side or end-to-end and it has the advantage of an anastomosis localization far distally in the arm.

This gives ample possibilities for reoperations more proximally, better vein length for use, and, as pointed out by the authors, probably carries less risk for cardiac strain. No prospective randomized comparison of patency rates versus the standard fistula is presented, which is unfortunate because of course we need to know that we are not depriving our patients of statistical chance to get a good working first fistula by the 'snuffbox' procedure. Still the results of the 'snuffbox' operation seem good enough and certainly such a comparison is not easy to do.

Everybody has experience with the shunts which have failed, and with the problems one runs into when trying to re-establish the vascular access in these patients. Moris and co-workers describe the use of elbow A-V fistulas in adults in a series of patients which to a large extent have had surgical procedures more distally or where there were other difficulties. The authors used the brachial artery for anastomosis to a perforating vein or to the basilic or cephalic vein. They had a difficult group of previously operated patients but in spite of this there were only 10% immediate failures. However, there were a large number of patients who had a steal syndrome or claudication and it seems logical that there should be more steal problems when the fistula is created to the brachial artery than to either of the two forearm arteries. I quite agree with Dr Moris that basilic veins on the upper arm should be surgically transposed to a more superficial position to facilitate later needling.

In a poster presentation by Dr K. Ono from Japan it is claimed that we should give our patients two A-V fistulas whenever possible, thereby diminishing the frequency of fistula punctures thus increasing fistula survival. This is somewhat contradictory to the feelings of at least our nephrology colleagues who seem to think that frequent haemodialysis use is good for a fistula. Perhaps the presented results should be interpreted with some caution as to my understanding the one- and two-fistula group patients were not randomized, rather the one-fistula patients were those that only had one available fistula site.

Few adjunctive methods to improve patency have been studied and used in vascular access surgery. I am thinking of platelet disaggregation drugs or drugs decreasing blood coagulability which seem logical in patients with high tendency to vascular occlusions. One of the reasons for the minute interest in this problem may be the fact that uraemics which represent the majority of these patients have a 'built-in' platelet function inhibitor, in other words uraemia *per se* inhibits platelet aggregation. This obviously is of considerable help in the management of these patients. However, as already mentioned, we now often create fistulas in non-uraemic, perhaps even hypercoagulable patients. We can, in a poster by Dr M. E. Thomsen, learn about such an adjunctive measure to facilitate vascular access surgery. Dr Thomsen shows that a preoperative intravenous regional sympathetic block with guanethidine significantly improves the blood flow in the arm, thus also in the fistula, thereby decreasing the failure rate. The technique is probably a helpful adjunct in the handling of patients with high tendency to fistula occlusions. It would be interesting to learn how long this sympathetic block remains postoperatively as the common practice alternative, of course, is to operate in a brachial plexus anaesthesia, thus in a temporary sympathetic block.

Dr Thomsen has informed me that the control patients had brachial plexus block and that the sympathetic block after such a procedure will last about 2 h as compared to about 2 days in guanethidine-treated patients.

In summary I think that this first section of our congress has pointed to several possible improvements in the handling of our patients which could diminish our fistula failure rates. I hope I have at least put some wood into the fire for a following general discussion. During this session I have realized that certainly among access surgeons there is an excess of different opinions.

Section II
Techniques for monitoring during long-term follow-up

7

Non-invasive assessment of the capacity of arteriovenous fistulas

J. A. van GERWEN, C. M. A. BRUYNINCKX, M. J. C. van GEMERT
AND P. G. G. GERLAG

INTRODUCTION

For efficient treatment by haemodialysis a surgically created arteriovenous
(A-V) fistula should fulfil two criteria:

(1) it must be easy to puncture (e.g. not too deep, not near an important
artery, etc.);
(2) the flow through the fistula should be great enough to enable an
adequate treatment in a relatively short time.

In order to fulfil this last criterion the flow through the artificial kidney
should be at least 200 ml/min. The total flow through the fistula should
exceed the flow through the artificial kidney by at least 50%. This extra flow
is needed to carry away the cleared blood and thereby prevent recirculation of
blood that has been cleared. We call this extra flow the carrier flow. This
means that the total flow through the fistula should be at least 300 ml/min
and preferably more than 400 ml/min. During a haemodialysis session the
flow through the artificial kidney and/or the carrier flow may appear too
small. Then there are two explanations possible:

(1) the total amount of blood flowing through the fistula is too small for
adequate dialysis treatment;
(2) the needle or needles with which access is gained to the circulation have
been placed wrongly.

It is of practical importance to distinguish between these well-known
clinical situations. In one case a simple replacement of the needles is all that is
needed to solve the problem. In the other case a revision of the fistula or

construction of a new fistula is required. Sometimes this can be a very demanding operation.

In other fields of vascular surgery it is known that the angiogram bears little relation to the haemodynamic capacity of the vessels[1]. The same applies for the fistulogram although this investigation is indispensable when a revision of the fistula is contemplated. That is why we looked for haemo-dynamic parameters of the functional capacity of surgically created A-V fistulas.

MATERIALS AND METHODS

In our vascular laboratory we examined 52 patients with a surgically created A-V fistula. All patients were at the time in the haemodialysis programme of the nephrologic department of our clinic (heads: Dr P. F. L. Deckers and Dr P. G. G. Gerlag). We measured the systolic pressure in the index finger non-invasively by the cuff occlusion technique (Figure 7.1). A specially constructed pressure cuff (width 2 cm) encircles the ground phalanx and a photocell is attached to the pulp of the finger. This photocell detects the finger pulse which is graphically depicted by the photoplethysmograph (PPG). The pressure cuff is inflated to suprasystolic pressures. This obliterates the finger pulse. The pressure cuff is then deflated gradually (2 mmHg/s). On the moment of the first return of the finger pulse the

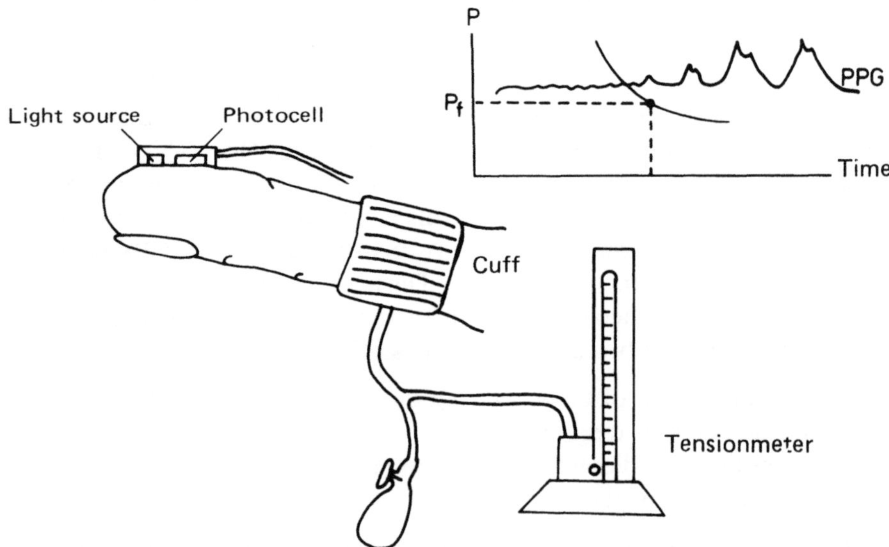

Figure 7.1 Method of measuring the systolic finger pressure. P = pressure in the cuff; Pf = cuff pressure at the moment of the return of the finger pulse; PPG=photoplethysmograph

pressure in the cuff is taken as the systolic finger pressure. The measurement is repeated twice and the mean of these three measurements is given as the systolic finger pressure with undisturbed fistula flow (PfO). This series of measurements is done again with digital compression of the efferent part of the A-V fistula by a second examiner. The mean of these measurements is given as the systolic finger pressure with occluded fistula flow (Pf●). The difference of these two pressures (Pf●-PfO), the so-called 'finger-pressure difference' has been studied.

Next we registered the Doppler signals of the brachial artery with undisturbed fistula flow (VO) and during digital compression of the efferent part of the fistula (V●). These signals were obtained with a commercially available Doppler apparatus (Versatone$^{®}$ bi-directional Doppler model D9) with zero-cross output. From a series of 10 registrations we calculated manually the mean frequency shift. Dividing this mean frequency shift obtained during undisturbed fistula flow by that obtained during compression of the efferent part of the fistula rendered the so called 'velocity index' ($\overline{V}$O/$\overline{V}$●).

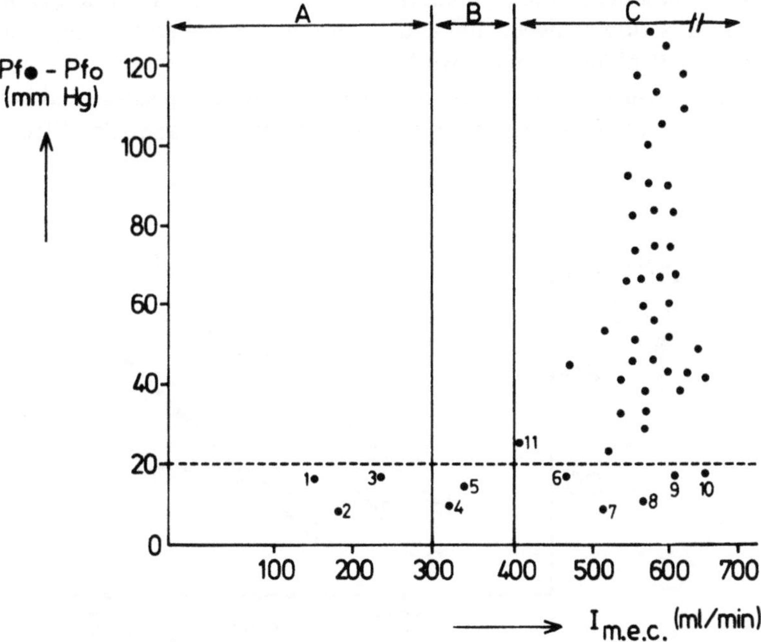

Figure 7.2 Relationship between the finger-pressure difference (Pf● −PfO) and the maximal obtainable extracorporeal flow (I$_{m.e.c.}$). Pf● =systolic finger pressure during compression of the efferent part of the fistula; PfO =systolic finger pressure during undisturbed fistula flow. I$_{m.e.c.}$ ⩽ 300 ml/min → poorly functioning fistula (← A →); 300 <I$_{m.e.c.}$ <400 ml/min → moderately functioning fistula (← B →); I$_{m.e.c.}$ ⩾ 400 ml/min → well-functioning fistula (←C—//→). Numbers 1 to 11 inclusive denote individual patients (see text)

In order to establish the value of the finger-pressure difference and the velocity index as parameters of the haemodynamic capacity of fistulas, we had to know the actual amount of blood that was flowing through these fistulas. Since we had no equipment to assess this fistula flow directly, we had to look for an indirect but reliable measure of fistula function. We decided upon the maximal flow that could be obtained briefly through the artificial kidney during three subsequent dialysis treatment sessions. This maximal flow was achieved by maximizing the capacity of the dialysis pump during a period of several minutes. The flow through the artificial kidney was exactly measured by the roller-pump flowmeter. We called this 'the maximal obtainable extracorporeal flow'.

RESULTS

Finger-pressure difference

In Figure 7.2 the finger-pressure difference is depicted on the vertical axis and the maximal obtainable extracorporeal flow on the horizontal axis. A maximal obtainable extracorporeal flow of more than 400 ml/min denotes a good fistula, a flow between 300 and 400 ml/min a moderate fistula, and a flow under 300 ml/min a poor fistula.

A finger-pressure difference of more than 20 mmHg was associated invariably with a good fistula function. Of the 10 patients with a smaller difference

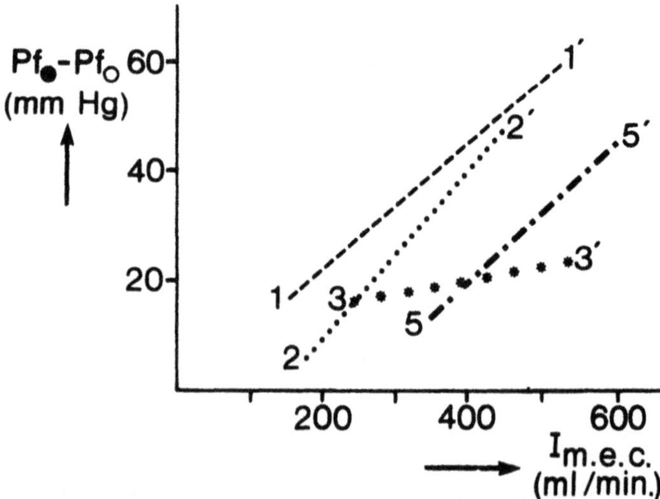

Figure 7.3 Changes in the finger-pressure difference (Pf●–PfO) and the maximal obtainable extracorporeal flow (Im.e.c.) in four patients with poorly functioning fistulas whose fistulas had been revised. Number, followed by a prime sign (') denote the situation after revision; numbers without this mark denote the situation before revision (see also Figure 7.2)

five had a well-functioning fistula. Four of the five patients with a more or less poorly functioning fistula were reoperated, e.g. their existing fistulas were revised. Figure 7.3 shows the results of these revisions on the finger-pressure difference and the maximal obtainable extracorporeal flow. There has been a substantial rise in the finger-pressure difference and a concomitant improvement of the total fistula flow.

Velocity index

Figure 7.4 represents the Doppler velocity curves of the brachial artery of a fistula arm. During the first six heart cycles the efferent part of the fistula has been compressed and during the last five cycles this compression was released. It can be seen that especially the diastolic flow increases substantially when the fistula is open. Figure 7.5 shows the relationship between the velocity index and the maximal obtainable extracorporeal flow. There is a very clear demarcation between the good fistulas on one side and the poorly and moderately functioning fistulas on the other side. Also patients 6 to 9 inclusive – who had a finger-pressure difference below 20 mmHg, but a good fistula function – are correctly defined by this index as having good fistulas.

DISCUSSION

Our results suggest that finger-pressure measurements have no clinical significance in patients with A-V fistula. This is not true. We observed five patients with complaints regarding their fingers which were suggestive of ischaemia. In all five patients the systolic pressure in the index finger of the fistula arm had an absolute value of less than 60 mmHg. It is known that a low intraluminal pressure in the arteries of the fingers can lead to a total spastic occlusion of the digital arteries, especially in the case of cold sensitivity[2]. By banding the efferent part of their fistulas we raised the finger

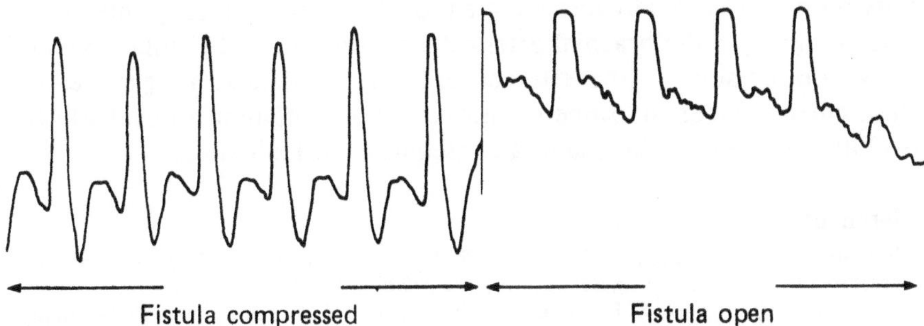

Figure 7.4 Original tracing of the transcutaneous CW-Doppler velocity waveforms during compression of the fistula and undisturbed flow through the fistula

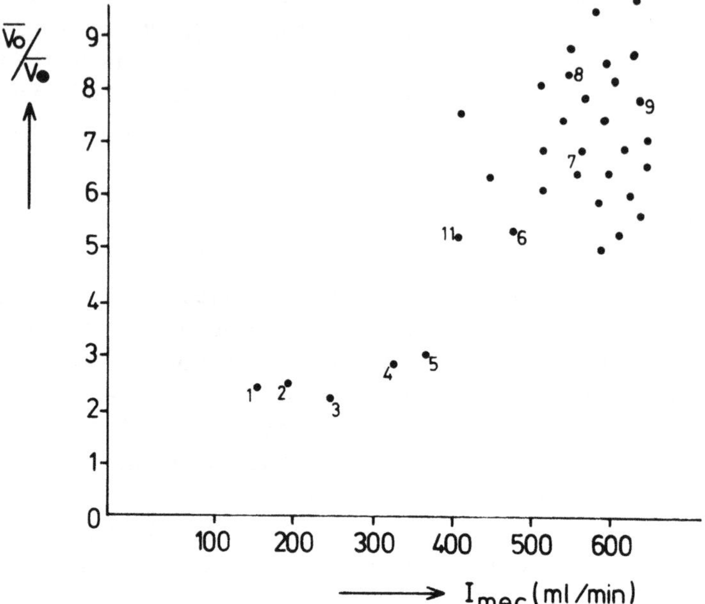

Figure 7.5 Relationship between the velocity index ($\bar{V}O/\bar{V}\bullet$) and the maximal obtainable extracorporeal flow ($I_{m.e.c.}$). $\bar{V}O$ = mean frequency shift of the Doppler signal of the brachial artery during undisturbed fistula flow; $\bar{V}\bullet$ as $\bar{V}O$ but with compression of the fistula. Numbers 1 to 11 inclusive denote individual patients (compare with Figure 7.2)

pressure, which was intermittently measured during the operation, to 90 mmHg or more. These patients were afterwards free of complaints while the flow through their fistulas remained adequate. In another paper the theoretical explanations for these observations have been elucidated[3]. For this very reason we consider the measurement of the systolic finger pressure with undisturbed fistula flow, and during compression of the efferent part of the fistula, mandatory in the work-up of patients with an A-V fistula.

The haemodynamic capacity of surgically created A-V fistulas can be assessed non-invasively by measurement of the mean frequency shift of the Doppler signal of the brachial artery during undisturbed fistula flow and during compression of the efferent part of the fistula. Finger-pressure measurements under the same circumstances are required to evaluate the possibility of finger ischaemia as a consequence of the fistula.

References

1 Brewster, D. C., Waltman, A. C., O'Hara, P. J. and Darling, R. C. (1979). Femoral artery pressure measurement during aortography. *Circulation*, **60**, (Suppl. 1) 120
2 Krähenbühl, B., Nielsen, S. L. and Lassen, N. A. (1977). Closure of digital arteries in high vascular tone states as demonstrated by measurement of systolic blood pressure in the fingers. *Scand. J. Clin. Lab. Invest.*, **37**, 71
3 Gemert, m. J. C. van and Bruyninckx, C. M. A. (1982). Hemodynamics of arteriovenous fistulas in the human arm. (In preparation)

8

A prospective study of the correlation between rheological factors and fistula failure

D. T. REILLY, R. F. M. WOOD AND P. R. F. BELL

INTRODUCTION

An increasing number of patients are being maintained on long-term haemodialysis for end-stage renal failure. The longest-lasting form of vascular access is the Brescia–Cimino radiocephalic fistula at the wrist, which may have a patency rate in excess of 65% at 4 years[1]. There is, however, a group of patients with recurrent fistula thrombosis which may be life-threatening if access proves impossible to maintain. In a prospective study of 157 patients undergoing fistula construction, although failure was more common when fistulas were constructed from small vessels, it was impossible to predict fistula failure from factors such as age, sex, vessel diameter, and time before use for dialysis[1]. Furthermore flow rates at the time of operation did not correlate with subsequent success or failure of the fistula[2]. The remaining possibility was that differences in thrombotic tendency might be detectable in patients with access problems.

At first sight, uraemic patients in end-stage renal failure should have few thrombotic problems; they have a low haematocrit and hence a low blood viscosity, and there is a well-known bleeding tendency in uraemia which has been related to a platelet defect[3]. However, shunts and fistulas often thrombose, and the reduction in failure rate by the use of sulphinpyrazone suggests that platelets may be implicated[4]. Whole blood viscosity or haematocrit has been found to be of importance in both arterial[5] and venous[6] thrombosis, and differences in viscosity might be a factor in fistula thrombosis. Similarly, low fibrinolytic activity has been demonstrated in venous thrombosis[7]. There are no published studies of prospective investigation of the reasons for fistula failure. This study is an attempt to examine differences in thrombotic tendency between patients undergoing fistula construction, and includes a retrospective study of patients on maintenance haemodialysis with and without past thrombosis.

MATERIALS AND METHODS

Patients

Twenty patients aged 23–60 years on maintenance home haemodialysis using an arteriovenous (A-V) fistula were studied on the day after dialysis. There were 10 patients with a mean follow-up time of 48.5 ± 25 months with no previous fistula thrombosis, and 10 patients with a mean follow-up of 34.5 ± 18 months, who had had two or more fistula thromboses. Forty-two patients in end-stage chronic renal failure aged 42 ± 12 years were studied on the day before construction of an arteriovenous fistula. Five had had previous access surgery. All fistulas were constructed by the same surgeon.

Methods

In both groups blood was taken for the following assays:

Platelet adhesiveness: Adeplat T glass-bead column (Immuno Ltd).
Platelet count: determined by light microscopy.

Table 8.1 Patients on maintenance haemodialysis: comparison between those with and without past thrombotic problems

	Past thrombosis ($n=10$)	No thrombosis ($n=10$)	Two-sample t-test (p value)	($=2\ \alpha$)
Age (years)	45.7	51.8		
Platelets ($\times 10^9/l$)	222 ± 64	217 ± 66	0.87	n.s.
Aggregation extent (%)	79 ± 7.6	69.5 ± 13.4	0.08	*
ADP threshold (μmol/l)	1.1 ± 0.7	1.9 ± 1.3	0.12	n.s.
β-Thromboglobulin (ng/ml)	176 ± 24	151 ± 22	0.04	*
Adhesion (%)	12.9 ± 14.3	13.6 ± 7.0	0.89	n.s.
Creatinine (μmol/l)	825 ± 182	698 ± 259	0.24	n.s.
Haematocrit (%)	32.5 ± 6.2	29.1 ± 8.6	0.33	n.s.
Whole blood viscosity (cps):				
$11.5\ s^{-1}$	7.70 ± 1.83	5.3 ± 2.4	0.03	*
$230\ s^{-1}$	3.48 ± 0.64	3.25 ± 0.65	0.43	n.s.
Fibrinogen (g/l)	4.2 ± 1.1	4.8 ± 0.6	0.16	n.s.
Fibrinolytic activity (ng ml^{-1} h^{-1})	254 ± 81	262 ± 81	0.83	n.s.
Plasma viscosity (cps)	1.73 ± 0.13	1.80 ± 0.11	0.23	n.s.
Red cell filtration index	0.45 ± 0.08	0.44 ± 0.13	0.87	n.s.

*Significant; n.s. = not significant

Platelet aggregability: in platelet-rich plasma: Aggregometer (H. Upchurch Ltd.), on the principle of Born[8]. Aggregation extent and the threshold level adenosine diphosphate (Sigma) causing a biphasic response were measured.

Plasma betathromboglobulin: radioimmunoassay (BTG-RIA, Amersham) by the method of Ludlam[9].

Whole blood viscosity at 37 °C: Wells–Brookfield microviscometer (Brookfield, Mass) at two shear rates, $11.5 \, s^{-1}$ and $230 \, s^{-1}$.

Plasma viscosity at 25 °C: Coulter–Harkness capillary viscometer.

Red cell deformability: filtration of 5% red cell suspension in autologous plasma through 5 μm pore-size polycarbonate filters (Nucleopore) by the method of Dodds[10].

Plasma fibrinogen: clot weight determination after recalcification of citrated plasma.

Fibrinolytic activity: a modification of the method of Moroz and Gilmore[11] using ^{125}I-fibrin labelled tubes prepared from human ^{125}I-fibrinogen (Amersham)[12].

Haematocrit and serum creatinine were also measured.

RESULTS

Patients on maintenance haemodialysis

An overall comparison between the thrombotic and non-thrombotic patients (Table 8.1) shows that despite a similar platelet count $(222:217 \times 10^9 \, l^{-1})$ the thrombotic group had a higher extent of platelet aggregation (79:69.5%) a lower threshold response to ADP (1.1:1.9 μmol/l), and a higher β-thromboglobulin level (176:151 ng/ml) although only the latter reached statistical significance ($p = 0.04$). Platelet adhesion was similar in both groups. Haematocrit and whole blood viscosity were higher in the thrombotic group; at low shear rates this was significant ($p = 0.03$) despite slightly lower plasma viscosity and fibrinogen levels. Fibrinolytic activity and red cell filterability were similar in both groups of patients.

Patients undergoing construction of an A-V fistula

The mean follow-up period after fistula construction was 8.7 months (1–18). Five patients with previous access surgery were excluded from analysis because of uncertainty as to whether previous thrombosis was related to surgical technique or to a thrombotic tendency. The outcome and patency of the 42 fistulas is shown in Figure 8.1. Of the 37 patients with first-time fistulas, nine without problems had been followed up for over a year and could be compared with the eight patients developing thrombosis within a year. The results of this comparison are shown in Table 8.2. There was no difference between the two groups in: age, sex, creatinine level, haematocrit, cause of renal failure, type of fistula, size of vessels, size of anastomosis, blood pressure, or type of suture material used.

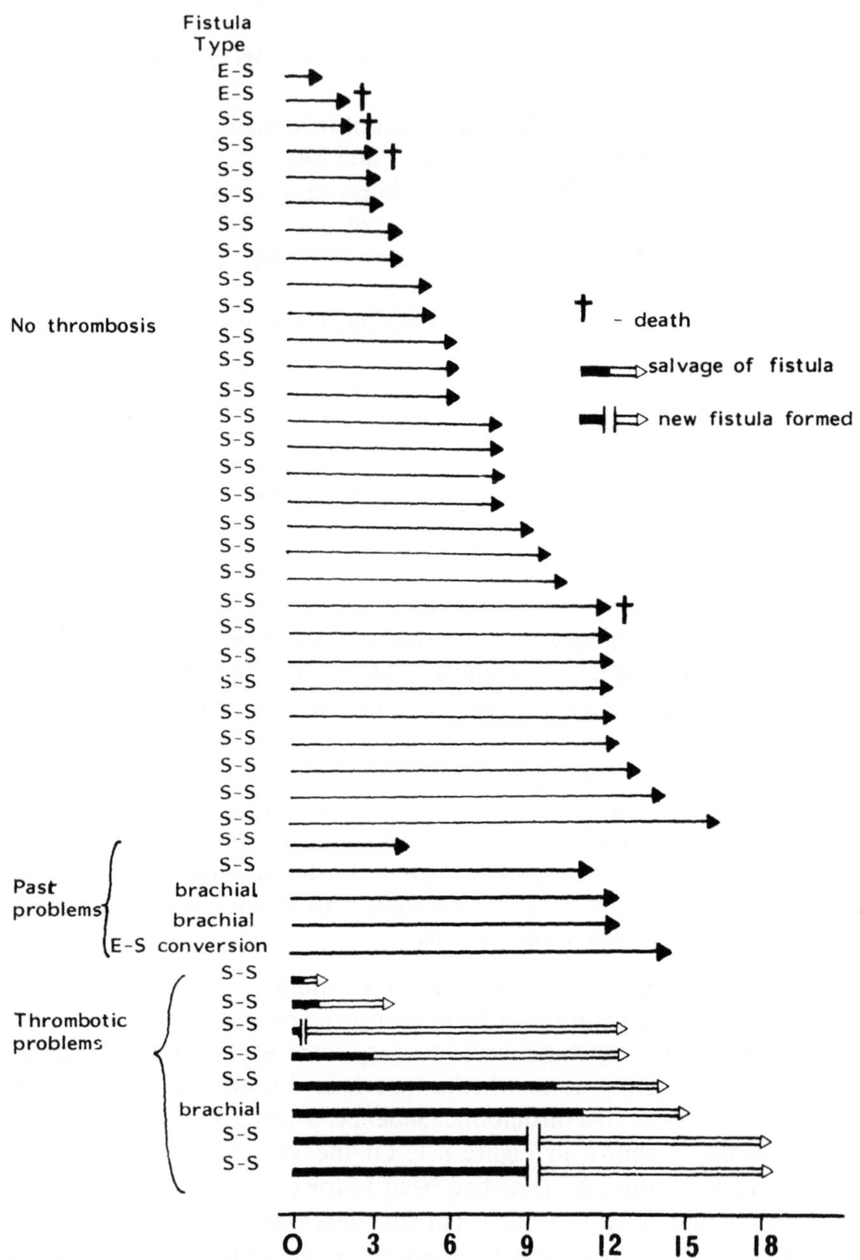

Figure 8.1 Patency of 42 consecutive A-V fistulas and outcome of complications. E−S: end-to-side; S−S: side-to-side

Table 8.2 Chronic renal failure patients followed up for over a year: comparison between patients with and without later thrombotic problems

	No thrombosis ($n=9$)	Thrombosis ($n=8$)	Two-sample t-test (p value)	($=2\,\alpha$)
Age (years)	43 ± 14	40 ± 15	0.7	n.s.
Platelets ($\times\,10^9/l$)	171 ± 55	277 ± 88	0.01	*
Aggregation extent (%)	72 ± 14	79 ± 14	0.35	n.s.
ADP threshold (μmol/l)	2.53 ± 1.69	1.28 ± 1.61	0.18	n.s.
β-Thromboglobulin (ng/ml)	90 ± 21	123 ± 65	0.27	n.s.
Platelet adhesion (%)	21 ± 14	14 ± 11	0.27	n.s.
Creatinine (μmol/l)	1039 ± 239	1012 ± 256	0.84	n.s.
Haematocrit (%)	25.8 ± 4.5	25.8 ± 5.5	0.99	n.s.
Whole blood viscosity (cps):				
$\quad$11.5 s^{-1}	5.36 ± 1.5	4.43 ± 1.62	0.24	n.s.
$\quad$230 s^{-1}	2.87 ± 0.32	2.71 ± 0.43	0.40	n.s.
Plasma fibrinogen (g/l)	4.87 ± 2.36	3.98 ± 1.38	0.46	n.s.
Plasma viscosity (cps)	1.74 ± 0.21	1.52 ± 0.1	0.03	*
Fibrinolytic activity (ng ml^{-1} h^{-1})	198 ± 102	291 ± 121	0.16	n.s.
Red cell filtration index	0.45 ± 0.15	0.37 ± 0.11	0.27	n.s.

*Significant; n.s. = not significant

Whole blood viscosity was lower in the thrombotic group at both low and high shear rates, although this did not reach significance. The patients with thrombosis had a significantly lower plasma viscosity ($p=0.03$) and a lower fibrinogen, although in contrast their fibrinolytic activity was raised ($291:198$ ng ml^{-1} h^{-1}). The results of the platelet function tests showed that there was apparently greater reactivity in the group that later suffered thrombosis; there was a higher extent of aggregation ($79:72\%$), a lower ADP threshold ($1.28:2.53\,\mu$mol/l) and a higher β-thromboglobulin level ($123:90$ ng/ml). Platelet adhesiveness, a very variable estimation, was lower in the thrombotic patients but not significantly so. The whole blood platelet count, however, was significantly higher in the thrombotic group ($p=0.01$).

In view of these differences an attempt was made to estimate the risk of thrombosis by multivariate regression analysis using the GLIM software computer program[13]. The program examines each variable for its value in discriminating between the patients with no problems and the patients with thrombotic problems. Having picked out the best discriminants, it assigns to each variable a certain weighting such that when the variables are added the maximum separation is achieved between the groups. The useful discriminants were whole blood platelet count, β-thromboglobulin level and plasma viscosity. These values were assembled into a formula which allowed the two groups to be separated without overlap:

$$x = 76.7 + 0.19 \text{ (platelet count)} - 100.6 \text{ (plasma viscosity)} + 0.43 \text{ (}\beta\text{-thromboglobulin)}.$$

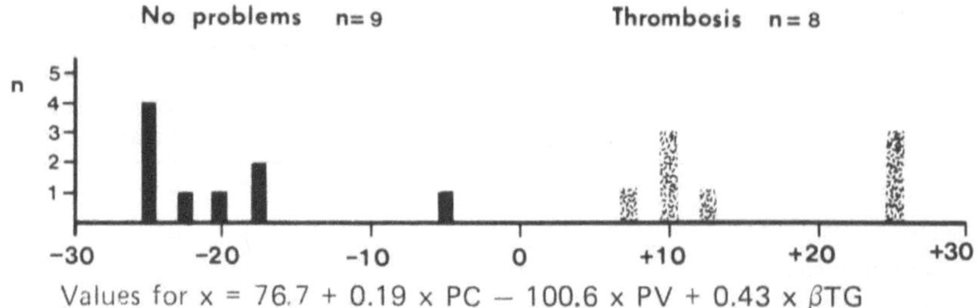

Figure 8.2   Graphical representation of separation of fistula patients into thrombotic and non-thrombotic groups using GLIM multivariate analysis. PC = platelet count, PV = plasma viscosity, BTG = β-thromboglobulin

The values of 'x' were calculated for each patient, and are shown in Figure 8.2.

DISCUSSION

On comparing rheological factors in dialysis patients with and without thrombotic problems, significant differences suggesting a tendency to thrombosis were found in the patients with previous access site thrombosis. These differences could be the result, rather than the cause, of thrombosis and a prospective study was therefore necessary to test the hypothesis that patients with 'thrombotic' blood tests were truly at risk of thrombosis. The final numbers available for analysis in the prospective study are small, because of the need for adequate follow-up before assigning a patient to the group at low risk of thrombosis. Despite the small numbers, significant differences emerged. In particular, the whole blood platelet count was more important than other parameters of platelet function. It seems reasonable that this should be taken into account; whole blood platelet count has been described as an index of thrombotic risk for example in peripheral vascular disease[5,14]. It is more difficult to explain the lower plasma viscosity of the thrombotic group. Plasma viscosity correlates strongly with fibrinogen but is also affected by other plasma proteins: fibrinogen was slightly lower in the thrombotic group, but other proteins were not measured. Although fibrinogen has been implicated as a risk factor for myocardial infarction[15], studies on the outcome of peripheral vascular reconstruction have shown no influence of fibrinogen[16]. The fact remains that it was possible to separate the thrombotic from the non-thrombotic patients without overlap using preoperative blood tests, something that was not possible in the previous study using technical factors such as vessel size[1].

The construction of a formula for thrombotic risk does not of course establish the validity of the supposed differences between the two groups; in order to prove the formula it should then be applied prospectively to a further group of patients to confirm whether thrombotic risk can be accurately predicted. This would allow prophylaxis of fistula thrombosis with platelet inhibitory agents in the small group of high-risk individuals and would avoid the drawbacks of drug therapy in the remaining patients.

References

1 Reilly, D. T., Wood, R. F. M. and Bell, P. R. F. (1982). Five year prospective study of dialysis fistulae: problem patients and their treatment. *Br. J. Surg.* (In press)

2 Reilly, D. T., Wood, R. F. M. and Bell, P. R. F. (1982). Arterio-venous fistulae for dialysis: blood flow, viscosity and long term patency. *World J. Surg.* (In press)

3 Rabiner, S. F. (1972). Uremic bleeding. In Spaet, T. H. (ed.) *Progress in Hemostasis and Thrombosis*. Vol. 1, p. 233. (New York and London: Grune & Stratton)

4 Kaegi, A., Pineo, G. F., Shimizu, A. *et al.* (1974). Arteriovenous shunt thrombosis – prevention by sulphinpyrazone. *N. Engl. J. Med.*, **290**, 304

5 Bouhoutsos, J., Morris, T., Chavatzas, D. and Martin, P. (1974). The influence of haemoglobin and platelet levels on the results of arterial surgery. *Br. J. Surg.*, **61**, 984

6 Dormandy, J. A. and Edelman, J. B. (1973). High blood viscosity: an aetiological factor in venous thrombosis. *Br. J. Surg.*, **60**, 187

7 Isacson, S. and Nilsson, I. M. (1972). Defective fibrinolysis in blood and vein walls in recurrent 'idiopathic' venous thrombosis. *Acta Chir. Scand.*, **138**, 313

8 Born, G. V. R. (1962). Aggregation of blood platelets by adenosine diphosphate and its reversal. *Nature (London)*, **194**, 927

9 Ludlam, C. A., Bolton, A. E., Moore, S. and Cash, J. D. (1975). New rapid method for diagnosis of deep vein thrombosis. *Lancet*, **2**, 259

10 Dodds, A. J., O'Reilly, M. J., Yates, C. J. P. *et al.* (1979). Haemorheological response to plasma exchange in Raynaud's phenomenon. *Br. Med. J.*, **2**, 1186

11 Moroz, L. A. and Gilmore, N. J. (1975). A rapid and sensitive ^{125}I-fibrin solid phase fibrinolytic assay for plasmin. *Blood*, **46**, 543

12 Reilly, D. T., Burden, A. C. and Fossard, D. P. (1980). Fibrinolysis and the prediction of postoperative deep vein thrombosis. *Br. J. Surg.*, **67**, 66

13 Nelder, J. A. (1975). *GLIM Manual: Royal Statistical Society*. (Oxford: Numerical Algorithms Group)

14 Morris-Jones, W. and Preston, F. E. (1981). Non-surgical management of peripheral vascular disease. *Br. Med. J.*, **282**, 317

15 Meade, T. W., North, W. R. S., Chakrabarti, R., Stirling, Y., Haines, A. P. and Thompson, S. G. (1980). Haemostatic function and cardiovascular death: early results of a prospective study. *Lancet*, **1**, 1050

16 Greenhalgh, R. M., Laing, S. P., Cole, P. V. and Taylor, G. W. (1981). Smoking and arterial reconstruction. *Br. J. Surg.*, **68**, 605

Acknowledgements

We are grateful to Eleanor Bolton for help with the red cell deformability tests and platelet counts, to the haematology laboratory at Leicester General Hospital for the fibrinogen and plasma viscosity determinations, and to Trent Regional Health Authority for a grant towards the ^{125}I-fibrinogen. Thanks are also due to Carol Jagger, David Clayton and John Woods of the Department of Community Health, Leicester Royal Infirmary, for help with the statistical analysis.

9

The role of angiography in vascular access surgery

R. F. SLIFKIN, M. HAIMOV, M. S. NEFF, A. EISER, A. BAEZ,
E. AMARGA AND S. GUPTA

Maintenance of reliable access to the circulation continues to be a vexing problem for haemodialysis patients and the medical staff responsible for their care. With the current dialysis population ageing[1,2] and the almost universal acceptance of elderly[3] and diabetic[4] patients for maintenance haemodialysis, preservation of existing access is vital. We found angiography to be a safe technique that is helpful in planning new access procedures and diagnosing problems in established access. This report will review the techniques utilized, list the indications for, and demonstrate representative findings in the angiographic procedures done in our dialysis population over the past 8 years.

MATERIALS AND METHODS

Seventy-five angiograms were done in 50 dialysis patients over an 8-year period. Techniques utilized included:

(1) *Brachial artery angiography*. The brachial artery was cannulated at the antecubital fossa utilizing an 18-gauge Teflon 'over the needle' catheter. Twenty millilitres of 60% diatrizoate meglumine and diatrizoate sodium injection USP (Renografin-60) was diluted with 40 ml of normal saline in a 60 cc syringe and injected by hand[5]. Serial films were taken with a rapid sequence film exchanger.

(2) *Graft angiograms*. Contrast was diluted as above and injected by hand via a 16-gauge haemodialysis needle placed in the graft close to the arterial anastomosis. A single film taken while injecting was usually

adequate. To visualize the arterial anastomosis the graft was occluded by hand or by blood pressure cuff while injecting.

(3) *Fistula angiograms.* Contrast was diluted as above and injected by hand via a haemodialysis needle placed at an appropriate point in the fistula depending upon the location of the lesion to be visualized. To visualize the arterial anastomosis the needle was placed in a vein close to the anastomosis and pointed towards the anastomosis. The outflow from this vein was occluded by hand or by tourniquet during the injection. In all cases the arterial vessel of the fistula was well demonstrated. In most cases a single film taken while injecting was adequate.

RESULTS

Table 9.1 lists the types of access visualized by angiography. The majority of the procedures were done for problems in grafts as opposed to arteriovenous (A-V) fistulas. The large number of problems in polytetrafluoroethylene (PTFE) grafts reflects the fact that this has been the graft material of choice in our programme during most of the period covered by this report.

Table 9.1 Arteriovenous access visualized by angiography

Grafts total		54
Bovine heterograft	16	
Polytetrafluoroethylene graft	37	
Dacron	1	
Fistulas total		17
Miscellaneous procedures		4

Table 9.2 Indications for angiography

Grafts	
High 'venous' pressure	23
Expanding aneurysms	3
Saline 'return' upon dialysis indication	6
Venous congestion of extremity	6
Sepsis − undetermined aetiology	5
Difficult cannulation	7
Repeated clotting	4
Fistulas	
High 'venous' pressure	2
Inadequate 'arterial' flow	5
Expanding aneurysms	1
Venous congestion syndrome	2
Cosmetic appearance	1
Ischaemic hand	6
Miscellaneous	
Ischaemic extremity after access closure	4

Table 9.2 lists the indications for angiography, and Table 9.3 the findings. Repeated clotting of a graft, high 'venous' pressure in the dialysis circuitry and saline 'return' via the 'arterial' needle upon initiation of dialysis were signs of venous stenosis either at the anastomosis of a graft or in the vein immediately draining the venous needle of a graft or fistula. Figure 9.1 demonstrates a graft angiogram with a venous anastomotic stenosis in a graft that had a high 'venous' pressure.

Table 9.3   Diagnosis at angiography

Grafts	
Total venous obstruction	6
Venous anastomosis stenosis	25
Proximal venous lesion or 'skip' lesion	6
Pseudoaneurysms	2
True aneurysms	3
Normal	12
Intraluminal obstruction	3
Fistulas	
Proximal arterial stenosis	1
Venous stenosis proximal to anastomosis	5
Ulnar steal	5
Tortuous complex of veins	1
Total venous obstruction	3
Proximal venous lesion or skip lesion	2
Miscellaneous	
Radial artery clotted from previous fistula – absent ulnar artery	4

Venous congestion of the access extremity and expanding aneurysms are almost always signs of complete occlusion of the main vein draining the access. With fistulas venous congestion was usually found in those constructed with a side vein anastomosis when the proximal limb of the vein became occluded. Figure 9.2 is a fistula angiogram of a fistula with an expanding aneurysm. The skin over this aneurysm was paper-thin. The main vein draining this area of the fistula is totally occluded. Figure 9.3 is a PTFE graft angiogram in an arm with massive venous congestion of the arm, forearm and hand. The congestion increased with each dialysis. The axillary vein is totally occluded well above the venous anastomosis. The collateral vein draining the graft developed a stenotic lesion leading to the venous congestion syndrome.

Inadequate arterial flow in a fistula usually indicated a stenosis in the main vein draining the fistula anastomosis or a lesion in the artery feeding the fistula. We did not find lesions directly at the fistula anastomosis that led to inadequate arterial flow. Ischaemia of the hand usually occurred in a radial artery fistula constructed as a side artery leading to a 'steal' syndrome from the ulnar circulation. Figure 9.4 is a brachial angiogram of a patient with an

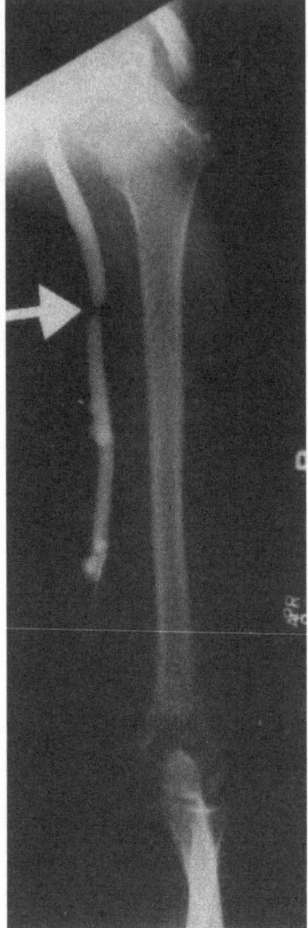

Figure 9.1   (See text) Arrow points to stenosis due to venous anastomotic hyperplasia

ischaemic hand due to a side artery fistula. It demonstrates blood flow directly from the ulnar artery into the fistula leading to a 'steal' from the ulnar circulation. This was treated by ligation of the distal radial artery.

Angiography in patients with sepsis and bacteraemia demonstrated infected pseudoaneurysms in two patients and an infected true aneurysm at the site of a branch ligature in a bovine heterograft. Two graft angiograms done in septic patients were normal.

Normal graft angiograms were found in all cases where the angiogram was done for difficult cannulation. However the X-ray demonstrated the course and depth of the graft to the staff and was a teaching aid for better cannulation of these grafts. Three normal graft angiograms were found where high 'venous' resistance was reported. This was probably due to less than optimal needle placement in these grafts.

Brachial angiograms were done in patients with ischaemic hands due to radial artery fistulas that had closed spontaneously or had been surgically

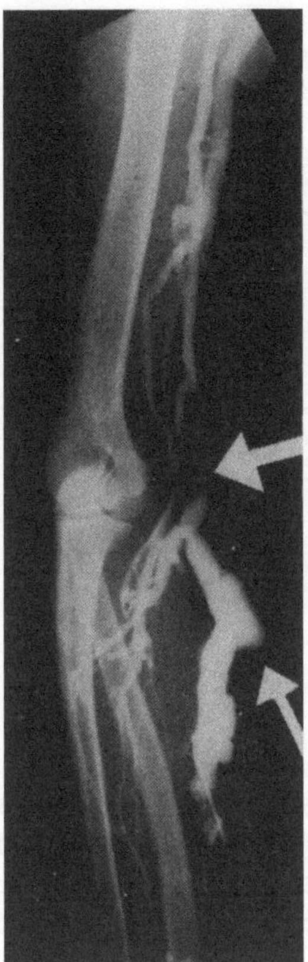

Figure 9.2　(See text) Large arrow points to occluded vein; small arrow points to expanding aneurysm

closed without complete relief of ischaemia. In all of these patients ulnar flow was absent or poor. In one patient a graft from the brachial artery to the distal radial artery stump alleviated the ischaemia.

The only complications were two perivascular injections in fistulas that occurred because the dialysis needle inadvertently was pushed into the back wall of the fistula vein while moving the patient from the dialysis unit to the radiology department. Other than pain immediately upon injecting there were no sequelae from these perivascular injections.

DISCUSSION

Access angiography has proven to be a valuable, safe and effective tool to demonstrate anatomic pathology in vascular access[6,7]. Graft and fistula angiograms can be done quickly via a dialysis needle utilizing the simplest of

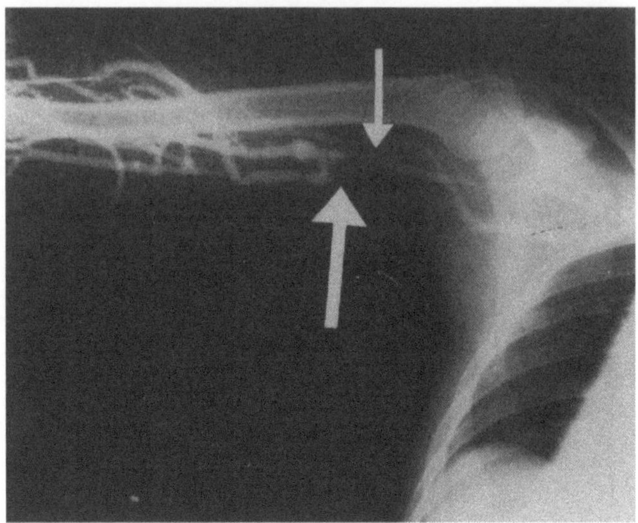

Figure 9.3 (See text) Large arrow points to occluded vein; small arrow points to stenotic collateral vein

radiographic techniques, a single film of the extremity. We found brachial angiograms with seqential films to be necessary in only two circumstances; when dynamic lesions such as 'steal' syndromes had to be demonstrated and when the anatomy had to be visualized for access planning. This was especially helpful in patients with extremities already ischaemic from previous access procedures and in diabetic or elderly patients who have a high incidence of peripheral arteriosclerotic lesions.

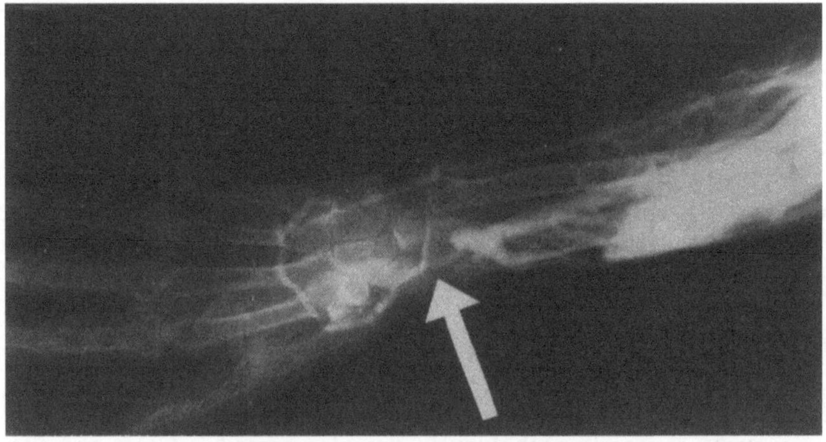

Figure 9.4 (See text) Arrow points to distal radial artery with flow from ulnar artery into fistula

When we demonstrated the presence of a normal access in patients with cannulation problems or unexplained sepsis we were able to avoid unnecessary access surgery. The angiogram was also useful as a teaching tool in these cases.

Specific surgical procedures or percutaneous transluminal angioplasty can be planned based on angiographic findings leading to access salvage. It is our recommendation that all clotted grafts that can be declotted have operative angiography immediately to demonstrate the arterial and venous anatomy. Any pathology found should be corrected at that time. We also recommend that angiography be done for the indications listed in Table 9.2. Demonstration of pathological lesions in fistulas and grafts can lead to intervention that may prolong the life of the access.

References

1 Lundin, A. P., Adler, A. J., Feinroth, M. V., Berlyne, G. M. and Friedman, E. A. (1980). Maintenance hemodialysis: survival beyond the first decade. *J. Am. Med. Assoc.*, **244**, 38
2 Neff, M. S., Slifkin, R. F., Baez, A., Gupta, S. and Eiser, A. (1981). Patient experience during ten years hemodialysis. (Abstract) *8th International Congress of Nephrology*, 7–12 June, Athens
3 Walker, P. J., Gunn, H. E. and Johnson, H. K. (1976). Long term hemodialysis for patients over fifty. *Geriatrics*, **31**, 55
4 Slifkin, R. F., Neff, M. S., Baez, A., Gupta, S., Mattoo, N. and Haimov, M. (1976). Maintenance hemodialysis in diabetic patients. *Proc. Eur. Dial. Transpl. Assoc.*, **13**, 377
5 Cohen, B. H., Chinitz, J. L., Soll, K. H., Ramirez, O., Onesti, G., Kim, K. E. and Swartz, C. (1970). Radiological contrast study of arteriovenous dialysis cannulae. *Radiology*, **94**, 603
6 O'Reilly, R. J., Hansen, C. C. and Rosental, J. J. (1978). Angiography of chronic hemodialysis arteriovenous grafts. *Am. J. Roentgenol.*, **130**, 1105
7 Anderson, C. B., Gilula, L. A., Sicard, G. A. and Etheredge, E. E. (1979). Venous angiography of subcutaneous hemodialysis fistulas. *Arch. Surg.*, **114**, 1320

10

Abstracts of posters in Techniques for monitoring during long-term follow-up

---

Spectral analysis of the Doppler signal in evaluation of arteriovenous shunts
J. M. VAN BAALEN, J. J. JAKIMOWICZ and J. A. FLENDRIG

Thrombosis of an A-V shunt is an important late complication that may result in loss of the access. Most often this is due to an obstruction at or just distal to the venous anastomosis. As the flow through a vessel will not be reduced unless the stenosis exceeds 90–95% narrowing of the lumen this obstruction will present itself at (near) occlusion. By means of non-invasive examination we tried to detect stenoses at an early stage.

In a pilot study we performed Doppler ultrasound examinations in 12 patients. A continuous-wave Doppler flowmeter (Medasonics Versatone D9) was used in combination with a real time spectral display of the frequency analysis of the Doppler signal (Unigon Angioscan). All patients had a PTFE (Gore-Tex) graft placed subcutaneously as an A-V haemodialysis access. The shunts were functioning from 1 to 54 months, mean 19.6 months. In all patients we tried to locate the arterial and venous anastomoses. In three patients we were unable to screen the arterial anastomosis as it was situated underneath the venous outflow traject. In the velocity profiles we compared the degree of spectral broadening and the peak velocities during systole and diastole as they were sampled over the anastomoses and the traject in between. In three patients a definite aberrant spectrum was found over the venous anastomosis with a sharp rise in peak systolic velocity and severe broadening of the Doppler spectrum. These patients were submitted to angiography. The non-invasively detected lesions were confirmed. In these patients both the site and the degree of stenosis could be predicted by non-invasive examination. This technique will be further evaluated in an already started prospective trial.

Transvenous serial-xeroarteriography (TSXA) – a new non-invasive angiographic method for arteriovenous fistulas in haemodialysis patients
K. KONNER, H. M. KARNAHL, J. EVERS and G. MEIDER

In order to avoid the risks and disadvantages of the commonly used angiographic methods in A-V fistulas a new non-invasive technique was evaluated.

Fifty-millilitre ioxotalamic acid are injected intravenously in the contralateral forearm. Using a cassette changer, TSXA allows visualization of both arteries and fistulated veins of the other arm, where 5% of the contrast medium injected arrive after the passage of heart and lung. A-V fistulas of 78 patients on chronic haemodialysis were examined. In all cases TSXA gave information about morphologic and functional alterations such as stenosis ($n=33$), aneurysms ($n=12$), reduced arterial output ($n=4$) etc. No side-effects were observed.

Transvenous serial xeroarteriography:
(1)   is largely free of risk, avoiding arterial puncture or catheterization;
(2)   shows the real haemodynamic situation of A-V fistulas, a pressure cuff not being necessary;
(3)   reliably identifies morphologic and functional alterations by a serial exposure technique;
(4)   makes surgical planning more precise, careful and time-saving;
(5)   can be performed 'prophylactically' before complications of A-V fistulas arise.

Phlebography in the management of fistula complications
D. T. REILLY, H. J. PEARSON, E. M. WATKIN and R. F. M. WOOD

The functional life of an arteriovenous fistula can be considerably increased by the recognition of remediable anatomical problems in the fistula. A radiographic technique described by Anderson *et al.* (1979) has been evaluated in a series of 36 consecutive fistula problems. The commonest abnormality shown was stenosis in the venous run-off (17) followed by thrombus (7), increased distal flow (3) and arterial stenosis (1). No abnormality was shown in eight phlebograms. In only three phlebograms was the information unhelpful, whereas in seven patients operation was avoided by the demonstration of a normal phlebogram. It is concluded that careful radiographic assessment of malfunctioning fistulas are an essential part of management.

The arteriovenous fistula on the upper limb: technique and follow-up
F. QUINTANA RIERA, F. CASTRO, R. LERMA, C. LISBONA,
R. MARTINEZ CERCOS, J. PUNCERNAU and
F. VIDAL-BARRAQUER

We present more than 400 A-V fistulas on upper limb carried out in the last 4 years. We describe the techniques used which preferably are end-to-side anastomosis between vena cephalica and arteria radialis. When it is not possible we use anastomosis between arteria brachialis and superficial veins of the elbow fold.

We comment on the complications arising because of the surgical technique and others shown up during the evolution of the A-V fistula. We comment also on the diagnostic methods used. Among them we point out some cases of distal ischaemia because of arterial insufficiency and oedema of the upper limb because of proximal venous thrombosis. As a conclusion we note:

(1) The efficiency of the A-V fistulas in the elbow fold when it is not possible to make them on the wrist;
(2) It is advisable to discard previously any ischaemic arterial pathology or venous thrombosis that, being asymptomatic, could expose the limb when we perform an A-V fistula on it;
(3) The strict control of the A-V fistula evolution permits the early diagnosis of the damage and its possible recovery.

Quantitative Doppler and ultrasound measurements in surgically created arteriovenous fistulas of the arm

L. FORSBERG, T. HOLMIN and E. LINDSTEDT

Arteriovenous (A-V) fistulas, surgically created between the radial artery and the cephalic vein according to the method described by Brescia *et al.* (1966) have been performed at our hospital for more than a decade to be used for dialysis and cytostatic infusion.

Eighty-three patients with well functioning fistulas were examined with 10 MHz directional, CW Doppler. Forty-five patients also with fistulas functioning well were examined, some at multiple instances giving 77 measurements in all with 5 MHz Doppler. Thirty-eight fistulas belonging to the latter group were also examined with 10 MHz. Sixty-three of the fistulas examined with 10 MHz and 56 of the fistulas examined with 5 MHz had diameter measurements performed with B-scan ultrasound of the feeding artery – the brachial artery – making possible volume flow measurements.

One hundred and ninety-eight (198) flow velocity measurements with directional CW Doppler of A-V fistulas of the arm made it possible to establish a 'normal' value of 50 cm/s (30–70 cm/s) in fistulas with adequate function. Diameter measurements performed with B-scan ultrasound using a 5 MHz transducer with an axial resolution of 0.3 mm make the volume flow measurements especially in patients with thin vessels less accurate, but the rapid developments in transducers will probably reduce this problem in years to come. Doppler flow velocity measurements with or without volume flow calculations are totally non-invasive and can be repeated without problems for the patients giving valuable information about the hemodynamic changes due to fistulas.

Prospective angiographic investigation of vascular access in haemodialysis
M. M. ELSEVIERS, A. M. DE SCHEPPER, H. A. VEREYCKEN,
R. VAN HEE, R. LINS, G. A. VERPOOTEN and M. E. DE BROE

A prospective angiographic investigation of vascular access (VA) in haemodialysis patients was started in November 1979. During this 26-month period 179 angiographies were performed in 79 patients, within the 2 months following the VA construction and repeated once a year ('routine' examination: 70%). Additional angiographies were performed, when clinical problems arose ('urgent' examinations: 30%): decreased flow, infection, haematoma. Immediate complication rate was 16%, mainly consisting of minor reactions due to contrast medium. In 9% a haematoma was observed. The results of the angiographies are summarized in Table 10.1. Table 10.2 represents the therapeutic consequences of these investigations.

Table 10.1 Observed abnormalities at different levels of VA

	Vas afferens		*Anastomosis*		*Vas efferens*	
	Routine ($n = 109$)	*Urgent* ($n = 45$)	*Routine* ($n = 109$)	*Urgent* ($n = 45$)	*Routine* ($n = 108$)	*Urgent* ($n = 48$)
Normal (%)	92	87	77	65	59	38
Abnormal (%)	8	13	23	35	41	62
Narrowing	6	5	15	7	32	19
Thrombosis	3	3	–	–	5	8
Aneurysm	–	–	2	1	2	–
Dilatation	–	–	–	1	9	4

Table 10.2 Therapeutic consequences

	Routine ($n = 145$) (%)	*Urgent* ($n = 99$) (%)
Unchanged use	82	44
Change of puncture side	9	13
Correction	4	13
New VA	5	30

To conclude, angiography of VA in haemodialysis patients has diagnostic and therapeutic relevance. The complication rate is acceptable. The clinical and prognostic importance of the high incidence of narrowing at the level of the vas efferens, observed in routine angiographies, needs further investigation.

11

Invited comment on papers and posters in Techniques for monitoring during long-term follow-up

P. MICHIELSEN

In his guest lecture at the opening ceremony, Dr B. Scribner mentioned the extremely important observation that in a small number of patients external A-V shunts can be tolerated during many years without problems. It is clear that, if it would be possible to determine why this subpopulation is protected against the usually occurring shunt problems, a major advance would be achieved in the prevention of these complications. In this line we have heard this afternoon an excellent paper of Dr. Reilly in which it is convincingly demonstrated that it is possible to predict which patients will be at risk of thrombotic complications of A-V fistulas. Thrombotic patients were found to have a greater extent of platelet aggregation and a higher β-thromboglobulin level before fistula construction. This opens the way for therapeutic trials designed to prevent thrombosis in the selected group of patients at risk. Thrombosis is, however, only a small part of the problems that can occur in patients with A-V fistulas. In Dr Reilly's series of angiographies the incidence was seven cases of thrombosis in 36 consecutive fistula problems. Stenoses at the venous outflow were far more frequent and the same was found by other groups. It would be important to extend the nice prospective studies of Dr Reilly to see if such stenoses occur more frequently in the subgroup of patients at risk of thrombosis.

The papers and posters concerned with monitoring of the A-V fistulas can be divided in two groups: those using the Doppler technique and those using angiography. Dr Bruyninckx presented elegant experiments in which he measured the influence of closing and reopening a fistula on systolic finger pressure and Doppler velocity ratios in the arteria brachialis. It is, however, disappointing to note that it was not possible with these techniques to determine reliably which fistulas had an adequate flow for efficient dialysis. Forsberg *et al.* did Doppler flow measurements on well-functioning fistulas. They found a normal flow velocity of 50 cm/s (30–70 cm/s) over the arteria brachialis. They were, however, unable to determine exactly the diameter of the vessels by B mode scan, so that the flow calculations were inaccurate. The major advantage of these non-invasive studies is that they can easily be repeated. At this time, however, it is not proved that they provide more information than the observation of the blood-flow through the dialyser during the dialysis procedure. An attempt to further improve this technique is presented by van Baalen *et al.* By real-time spectrum display of the frequency analysis of the Doppler signal they were able to detect a stenosis at the site of the venous anastomosis. This result was obtained in patients with a PTFE (Gore-tex®) graft which is a special situation; there is no indication that this technique could be used for the localization of stenoses in standard A-V fistulas.

If the practical significance of Doppler flow velocity measurements seems thus very limited, angiography is already well introduced in clinical practice. There seems to exist a general agreement on the fact that angiography is useful for preoperative investigation of difficult cases and for diagnosis in fistula problems. Both the presentation of Slifkin and the poster of Reilly are convincing arguments in favour of the selective use of this technique in patients with fistula problems. Is it also useful to perform angiographies in patients with well-functioning fistulas? This is suggested in the posters of Quintana Riera *et al.* and of Konner *et al.* These last authors performed 24 prophylactic angiographies which led to 10 surgical revisions. From these and the following data it is clear that even in patients with well-functioning fistulas angiography can disclose localized stenoses, generally located at the outlet. To justify routine prophylactic angiographies it must, however, be demonstrated that these stenoses are progressive and that early operative repair is superior to a delayed operative repair once inadequate blood flow during dialysis has occurred. Such a question could be resolved only by a well-controlled prospective trial. After informed consent is obtained patients must be randomly allocated to a group in which routine prophylactic angiographies are performed and a group with selective angiographies only. This is the only way to determine if early diagnosis is useful and if the advantages outweigh the side-effects of the investigation. To submit dialysis patients with a well-functioning fistula to a series of routine angiographies is a difficult decision which raises ethical problems. It is therefore highly regrettable that the group of Elseviers' submitted 79 patients to 145 routine angiographies without a control group. This considerable and impressive effort cannot thus answer the fundamental question of the therapeutic relevance of routine angiography. This study only confirms the high evidence of unsuspected abnormalities in well-functioning fistulas. In this study the contrast medium was injected in the arteria brachialis and the complication

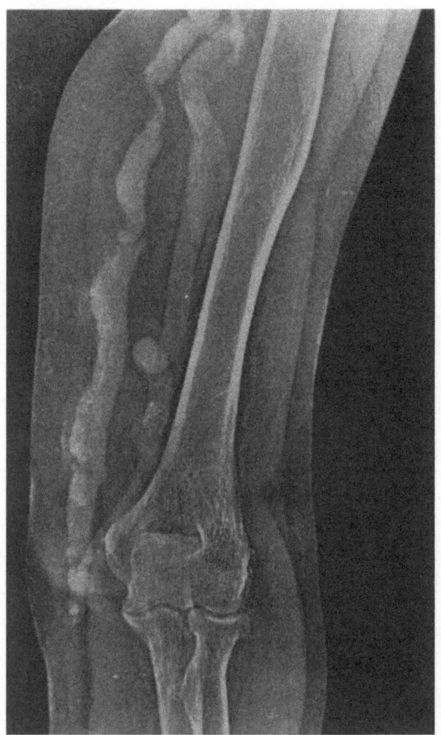
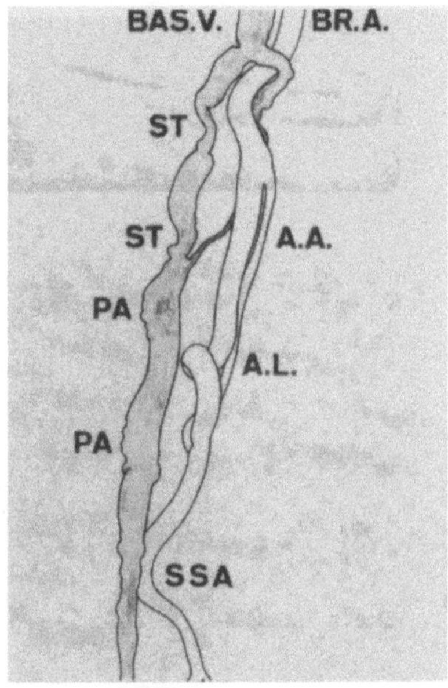

Figures 11.1 and 11.2   Side-to-side anastomosis (SSA) between brachial artery (BRA) and basilic vein (BASV) with superficial repositioning of the vein 3 years after surgery. ST = stenosis; PA = puncture area; AA = accessory artery; AL = arterial loop

rate was 16%. The Andersen technique was used to obtain the data presented in the poster of Reilly. From the discussion it was apparent that there was no consensus as to which technique is to be preferred. An interesting new technique is presented in the poster of Dr Konner *et al.* Using Xerox films in a special cassette changer he injects the contrast medium intravenously in the contralateral arm and obtains beautiful pictures of the fistula vessels (Figures 11.1 and 11.2). In 78 patients no side-effects were observed – but 50 ml of contrast medium is still needed for angiography with this technique. Another more recent technique which also allows injection of low doses of contrast medium in a vein in the opposite arm is intravenous digital subtraction angiography[1]. This is a computer angiography with a high-resolution TV system. The radiation image is converted in an analogue video signal which is taken to a digital converter and stored. During angiographic examination two pictures are 'frozen'. The first store contains a picture before the contrast medium has reached the arteries; the second the picture with contrast medium. After digital subtraction of the two pictures, the low contrast levels remaining are amplified. Figure 11.3 illustrates the results obtained in a

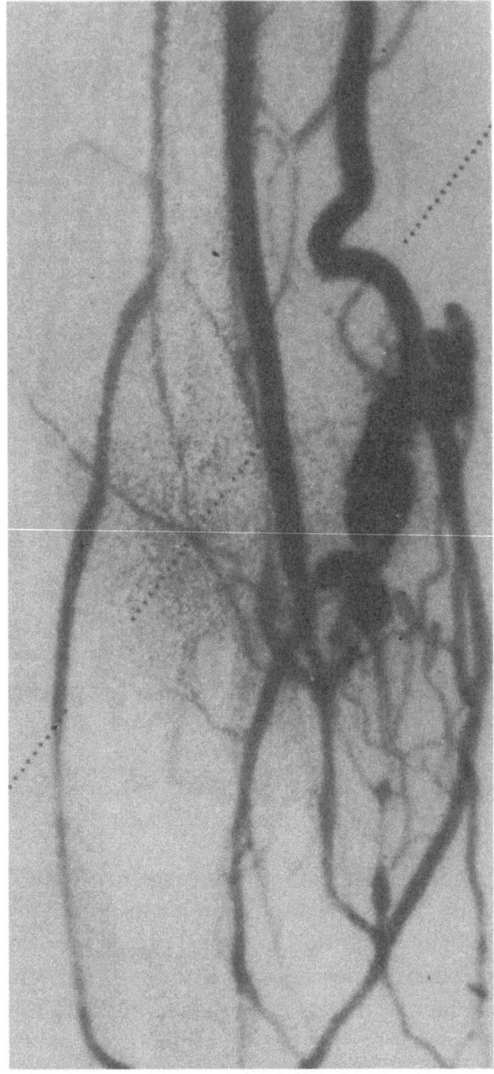

Figure 11.3 Elbow A-V fistula between arteria brachialis and vena basilica. Intravenous digital subtraction angiography (courtesy Professor A. Baert)

fistula at the elbow. It is likely that this method will progressively replace the previous ones. A decrease in the incidence of side-effects and an improvement in the quality of the image will certainly broaden the indications for angiography in the long-term monitoring of access vessels.

References

1 Baert, A. L., Wilms, G., Marchal, G. and Ponette, E. (1981). Intravenous digital subtraction angiography. *Eur. J. Radiol.*, **1**, 97

Section III
Access in children

12

Access surgery in children: a big problem?

F. G. M. BUSKENS, S. H. SKOTNICKI, H. REINAERTS AND
M. C. J. de JONG

INTRODUCTION

Encouraged by more than 10 years experience with haemodialysis and
consequently with vascular access in adults, a department for dialysis in
children was started at the Radboud Hospital of the University of Nijmegen
in July 1977. Up to December 1981, our experience with vascular access in
children covers a period of 4½ years. We approached this kind of surgery
with some reluctance especially because the results, described in the literature
at that time, were not very encouraging. Now, looking back after 4½ years,
in this group of young patients most of the problems seem to have been
overcome and the results have not been as bad as expected.

PATIENTS AND RESULTS

From July 1977 until December 1981, 42 children were presented for haemodialysis. Of these children 14 were suffering from acute renal failure and 28
from chronic renal failure. The indications for urgent dialysis in the above-
mentioned 14 children are presented in Table 12.1. Three patients died: two
post-traumatic and one after an orthopaedic operation (reconstructive
osteotomy). The duration of acute dialysis ranged from 4 to 56 days with a
mean of 18 days. In all instances a Scribner shunt was used, situated in one of
the lower legs. In six of the 14 patients a revision of the shunt was necessary
within 2–8 days, and four of them needed more than two shunts and one
patient had to be operated five times.

The group of 28 patients with chronic renal failure consisted of 16 boys and
12 girls. The age of these 28 children at the time of the construction of the first

Table 12.1 Causes of acute renal failure in 14 children

Trauma with intra-abdominal bleeding	5

Extensive surgery
  open-heart surgery
  laparotomy for malignancy
  reconstructive osteotomy
	3

Haemolytic uraemic syndrome	2
Angiography	1
Cytostatic drugs	1
Poisoning by paraquat	2

vascular access ranged from 3 to 16 years with a mean of 11.8 years. In 21 of the 28 children, who were considered for regular haemodialysis, a primary A-V fistula, according to Cimino–Brescia, was created in the non-dominant forearm. The fistula was made either end-to-side at the wrist or side-to-side at the elbow. In seven patients the first vascular access was a Scribner shunt in the lower leg constructed at the acute onset of the renal failure. Later on an A-V fistula was created. The time between construction of the A-V fistula and its successful use for dialysis varied from 5 to 12 weeks.

In 25 children an attempt for an A-V fistula according to Cimino–Brescia was made. In 15 cases this was successful and a useful fistula resulted (60%). Out of the 16 Cimino fistulas performed at the wrist, 10 were still functioning when transplantation took place or were still patent up to the time of the end of the follow-up (5–24 months). In the cases of primary failure of the Cimino fistula, a second attempt was made twice direct postoperatively and twice after 8 and 12 months. These four A-V fistulas were still functioning up to the time of transplantation (5–26 months). In one patient with a primary failure a saphenous vein graft was inserted in a U-shape in the forearm. This attempt was unsuccessful and necessitated repeated surgery to obtain vascular access. The patient ultimately died from uraemic pericarditis. Another patient in this group also proved to be very difficult to help. A second A-V fistula failed and a bovine graft in the upper leg was constructed. Revision of the venous anastomosis was necessary at 3 months and several times afterwards, however without satisfactory result. Recently another bovine graft has been implanted in the contralateral upper leg.

In five patients primary vascular access was attempted at the elbow site. Two of these A-V fistulas were still functioning at transplantation. In one case a Cimino fistula was created in the other arm with good result. In two patients a bovine graft was implanted in the upper leg. One was functioning well until transplantation (10 months later) and one is still being used at the end of the follow-up (7 months).

Out of the seven patients with an acute onset of chronic renal failure, who had received primary a Scribner shunt in the lower leg, three received at a later stage an A-V fistula at the wrist and another three a bovine graft in the upper leg. One bovine graft developed an aneurysm and was ligated. After a temporary Scribner shunt a useful Cimino fistula was made. In the last patient of this group a third attempt to make an A-V fistula was successful.

Early or late thrombosis of the primary A-V fistula was seen in 11 patients. One patient developed cardiac failure, due to massive shunting. Problems with venous hypertension or ischaemia were not observed. There were no postoperative infections. Infection at the site of puncture occurred three times. One of these fistulas with a mycotic aneurysm was lost. In one occasion an aneurysm was observed in a bovine graft a few weeks after the start of dialysis. Ligation of the graft was performed. Intimal hyperplasia at the venous anastomosis of a bovine graft, frequently seen in adults, was encountered once in a boy of 9 years. Repeated reoperations could not save the fistula in the long run. Recently, in this patient, another bovine graft fistula in the contralateral upper leg was successfully performed.

DISCUSSION

When considering the above results and comparing them with reports from the literature, the result of our vascular access in children seems quite satisfactory. This may be favourably influenced by the fact that the children in Nijmegen were transplanted quite early in the course of their disease. The time between the first dialysis and transplantation ranged from 5 to 26 months with a mean of 11.3 months. There are few surgeons, who opt in the first instance for an A-V fistula, as we do. Gagnadoux[1,2] from Paris and Sicard[3] from St Louis follow the same policy. They also opt primarily for an A-V fistula in the forearm. L'Opez Uriate[4] from Mexico prefers a saphenous loop in the forearm. As an alternative he makes an anastomosis between femoral artery and saphenous vein, just above the knee, but these fistulas are not very useful, because of the deep position of the vein. Knaepen et al.[5] prefer the saphenous-vein loop as primary access procedure. They assert that in a Cimino fistula the flow through the small vessels is too low and that consequently the enlargement of the forearm veins, necessary for easy percutaneous cannulation, is often delayed for a long period. We acknowledge their argument, but if it is possible to make the fistula a long time before use – and that means at least 6–9 weeks before dialysis treatment – one will have a good fistula. It is therefore important that the nephrologist presents the patients at the earliest possible moment.

Other authors, including VanderWerf[6] and Wellington[7], prefer in children the use of artificial material like bovine or PTFE grafts. On the assumption that the cephalic vein is too small for a good flow through the fistula. However, since the results of vascular access by various surgeons with their various techniques are not better than our results, we intend in the future to follow the same protocol. Our first choice for vascular access will remain an A-V fistula according to Cimino, also in children.

References

1 Gagnadoux, M. F., Degoulet, P., Pascal, B. and Bourquelot, P. (1978). L'Abord vasculaire chez l'enfant traité par hémodialyse périodique. *J. Urol. Nephrol.*, **84**, 935
2 Gagnadoux, M. F., Pascal, B., Bronstein, M. and Bourquelot, P. (1978). Arterio-venous fistula in small children. *Proc. EDTA*, **15**, 573
3 Sicard, G. A., Merrell, R. C., Etheredge, E. E. and Anderson, C. B. (1978). Subcutaneous arteriovenous dialysis fistulas in pediatric patients. *Trans. Am. Soc. Artif. Intern. Organs*, **24**, 695
4 L'Opez Uriarte, A., Ledon Valenzuela, S. and L'Opez G'Ames, C. (1978). Arteriovenous fistula for pediatric hemodialysis. Experience of 9 years. *Bol. Med. Hosp. Infant Mex.*, **35**, 695
5 Knaepen, P., de Geest, R., Donckerwolcke, R. and de Jong, R. (1977). *Vascular Access for Regular Hemodialysis in Children*. Proceedings of the Symposium: Access and reconstructive vascular surgery, Nijmegen, 1976
6 VanderWerf, B. A., Kumar, S. S., Rattazzi, L. C. and Katzman, H. E. (1978). Experience with bovine heterografts in A-V fistulas for dialysis access. In P. N. Sawyer and M. J. Kaplitt (eds.). *Vascular Grafts.* (New York: Appleton–Century–Crofts)
7 Wellington, J. L. (1978). Expanded P.T.F.E. prosthetic grafts for blood access in patients on dialysis. *Can. J. Surg.*, **21**, 420

13

Conversion of Teflon–Silastic shunts to A-V fistulas in small children with chronic renal failure

A. E. DAUL, N. GRABEN, R. WINDECK AND K. PISTOR

INTRODUCTION

Access to blood is still the most important determinant for continued well-being of patients with end-stage renal failure, maintained on haemodialysis (HD)[1-3]. The two types of vascular access used most frequently are the internal arteriovenous fistula as introduced by Brescia–Cimino and the external Teflon–Silastic shunt of Quinton–Scribner[4,5]. For chronic HD treatment the internal fistula represents the vascular access of choice, whereas in acute renal failure HD is started via a Scribner shunt in many centres[2,6]. In paediatric nephrology an immediate start of HD often becomes necessary because of acute onset of renal failure with rapid and – unfortunately often irreversible – deterioration of renal function. In this situation the A-V fistula is unsuitable since, particularly in children, many weeks or months may pass before an accessible vessel has matured. Therefore in these cases a Scribner shunt is used most commonly, later being abandoned in favour of a Cimino fistula on the contralateral forearm[6]. By this procedure, valuable vascular access sites are already wasted in the first weeks of dialysis treatment.

In order to conserve vessel resources, we endeavoured to convert external shunts to internal A-V fistulas. After studying the literature we found that little thought had been given in the past to the problem of shunt conversion. We came up with only three reports with a total of 43 cases with shunt conversion, all being performed in adults[7-9]. Since we already had gathered good results with shunt conversion in 62 adults, we felt encouraged to try this procedure also in children.

TECHNIQUE

For acute HD we insert exclusively a straight in-line A-V shunt between the radial artery and the cephalic vein[10]. In children who need subsequent HD treatment we attempt shunt conversion as soon as a dilated and accessible vein is visible. Under local anaesthesia we begin with a 3–4 cm straight skin incision proximal to the skin outlets of the Silastic tubes and between both cannulated vessels.

Proximal to the vessel tips the radial artery and the dilated cephalic vein are mobilized, freed of connective tissue and adapted side to side. After that a 15–18 mm anastomosis is constructed by side-to-side technique (Figure 13.1). We use this technique in order to create a large anastomosis and to obtain sufficient blood flow even through small vessels. Prior to completing the anterior suture line, fistula function is examined by relieving the arterial occlusion, followed by instillation of heparinized saline into the vein. After complete closure the appearance of a typical thrill is awaited before the vessels distal to the fistula are ligated. Finally the vessel tips are removed by external traction through their original skin outlets, thereby avoiding contamination of the wound. Then the skin incision is closed. The patients are observed in the hospital overnight and the fistula is used within 1–2 days.

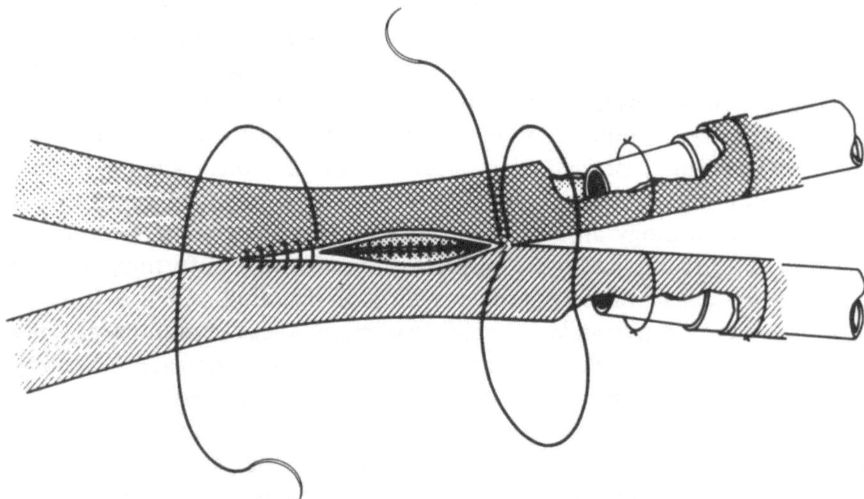

Figure 13.1 Shunt conversion is shown before closure of the anterior suture line of the anastomosis. Vessel tips are still in position. Proximal to the anastomosis both vessels are occluded by a rubber loop

PATIENTS AND RESULTS

Between January 1979 and March 1982 in our unit 251 Teflon–Silastic shunts were inserted and 241 Cimino fistulas were created. Out of these in 74 patients A-V fistulas were constructed, using the dilated vessels of previous external shunts. In children this has been achieved in 12 cases so far. This group consisted of six girls and six boys aged 4–14 with a body weight between 11.5 and 56 kg; 10 of them had a body weight under 30 kg.

The time interval between construction of external shunts and conversion to A-V fistulas was between 29 and 194 days, with a mean of 73 days. Conversion was successful in 11 of 12 attempts and the newly created A-V fistulas were accessible within 1–2 days. In one child early thrombosis occurred subsequent to local infection. Uncomplicated wound infection was seen in another child. In April 1982 11 of 12 fistulas were still functioning with a lifespan of 140–1127 days.

DISCUSSION

A-V fistulas can be considered to be suitable as vascular access of choice in children, if chronic HD treatment becomes necessary[6,11,12]. Only in a few paediatric nephrology centres are external shunts preferred in order to avoid frequent venipunctures with the associated pain and psychological pressure[13]. A-V fistulas must be constructed early in the course of the disease, i.e. weeks or months before HD treatment becomes unavoidable. However, under certain conditions it may become absolutely necessary not to wait until a fistula has matured. In these cases one may be forced to use an external Teflon–Silastic shunt[6,14]. Intermittent use of Sheldon catheters or peritoneal dialysis has proved to be less favourable in our experience.

Our results show that this external Teflon–Silastic shunt between radial artery and cephalic vein can successfully be converted into an A-V fistula. Since the diameter of the cannulated vein increases considerably through arterial blood flow, it may be immediately punctured for subsequent chronic HD treatment after conversion.

Previous use as an external shunt does not adversely influence the outlook for later functioning of the fistula. From our experience, as well as from other vascular surgeons, one may expect that function of converted shunts in small children is better than that of primary constructed A-V fistulas. We attribute this to previous dilatation of the vessels. Although there is the imminent danger of wound infection, among our patients this never became a prevailing problem. Only in two patients did localized wound infection occur, caused by *Staphylococcus aureus*. To avoid these complications, it is necessary to convert only those external shunts which show no signs of infection. If shunt infection is suspected it is essential to await the success of antibiotic treatment. After a 1–2-week interval free of recurrence, shunt conversion can be planned.

An important prerequisite of successful shunt conversion is to construct the external Teflon–Silastic shunt as an in-line version. This variation of the original Scribner shunt offers some notable advantages in children: less foreign material is implanted, which may favour wound healing and diminish the risk of wound infection[10,15]. Particularly in small children with small upper extremities pressure necrosis of overlying tissues will be avoided. In addition, better blood flow properties are obtained by avoiding the curved shape of the original Scribner shunt[10,15]. Shunt clotting occurs less frequently in in-line shunts, and in such cases mechanical or fibrinolytic declotting is easier. Last but not least the in-line shunt can be constructed further distal in the course of the vessels, thereby conserving the more proximal segment for future shunt surgery. Although the use of the hand may be reduced temporarily, this must be weighed against optimal use of vascular resources. By our technique of shunt conversion in children, we obtain optimal access from the same vascular site for acute and for subsequent chronic HD treatment, thereby conserving alternative vessel sites for the future.

References

1 Butt, K. M. H. (1978). Blood access. *Clin. Nephrol.*, **9**, 138

2 Haimov, M. (1975). Vascular access for hemodialysis. *Surg. Gynecol. Obstet.*, **141**, 619

3 Hirschmann, G. H., Wolfson, M., Mosimann, J. E., Clark, C. B., Dante, M. L. and Wineman, R. J. (1981). Complications of dialysis. *Clin. Nephrol.*, **15**, 66

4 Brescia, M. J., Cimino, J. E., Appel, K. and Hurwich, B. J. (1966). Chronic hemodialysis using venipuncture and a surgically created arteriovenous fistula. *N. Engl. J. Med.*, **275**, 1089

5 Quinton, W. E., Dillard, D. and Scribner, B. H. (1960). Cannulation of blood vessels for prolonged hemodialysis. *Trans. Am. Soc. Artif. Intern. Organs*, **6**, 104

6 Bell, P. R. F. and Calman, K. C. (1979). Vascular access in dialysis. In Drukker, W., Parsons, F. M. and Maher, J. F. (eds.). *Replacement of Renal Function by Dialysis*, pp. 182−198. (The Hague: Martinus Nijhoff)

7 Buselmeier, T. J., Rynasiewicz, J. J., Howard, R. H., Sutherland, D. E. R., Davin, T. D., Lynch, R. L., Hodson, E. H., Simmons, R. L., Najarian, J. S. and Kjellstrand, C. M. (1977). Fistulisation of shunt vasculature: a unique approach to fistula development. *Br. Med. J.*, **2**, 933

8 Sigley, R. D., May, K. J. and Mack, R. M. (1979). Scribner shunt conversion to arteriovenous fistula. *Am. J. Surg.*, **137**, 423

9 Simonian, S. J., Stuart, F. P., Hill, J. L. and Mahajan, S. K. (1977). Conversion of a Scribner shunt to an arteriovenous fistula for chronic dialysis. *Surgery*, **82**, 448

10 Höffler, D., Kaltenbach, Th., Quellhorst, E., Scheler, F. and Wigger, W. (1965). Erfahrungen mit einem Silicon-Teflon-A-V-Shunt bei der Hämodialyse. *Dtsch. Med. Wochenschr.*, **90**, 1824

11 Hardy, M. A., Schneider, K. M. and Levitt, S. B. (1974). An improved technique for the construction of internal arteriovenous fistulas in uremic children. *J. Pediatr. Surg.*, **9**, 465

12 Wander, J. V., Moore, E. S. and Jonasson, O. (1970). Internal arteriovenous fistulae for dialysis in children. *J. Pediatr. Surg.*, **5**, 533

13 Baillod, R. (1975). Eight years experience in home dialysis in children under the age of 15 years. In Bulla, M. (ed.). *Probleme der Kinderdialyse*, pp. 97−106. (Melsungen: B. Braun)

14 Buselmeier, T. J., Santiago, E. A., Simmons, R. L., Najarian, J. S. and Kjellstrand, C. M. (1971). Arteriovenous shunts for pediatric hemodialysis. *Surgery*, **70**, 638

15 Graben, N., Cremer, W. and Merguet, P. (1976). Der In-Line-Shunt als optimale Modifikation des Teflon-Silastic-Shunts. *Nieren- und Hochdruckkrankheiten*, **7**, 177

14

Central venous catheter for total parenteral nutrition in small children

R. DEREERE, J.-M. BOUTON AND P. DECONINCK

INTRODUCTION

Total parenteral nutrition (TPN) has contributed a great deal to recent progress in pediatric surgery, particularly in neonatal surgery[1]. Neonates, and even more so premature infants, have a low calorie reserve[2] and tolerate poorly suboptimal conditions. Therefore, a steady infusion of the correct amount of TPN is important in that age group. The peripheral venous network is quite rapidly exhausted if used for this purpose as well as for the intravenous administration of several drugs, for blood and/or plasma transfusions. A central venous catheter seems to be an efficient way to administer TPN for long periods of time in satisfactory conditions. Thus the peripheral network remains available for intravenous antibiotics, blood, etc. The risk of skin necrosis by subcutaneous infiltration, as may be seen occasionally when infusion pumps are used, is avoided. Finally the patient is more comfortable, not being submitted to repeated venipunctures.

This chapter will deal with a few technical aspects only. An important point is the choice of the right catheter. Because this catheter will be implanted for a long time, it should not irritate the venous wall, nor should it be thrombogenic. It is generally accepted that Silastic and other silicone catheters are the best[3].

MATERIALS AND METHODS

Between January 1980 and February 1982 we inserted a total of 82 central venous catheters: 46 infant-sized Vygon catheters and 36 Silastic catheters. Seventy-eight catheters were introduced in the superior vena cava (Table

14.1), most often through the internal jugular vein, less frequently through the external jugular vein or the greater superficial arm veins. Only four catheters were put in the inferior vena cava, through the great saphenous vein or the epigastric vein[4]. The greater risk of venous thrombosis and/or infection through this route explains why so few cases had a central venous catheter in the inferior vena cava.

Table 14.1 Choice of access vein

Superior vena cava	78	
jugularis interna		61
jugularis externa		6
basilica-cephalica		11
Inferior vena cava	4	
saphena magna		2
epigastrica inferior		2

After the patient is intubated and anaesthetized, all catheters are placed by the same surgeon. A standardized technique is used. The operative field is widely disinfected with iodophore solution and carefully draped. A 1½ cm incision is made at the level of the internal jugular vein, which is easily exposed between the sternal and clavicular heads of the sternocleidomastoid muscle. The jugular vein is dissected over 1 cm. Between two stay sutures, which are used for control of bleeding, a small circular 6/O suture is put on the anterior surface of the vein. In its centre, a punctiform incision is made and an infant-sized silicone tube, flushed with saline, is inserted under X-ray control for positioning of the tip at the entrance of the right atrium. The circular suture is tied and the stay sutures are removed. Catheter tube and connecting device are separated and tunnelization to the nipple areola is carried out, making sure that the catheter is not kinked in front of the jugular vein. Retro-auricular tunnelization is avoided to allow free access to the venous network of the scalp. Tunnelization from the great saphenous or from the inferior epigastrica is on the abdominal wall. The two-piece connecting device with a conical tightening system is then secured to the catheter tube, which is cut at the desired length to allow correct dressing.

A catheter prolongator, flushed with saline, is also attached. A non-adherent dry dressing is put around the catheter exit. Catheter and dressing are fixed to the skin with ½ inch (12 mm) wide Steristrips and covered with a dry gauze dressing. A loop of catheter tube is brought on top of this dressing, fixed again with Steristrips and covered with another dry gauze. On top of this comes the connecting device, which is fixed with Steristrips and covered with a large dry gauze, hiding the Steristrips entirely. This entire dressing is now covered and fixed to the skin with Steridrape, reinforced with Steristrips at the borders and occasionally with Kling bandage. This dressing should not be changed and should guarantee excellent fixation and sterility. Catheter prolongator and sterile intravenous fluid administration set are connected with a 0.2 μm bacterial filter in between. This connection is covered with an iodophore-saturated dressing and changed daily by one of the surgical residents in operating room dress.

TPN solution is prepared daily by a specialized team under a laminar flow hood, everything being kept sterile until connected to the catheter prolongator by the surgical resident. In this manner, 82 central venous catheters were introduced in 61 patients: 40 males and 21 females. The total duration of TPN was 2004 days, with a mean of 33 days and a maximum of 210 days. Age distribution is shown in Table 14.2.

Table 14.2 Weight and age distribution of children who underwent TPN

22 prematures		1−30 days	32
under 1000 g	3	1−6 months	12
1000−1500 g	4	6−12 months	5
1500−2500 g	15	1−12 years	12
TOTAL			61

Indications were gastrointestinal-tract surgery in 37, cardiac surgery in 10, malignancies in five and miscellaneous in nine. Eleven patients had two or more catheters, with a maximum of six catheters in one patient. This was a premature infant with a birth weight of 1100 g and presenting with necrotizing enterocolitis (NEC) at 2 weeks of age. The first catheter was removed 2 months later, after the patient had recovered. A new episode of NEC made TPN again necessary. The patient had several complications such as sepsis, superior vena cava syndrome and inferior vena cava syndrome. Eventually she did well and is now thriving on a normal diet. The complications are listed in Table 14.3.

Table 14.3 Catheter complications

Accidentally or erroneously removed	6
Plugging of catheter	7
Catheter infection with sepsis	2
Removed for suspicion of sepsis (negative catheter tip culture)	5
Superior vena cava syndrome	2
Inferior vena cava syndrome	1
TOTAL	23

DISCUSSION

In several instances sepsis was suspected and the catheter removed. Most often, culture of the catheter tip failed to show any growth. Obviously, nursing care is critical in TPN. Accidental or erroneous removal and plugging of the catheter should be avoided. Vena cava syndrome occurred in two patients in whom a new type of Vygon catheter was used. This material was therefore abandoned. In conclusion, a central venous catheter seems to be the preferred route for TPN, especially in small children with a life-threatening condition. To achieve an acceptable morbidity and a good reliability, a sufficient turnover and a whole team, with surgeons and pediatricians, dieticians, pharmacists and high-level nurses are necessary. A chain is as strong as its weakest link.

References

1 Dudrick, S. (1968). Long-term parenteral nutrition with growth, development, and positive nitrogen balance. *Surgery*, **64**, 134
2 Heird, W. C. (1972). Intravenous alimentation in pediatric patients. *J. Pediatr.*, **80**, 351
3 Broviac, J. W. (1973). A silicone rubber right atrial catheter for prolonged parenteral alimentation. *Surg. Gynecol. Obstet.*, **136**, 602
4 Donahoe, P. K. and Kim, S. H. (1980). The inferior epigastric vein as an alternate site for central venous hyperalimentation. *J. Pediatr. Surg.*, **15**, 737

15

Abstracts of posters in Access in children

Arteriovenous fistula in children using a pre-arterialized vein
F. CERIATI, I. R. MARINO and C. CAVICCHIONI

In paediatric hemodialysed patients it is often very difficult to realize a lasting vascular access with a balanced flow rate. To perform an effective surgical management without a serious injury to the vessels of the arm, and without causing cardiac failure, we have realized twelve A-V shunts between ulnar artery and cephalic vein in the forearm. This vascular access allows us to dialyse the patients and, at the same time, we can obtain the arterialization of the cephalic vein. About 60 days afterwards, we performed an A-V fistula between brachial artery and the pre-arterialized cephalic vein, by continuous silk suture. At the same time, using another forearm vein, we performed a new external shunt to continue the dialysis treatment, waiting for wound healing of the A-V fistula. By this method we obtained good results, without complications.

Access surgery in childhood
H. ERASMI, S. HORSCH, R. SCHMIDT and H. PICHLMAIER

With the ever-increasing number of dialysis-dependent children shunt surgery has become more important. At the University Hospital of Cologne between 1972 and 1981, 69 internal blood accesses were created in children with a mean age of 11 years. We have distinguished 43 Cimino and 17 brachial fistulas; nine bovine heterografts were also implanted.

The complications and function of different fistulas were compared. It is shown that Cimino fistulas are the most successful. The brachial fistula has a higher rate of complications: development of aneurysms and difficulties in puncture. Therefore, in situations where the peripheral vessels are unsuitable for a direct anastomosis between artery and vein a bovine heterograft should be implanted.

Angioaccess in small children hemodialysed for acute or chronic uraemia
L. BERARDINELLI, G. STORELLI, L. MILITANO and A. VEGETO

Paediatric or adult patients weighing less than 25 kg coming from five Italian centres were treated for uraemia. An external femoral shunt was prepared by us in almost all cases of immediate necessity of haemodialysis in very small children. An end-to-side anastomosis of the Dacron knitted portion of an Allen-Brown shunt has always been constructed on a superficial artery considering the possibility of complications and eventual necessity of surgical replacements. An alternative useful technique adopted by us particularly in small children needing immediate dialysis is the composite shunt. This consists of the anastomosis of a venous homograft end-to-side to an artery. A Ramirez Teflon–Silastic cannula is then placed in the free end of the venous graft. Two principal patterns of internal arteriovenous fistulas were used for chronic patients: side-to-side proximal fistula between the brachial artery and an antecubital vein, and angioaccess with organic prostheses (homologous vein or bovine carotid graft). The proximal fistulas were performed either for direct utilization or for preparing the vascular bed for graft interposition. In the cases of unsuitable upper limb vessels vascular grafts were inserted in the thigh with high success rate.

Use of arteriovenous fistulas for long-term parenteral nutrition in children
Y. RÉVILLON, D. BOUGLÉ and C. RICOUR

In order to allow the vascular access required by long-term cyclic parenteral nutrition (PN) a programme of arteriovenous (A-V) fistulas has been developed in children. There were 17 children aged from 5 months to 18 years, with large intestinal resections or chronic adynamic bowel disease. 30 A-V fistulas were performed: humeral: 17, femoral: 13. Six could not be achieved and spontaneous thrombosis occurred in seven cases before use. The last 17 had been used for total ($n=4$) or partial ($n=13$) cyclic PN. Parenteral intakes varied from 12 to 80 kcal kg^{-1} day^{-1} (glucose 70%, lipid 30%) and from 90 to 600 mg N kg^{-1} day^{-1}.

Normal growth was observed in all but two of the children. Septic, trophic or haemodynamic complications did not occur. Six A-V fistulas thrombosed after 10 ($\pm$1) months of use, mainly in younger children; nine others are functioning after 4 months to 3 years.

These results show that: (1) so far the creation of A-V fistulas in infants less than 1 year old is not valid; (2) the long life of A-V fistulas without side-effects makes them an appropriate alternative to central catheters for long-term PN.

Single needle haemodialysis (SND) via subclavian vein
C. D. MISTRY, R. GOKAL and N. P. MALLICK

Adequate vascular access is essential for patients requiring haemodialysis. This is usually achieved by the use of a fistula or the Scribner shunt. In situations where temporary but immediate vascular access is required, the use of the subclavian vein catheter technique with SND has major advantages over the Scribner shunt.

Using this technique 12 patients (five male, seven female) were dialysed for a mean period of 4 weeks (range 1–9 weeks). Indication for the use of this technique were thrombosis or lack of an A-V fistula (6), and CAPD patients without vascular access requiring short-term haemodialysis (5). Nine patients had more than one subclavian puncture for exit site infections (4), cannula thrombosis (3), inadequate blood flow (1), leakage from the cannula site (1).

A major problem was that of catheter exit site infection (12 episodes) and one episode of septicaemia. These were successfully treated. Catheter patency was maintained by heparin infusion through the catheter (500 units in 5 ml normal saline 6-hourly), which the patients were able to perform themselves. Five patients were able to go home with the catheter *in situ* after a median inpatient stay of 8 days. There was no morbidity associated with catheter insertion and adequate biochemical control and blood flows were obtained.

Subclavian vein catheterization provides immediate and adequate access for dialysis, preserves a vascular access site and has a very acceptable morbidity. SND using this access provides good biochemical and fluid control and appears to be superior to the Scribner shunt.

Subclavian vein catheterization in infants
J. H. BERGMEIJER, N. M. A. BAX, F. W. J. HAZEBROEK and
J. C. MOLENAAR

From January 1981 till January 1982 a subclavian venipuncture procedure for parenteral alimentation was carried out 19 times in 14 surgical patients under the age of 1 year. Five patients underwent the intervention twice. Ages ranged from 5 weeks to 7 months. Mean weight was 3060 g, ranging from 1690 to 7000 g. The subclavian route was successful in nine cases, in five cases a line was introduced in the jugular vein, in three cases in the femoral vein and in the remaining two cases a peripheral vein was used. No serious complications occurred in connection with the puncture. Reposition of the catheter was required on five occasions. Pneumothorax did not occur, one infant developed a hydrothorax. Catheters remained in position an average of 14 days, the longest for 1 month. Most catheters were removed on suspicion of sepsis. This was confirmed in only two cases.

16

Invited comment on papers and posters in Access in children

P. KINNAERT

Vascular access in young children remains a challenge for the surgeon. However, the various papers and posters of this symposium show that in the last few years some solutions have been found and that surgeons try continuously to improve their techniques. Buskens, Skotnicki, Reinaerts and De Jong ('Access surgery in children: a big problem?') created A-V fistulas in 28 children with a 60% immediate success rate. In the cases where the primary procedure failed, they succeeded in constructing another access device during a second operation. They conclude that the A-V fistula is the first choice in children who must be treated by haemodialysis. They favour the side (artery) to end (vein) anastomosis which should always be preferred to the end-to-end anastomosis because the flow through the fistula is 30% higher when the distal portion of the artery remains patent[1]. Thus, we hope to decrease the immediate failure rate and ameliorate the late patency rate of these devices. If a steal syndrome occurs it is always possible to ligate the distal radial artery. This technique avoids also the venous hypertension in the hand sometimes seen following side-to-side A-V fistulas at the wrist. Daul, Graben, Windeck and Pistor ('Conversion of Teflon–Silastic shunts to A-V fistulas in small children with chronic renal failure') and Ceriati, Marino and Cavicchioni ('Arteriovenous fistula in children using a pre-arterialized vein') describe ingenious techniques to convert an external A-V shunt into an A-V fistula, the idea being to dilate the veins with the shunt and construct an A-V fistula more easily when the vessels are larger. These procedures are interesting to know for children who present themselves with a shunt already in place because they preserve other vascular access sites. However, I am reluctant to systematically insert cannulas in the vessels of small children. Indeed, with proper technique, A-V fistulas can be constructed when the veins are large enough to be cannulated by paediatric vessel tips. Eventually we can use microsurgical techniques as shown by Bourquelot[2]. Incidentally we always use at least magnifying glasses when we construct a fistula (even in adults). In our earlier experience with external A-V shunts there was a high incidence of clotting of cannulas, moreover infection was not infrequent. These complications would prevent the use of the same vessels for construction of the subsequent A-V fistula. Moreover, because of the length of the cannula, the necessity to create a subcutaneous tunnel and the fact that the anastomosis must be performed above the tip of the cannulas, one may lose, in the smallest children, as much as one-third of the length of the vessel.

Berardinelli, Storelli, Militano and Vegeto ('Angioaccess in small children hemodialysed for acute or chronic uraemia') favour the A-V fistula constructed in the antecubital fossa. We have also used this device in small children with very satisfactory results[3]. When the operation is well planned the fistula can be made without altering the venous drainage of the forearm. The veins of the forearm can be utilized later on for the creation of a fistula if needed when the child grows up. When haemodialysis has to be instituted quickly, Berardinelli *et al.* recommend the Allen–Brown shunt in the thigh or a composite shunt, the arterial branch of which is composed of a venous homograft anastomosed to an artery and intubated with a Ramirez Teflon–Silastic cannula. These interesting techniques should not be used systematically. One should keep in mind that it is rather difficult to keep the orifices around the cannulas in the thigh clean, especially in small children, because of the proximity of the perineum. If treatment is required immediately, peritoneal dialysis should be tried first in the younger patients and an A-V fistula should be planned only when blood chemistry and haemodynamics are stabilized. In the biggest children (weighing more than 20–25 kg), single needle haemodialysis (SND) via the subclavian vein as described by Mistry, Gokal and Mallick in adults is another possible method. It preserves all the vascular access sites. In order to maintain the patency of the catheter, the authors inject heparinized saline every 6 hours. In our unit we infuse heparinized saline through the catheter only at the end of each dialysis session and put the whole device under a sterile dressing. The patient is instructed not to touch this dressing between dialysis sessions. Since we adopted this protocol there has been no increase in the frequency of clotting episodes but the morbidity due to infections has diminished substantially.

Erasmi, Horsch, Schmidt and Pichlmaier ('Access surgery in childhood') report their experience with 69 internal blood access devices. Brescia–Cimino fistulas gave the best results but it should be mentioned that this type of fistula is usually performed in the children with the best vascular supply. Brachial fistulas were more difficult to puncture and aneurysms developed. In her abstract, Mrs Erasmi concludes that bovine heterografts should be implanted when distal vessels are unavailable. Fortunately, this statement has been corrected in the poster where the bovine graft is considered to be the last choice. .Indeed, pseudo-aneurysms have been described with this material[4] and there is an increased risk of infection due to repeated puncture of foreign material and problems may arise with grafts in straight position because of the presence of a non-growing conduit in a growing limb.

Vascular access for hyperalimentation is another challenge for the surgeon. Dereere, Bouton and Deconinck ('Central venous catheter for TPN in small children') used the classical central venous catheter inserted surgically through various veins (jugular, basilic, internal saphenous or epigastric vein). With careful surgery and rigid asepsis during subsequent manipulation of the catheter, they obtained satisfactory results. Bergmeijer, Bax, Hazebroek and Molenaar ('Subclavian vein catheterization in infants') report a shorter series of catheters inserted percutaneously with similar results. However, the main and most dangerous complication of these catheters remains infection. Therefore, other solutions were searched for. Révillon, Bouglé and Ricour ('Use of arteriovenous fistulas for long-term parenteral nutrition in children') tried to create A-V fistulas for hyperalimentation. While most of the children with renal failure have a series of features which facilitate the creation of an A-V fistula (low haematocrit, alterations in the coagulation system, increased plasma volume, high cardiac output) the patient who needs hyperalimentation has usually a normal or nearly normal haematocrit, a normal or low blood pressure and he may be slightly dehydrated. Consequently, the creation of a functioning A-V fistula is not an easy task for the surgeon. Révillon *et al.* report an immediate failure rate of 43%. Moreover, the hyperalimentation mixture favours thrombosis which occurred in six of the 15 fistulas that were used. However, the most important point in their work is that no septic episode was recorded. Therefore, the technique should be explored further.

In conclusion, the conditions that should be fulfilled by an ideal vascular access are:

(1) It should preserve as much as possible the vascular supply of the child.

(2) It should not prevent normal activities. This means that we should avoid external devices that destroy vascular access sites. Because of the risk of disconnection or the risk of infection by soiling of the dressings, the children are not allowed to play normally. The external device always reminds them of their disease. Psychological problems can occur not only in children but also in parents[5].

(3) It should be easy to use, which means that the fistula should be easy to puncture and that its flow should be high enough to allow adequate dialysis. Therefore, we have not investigated the distal fistulas in small children because in our experience they take a very long time to mature and we prefer the elbow fistula in these situations.

(4) The complication rate should be low and the late patency rate high. This is best obtained by internal access devices constructed with the child's own vessels.

(5) One very important point is that the vascular access device should be used correctly. This means that the surgeon is not only involved in the creation of the A-V fistula but that he should supervise its utilization by regularly meeting the nurses and the paediatricians in order to discuss the vascular access problems. I am convinced that it is only by such teamwork that we will be able to improve our results in the future.

Finally it should be stressed that kidney transplantation is the only acceptable treatment of renal failure in childhood and that the haemodialysis or peritoneal dialysis period should be as short as possible.

References

1 Anderson, C. B., Etheredge, E. E., Harter, H. R., Graff, R. J., Codd, J. E. and Newton, W. T. (1977). Local blood flow characteristics of arteriovenous fistulas in the forearm for dialysis. *Surg. Gynecol. Obstet.*, **144**, 531
2 Bourquelot, P., Wolfeler, L. and Lamy, L. (1981). Microsurgery for haemodialysis distal arteriovenous fistulae in children weighing less than 10 kg. *Int. J. Microsurg.*, **3**, 187
3 Kinnaert, P., Janssen, F. and Hall, M. (1982). Elbow arteriovenous fistula (EAVF) for chronic hemodialysis in small children. *J. Pediatr. Surg.*, (Accepted for publication)
4 Rosenberg, N., Thompson, J. E., Keshishian, J. M. and VanderWerf, B. A. (1976). The modified bovine arterial graft. *Arch. Surg.*, **111**, 689
5 Raimbault, G. (1973). Psychological aspects of chronic renal failure and haemodialysis. *Nephron*, **11**, 251

Section IV
Graft material

17

A comparative study in angioaccesses for haemodialysis using homologous saphenous vein, bovine and PTFE graft

L. BERARDINELLI, C. BERETTA, E. POZZOLI AND A. VEGETO

Interposition of prosthetic material for arteriovenous communications became an indication for access surgery if there are no possibilities to construct a direct arteriovenous fistula. This study will describe and analyse the results of 202 arteriovenous and graft fistulas out of a total experience of 684 vascular access procedures. The frequency of complications and the outcome of reoperations of homologous saphenous vein, bovine carotid and extended PTFE grafts are specially compared.

MATERIALS AND METHODS

Between 1968 and 1981, 684 new vascular access procedures and 172 reoperations have been performed on 471 patients by the same surgical team. No patients had vessels suitable for construction of a regular Brescia—Cimino forearm fistula.

From 45 dialysis centres in Italy 245 men and 226 women, aged from 6 months to 83 years, came to our hospital. All patients had been operated elsewhere, for an average of seven arteriovenous vascular procedures. All operations were done using local anaesthesia, with minimal patient discomfort.

Prior to the insertion of a graft the patency of the venous outflow was ascertained by phlebography. The grafts were indifferently placed across the joints, if necessary. Grafts were not cannulated for at least 3 weeks after insertion and the technicians were not aware of the nature of the graft. Only in one case was the patient's own saphenous vein used as a graft. The homologous saphenous veins, obtained from routine saphenectomy and preserved in an ordinary refrigerator, were used as graft in 130 cases. In the last

5 years the veins have been chosen based only on their integrity and sterility, without regard to the major ABO blood group compatibility. In 59 cases there was no suitable vein available and a bovine graft interposition was performed. We now use bovine carotid grafts with a larger diameter than we used originally.

In comparison with a venous graft we double the amount of heparin to prevent clotting due to the lack of an endothelial layer in the bovine graft during the anastomosis of this graft. We also found it technically useful to grease the external surface of the carotid graft with sterile Vaseline oil for easier passage through the subcutaneous tunnel. Expanded PTFE was used in nine, and human umbilical vein graft (Dardik) in three, cases. The grafts were placed at the upper or lower limb, indifferently in straight or loop-shaped tunnel position. All patients were dismissed with platelet disaggregating agents.

RESULTS

The best surgical results were observed with the homologous saphenous vein graft, with a mean function time of 13 months and a maximum function of 6 years. The bovine graft has a mean function time of 5.6 months (maximum 35 months). The worst clinical results were noted with artificial material: in fact only one PTFE graft is still functioning after 3 months (mean survival time 1.7 months). The tolerance for repetitive punctures is better for all biografts, if compared with the artificial graft.

Table 17.1 Functioning of vascular grafts

	Allografts	Bovine	PTFE
Number of vascular accesses	130	59	9
Mean life (months)	13.9	5.6	1.7
Number of reoperations	46	28	5
Mean prolongation of graft life after reoperation (months)	6.4	1.2	1.1

No serious vascular insufficiency, nor arterial steal syndrome, were noted in our cases. We believe that this complication depends on the surgical technique and size of the anastomosis, rather than on the graft material itself.

The immediate thrombosis observed in the first month after operation was seen seven times in 130 homologous venous grafts (5.3%) and five times in 59 bovine carotid grafts (8.4%). In our experience a stenosis at the venous end of the bovine graft occurs frequently about the 5th–6th month of function. A phlebography is recommended when the venous pressure arises during haemodialysis. On the other hand dilatation is the most frequent complication in the venous graft at the arterial side. Eight aneurysms were seen (6.1%), four of them successfully corrected later. No aneurysm was seen in 59 bovine grafts, but we have had the opportunity of resecting aneurysms in grafts installed by other surgeons.

Rare episodes of early infection were seen by well-controlled biografts, without loss of function of the fistula.

In six venous grafts (4.6%) and three bovine grafts (5%) we later lost the fistula due to infection. After reoperation there was an increase in function time of 6.4 months for homologous vein grafts, 1.2 months for bovine grafts and 1.1 months for PTFE grafts. Due to the infection risk of the thrombosed graft, most of the PTFE grafts must be totally removed, while all except one biograft could be left *in situ* after thrombosis. The experience with umbilical vein graft (Dardik) was too short, but we saw late erosions of the overlying skin in patients with a small amount of subcutaneous tissue.

DISCUSSION AND CONCLUSIONS

Intimal hyperplasia at the venous anastomosis of bovine graft has often been reported[1-3]. However, our experience with heterograft is satisfactory. Investigations in the problems of the tensile strength could lead to improvement in the quality of this biograft. We cannot explain the disappointing results obtained with PTFE grafts in contrast with other authors[4,5]. Neither intraoperative contamination nor contact with Betadine or alcohol were confirmed[6]. The main factor responsible for this unsatisfactory outcome could be the 'prefilling' of the PTFE graft with blood, as we usually do, in order to prevent twisting.

The best results were obtained with homologous saphenous grafts, whose advantages, at least in our opinion are: lowest cost of preservation, free availability in a vascular surgery division, absence of legal problems and excellent functional results[7].

References

1 Hammil, F. S., Johnston, G. C., Collins, G. M., Halasz, N. A., Dilley, R. B. and Bernstein, E. G. (1980). A critical appraisal of the changing approaches to vascular access for hemodialysis. *Dial. Transplant.*, **9**, 325

2 Latimer, R. G., Gebhart, W. F., Freidell, H. V., Murray, J. J. and Fisher, M. B. (1980). Comparison of chronic hemodialysis angio-access procedures. *Dial. Transplant.*, **9**, 499

3 Giacchino, J. L., Geis, W. P., Buckingham, J. M., Vertuno, L. L. and Bansal, V. K. (1979). Vascular access: long-term results, new techniques. *Arch. Surg.*, **114**, 403

4 Owens, M. L., Stabile, B. E., Gehr, J. A. and Wilson, S. E. (1979). Vascular grafts for hemodialysis: an evaluation of sites and materials. *Dial. Transplant.*, **8**, 521

5 Lawton, R. L. (1980). Vascular access: always one more arrow in the quiver. *Dial. Transplant.*, **9**, 10

6 Gupta, S. K. and Veith, F. J. (1980). Three years experience with expanded PTFE arterial grafts for limb salvage. *Am. J. Surg.*, **140**, 214

7 Vegeto, A., Berardinelli, L. and Malan, E. (1977). Use of homologous vein grafts for chronic hemodialysis. *J. Cardiovasc. Surg.*, **18**, 501

18

Bovine xenograft – a useful tissue for construction of arteriovenous fistulas for chronic haemodialysis

M. DECURTINS, G. K. UHLSCHMID, P. BUCHMANN,
S. GEROULANOS AND F. LARGIADÈR

Haemodialysis, performed for the first time in 1943, has since 1960 become a successful method of treatment of chronic renal insufficiency. In 1978 there were 8000 patients on chronic haemodialysis in Switzerland and in the same year one new patient in 20 000 inhabitants needed haemodialysis.

For the performance of routine haemodialysis adequate vascular access is one of the most important prerequisites[1]. The great number of operative techniques and materials described since the first creation of an A-V fistula illustrates the fact that the individual vascular situation is to be considered for the construction of such access.

In accordance with various authors we can only agree that the best long-lasting results can be achieved with a simple arteriovenous (A-V) fistula on the forearm (Brescia–Cimino)[2-4]. Between 1975 and 1980, 181 such fistulas were performed at our department.

In cases where a simple A-V fistula was impossible to construct, or where immediate onset of haemodialysis was indicated, graft fistulas were constructed by the interposition of autologous veins[5] or in recent years in an increasing number of patients with xenogeneic or allogeneic material. In the present chapter we summarize our results with xenogeneic materials used for the construction of graft fistulas.

MATERIAL AND METHODS

Between 1975 and 1980 in 81 patients (46 females and 35 male) with a mean age of 44 years (6–68 years) an overall number of 115 arteriovenous graft fistulas using non-human material were constructed. The bovine xenografts are prepared from denatured calf carotid arteries with diameter 4–5 mm and an approximate length of 10–30 cm (Solco–Graft®) treated with dialdehyde. Artificial vascular prostheses were prepared from polytetrafluorethylene (PTFE) (Gore-tex®).

The construction of the graft fistula was done in the majority of cases in local anaesthesia using lidocain 2% with an addition of adrenalin; in infant patients usually under general anaesthesia. Depending on the vascular conditions of the patients a straight graft from the radial artery to one of the superficial veins distal or proximal of the fossa cubiti was used or if necessary connected to one of the deeper cubital veins accompanying the artery. In cases of insufficient flow in the radial artery the graft was connected to the cubital artery and pulled through a subcutaneous channel U-shaped to one of the veins in the fossa cubiti. In cases where the graft had to be positioned on the upper arm, a straight graft was used between the cubital artery and one of the veins of the upper arm or a graft was drawn from the brachial artery in the bicipital sulcus U-shaped to one of the accompanying veins in the bicipital sulcus (Table 18.1).

Table 18.1 Localization and shape of the A-V graft

		Straight graft	*Curved graft*
Forearm	($n = 85$)	60	25
Upper arm	($n = 13$)	9	4
Thigh	($n = 1$)	—	1

On the arterial side a side-to-end anastomosis, on the venous side an end-to-end or end-to-side anastomosis was performed using synthetic suture materials (Tevdek, Prolene) of 6/O or 7/O strength. Postoperatively a drainage of the anastomotic region for 24 h was established and the arm was kept elevated for 2–4 days. For thromboprophylaxis a single intraoperative dose of 5000 units of heparin (liquemin) intravenously followed by the same dose every 6 h for 24 h was applied. Chronic thromboprophylaxis with thrombocyte inhibitors will be discussed later. Statistical evaluation is performed using the χ^2-test. The experimental set-up and the preparations for scanning electron microscopy are described in another publication[6].

RESULTS

Bovine xenograft

After an observation period of 1–48 months, 33 of the 99 xenografts were still used for haemodialysis access. During the same period 21 patients died with functioning graft fistula and in six patients the xenograft A-V fistula was

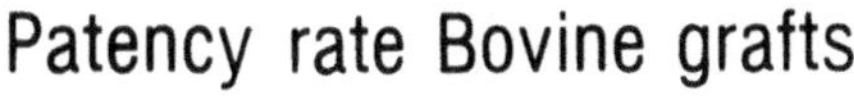
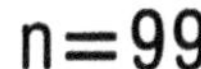
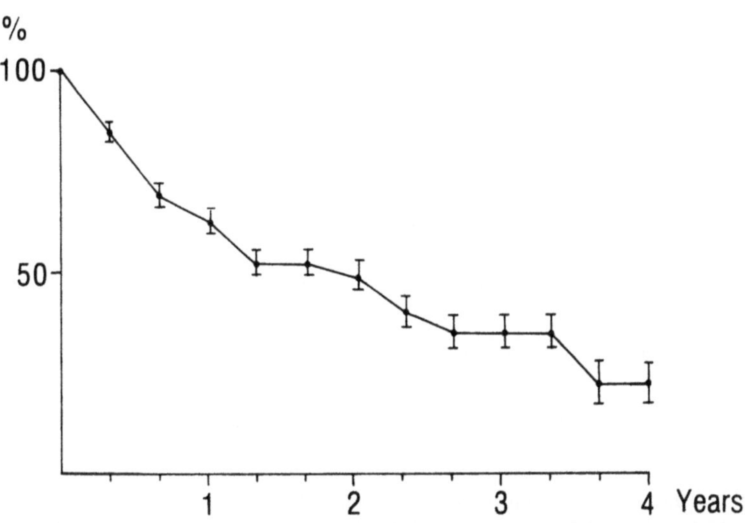

Figure 18.1 Cumulative, actuarialized overall-graft function rate (xenograft)

unnecessary after successful renal transplantation. Altogether 39 fistulas had to be abandoned in this period and replaced by new constructions.

The cumulative rate of function of our **99** graft fistulas is shown in Figure 18.1. For the first 12 months the risk of fistula failure of 38% has been calculated from this curve.

A clear-cut dependence of the function of a graft fistula from its geometric course (straight or curved) was not found. In the curved types of grafts, however, significantly less thromboses were found compared to the straight grafts ($p < 0.05$) (Table 18.2).

Table 18.2 Occurrence of complications in straight and loop grafts

		Straight graft ($n = 69$)	*Curved graft* ($n = 30$)
Thrombosis	($n = 41$)	33	8*
Infection	($n = 8$)	7	1
Aneurysm	($n = 10$)	7	3
Haemorrhage	($n = 2$)	—	2

*$p < 0.05$

Thromboses of a xenograft fistula are the most frequent complications in this type of vascular prostheses. Reason for thrombosis could be found in 62% ($n = 26$) of these complications. In 19 cases intraoperatively or by pre-operative phlebography a localized long stenosis, approximately 1 cm long,

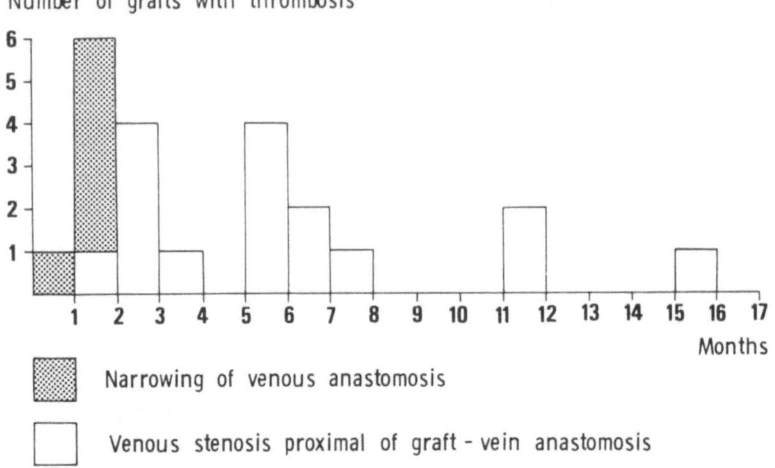

Figure 18.2 Peak period of occurrence of graft thrombosis for stenosis at the graft–vein anastomosis and thromboses caused by narrowing of the vein above the graft–vein anastomosis

in the region of the draining vein immediately proximal to the venous anastomosis with the graft could be found. The majority of these 19 fistulas had once or repeatedly been thrombectomized before the stenosis had been diagnosed. It becomes obvious from Figure 18.2 that at least 2 months, and in the mean 8 months, passed between the construction of the fistula and the first symptoms of venous narrowing. In six cases where the stenosis was at the venous anastomosis, the thrombosis of the fistula occurred within the first 2 months (Figure 18.2).

The reason for thrombosis of the fistula could not be elucidated in 38% ($n = 16$), even though a narrowing of the entire A-V system could be excluded by intraoperative revision. More than half of these thromboses occurred in the first month after construction of the fistula. Another frequently observed complication was the formation of aneurysms ($n = 10$). In seven cases this was an aneurysm of the spurium type, in two cases an aneurysma verum at the arterial anastomosis and once a dissecting aneurysm arising from a point of repeated puncture. Eight of these 10 aneurysms could be corrected successfully by operation.

In all eight cases of graft infection the xenograft had to be removed for effective treatment of the infection. In three cases an infection became evident a few days after revision of the xenograft; in one case a xenograft infection occurred in the frame of an acute cholecystitis with septicaemia.

In two cases revision of a xenograft for massive haemorrhage was necessary. Untreatable haemorrhage from a puncture channel after haemodialysis and once from the arterial anastomosis made surgical intervention successfully necessary.

Of the patients with a xenograft A-V fistula 51% ($n = 51$) were treated postoperatively with a daily application of thrombocyte aggregation inhibitors (Colfarit), 29% ($n = 29$) received dicoumarol derivatives (Sintrom or Marcoumar) and in 19 patients no medical thromboprophylaxis was performed. In those patients receiving thrombocyte aggregation inhibitors significantly less thromboses ($p < 0.05$) were observed compared to those on chronic anticoagulation or without thromboprophylaxis (Table 18.3).

Table 18.3 Occurrence of graft thromboses related to type of thromboprophylaxis

		Thromboses (n)
Thrombocyte agglutination inhibition	($n = 51$)	11*
Anticoagulation	($n = 29$)	13
No thromboprophylaxis	($n = 19$)	9

*$p < 0.05$

On average the 99 xenografts were punctured for the first time for haemodialysis on the 5th postoperative day. Only 10 grafts developing aneurysms between 6 and 52 weeks after the first puncture were used on the 2nd postoperative day. Otherwise no connection between an early puncture of the graft fistula and any other complications could be found.

The artificial vascular prosthesis
Of the 11 artificial vascular prostheses, five (45%) had to be removed after 3 months due to infection, five because of thrombosis after an average of 6 months after implantation. One patient died 1 month after construction of a graft fistula due to cardiac insufficiency.

Allogeneic umbilical vein grafts
Of the five allogeneic umbilical vein grafts three thrombosed irreversibly within the first 3 months and one graft had to be removed because of infection after 1 month. One umbilical graft is still used for haemodialysis 21 months after implantation, however, following thrombectomy after 17 months.

A new xenograft (Solco-P®)
Recently we have implanted a new type of bovine xenograft treated with adipin acid and digested with ficine in five patients. By this new preparation of the graft an additional elasticity of up to 20% of its original length can be achieved, which is especially important for the avoiding of kinking in curved xenografts. Comparative experimental examinations (Table 18.4) with this new type of graft showed it to be less thrombogenic. In contrast to other

grafts examined its inner surface is still recognizable after 6 weeks or covered by a neoendothelium which grows onto the inner surface of the new type xenograft starting from both suture lines. Histologically no eosinophilic or histiocytopathic proliferation was observed. The occlusion rate after 6 weeks is 29%, significantly lower than in the conventional bovine xenografts[6].

Table 18.4 Results of canine experiments listing the frequency of thromboses for different graft types after 6 weeks[6]

Occlusion rate after 6 weeks		n	%
PTFE	($n = 34$)	34	100
Umbilical vein	($n = 12$)	12	100
Dacron	($n = 34$)	26	77
Old bovine CA	($n = 32$)	21	66
New bovine CA	($n = 36$)	14	39

CA = carotid artery

From a clinical point of view it is too early for a definite judgement of this new material. We can, however, say that this type of material is much easier and smoother for suturing.

DISCUSSION

Since 1975 we have used allogeneic, xenogeneic or synthetic materials for the construction of A-V fistulas for chronic haemodialysis in cases where a direct conventional A-V fistula was impossible to construct. In recent years, however, the importance of such grafts has diminished as patients with bad vascular conditions are better treated by chronic ambulant peritoneal dialysis.

Because of the poor experiences with allogeneic umbilical vein (high rate of thrombosis) and synthetic vascular prostheses (high rate of infections) bovine xenograft proved to be the best alternative. Concerning the synthetic vascular prosthesis, however, we have to admit that our material is too small for statistical relevance. Other authors have experienced excellent results with this type of graft[5,7]. Among the prerequisites for achieving good results with this type of graft are special septic conditions and a particular technique of puncture. These conditions seem, however, not to be fulfilled in our institution as we are performing the surgical service for a great number of dialysis stations.

Autologous veins, especially the great saphena vein, achieve at least as good long-term results as xenograft interpositions[5]. A major disadvantage of this type of graft is the relatively long hospitalization of at least 1 week due to the removal of the vein and the high rate of complications when puncture is performed too early. Therefore we use autologous veins only in rare cases.

The cumulative, actuarialized risk for a definitive failure of the bovine xenograft fistula in our patients within the first 12 months was 38%. This is between the failure rate of 14 and 63% reported by other centres[4,8].

Thromboses are the most frequent reasons for the loss of function of xenograft fistulas. Interestingly enough straight grafts show thrombosis significantly more frequently than do curved grafts ($p<0.05$). The reason for these thromboses could be found in 60%. In 19 cases a venous stenosis or narrowing a few centimetres cranially of the venous anastomosis with the xenograft was the reason for such a thrombosis, in six cases a narrowing of the venous anastomosis was the reason for the thrombosis. The time of occurrence of these two complications is important. The narrowing of the venous anastomosis occurred exceptionally after the first 2 months. The stenosis or narrowing of the efferent vein occurred always later than 2, in the average 8, months after the construction of the fistula. Therefore, thrombosis occurring after the first 8 weeks should always be a warning of a narrowing of the draining vein, and always needs angiography or immediate intraoperative revision of this part of the graft fistula.

The cause of this narrowing of the vein is not clear[9]. Among others, haemodynamic factors are considered causative for the appearance of intimal hypertrophy or deposits of fibrin in the region of the draining vein[10,11]. It is obvious that in our material this type of venous narrowing occurs significantly more frequently in straight graft fistulas ($p<0.05$) which might support the above hypothesis.

After various periods of use for chronic haemodialysis 10% of our xenograft fistulas developed aneurysms. This frequency is comparable with that of other reports[12,13]. In over 80% of these cases the complications could be corrected successfully by surgery.

Xenograft infection, on the other hand, necessitated removal of the graft in all cases. Our rate of 8% xenograft infection is comparable with the rate of 4–25% reported by other authors[14,15].

Of the other complications described after graft fistula construction, such as oedema of the arm, ischaemia, steal syndrome or cardiac decompensation due to a high A-V shunt volume, could not be found in our material[10,11,14].

The question of thromboprophylaxis in patients with xenograft fistulas is not answered conclusively in the literature. In our patients we found a significantly lower rate of thrombosis under thrombocyte aggregation inhibitors as compared with the group treated with chronic anticoagulation or the group without any medical thromboprophylaxis ($p<0.05$). A possible explanation of this fact might be the easier application of aggregation inhibitors.

As we see one of the principal advantages of xenograft fistulas in the possibility of its early use, we consider an interval of 2–3 weeks between construction and use of xenograft fistulas as advocated by other authors[1,11] not necessary. From our observations we cannot find any influence of the time of first puncture of the graft on its function.

The new type of bovine xenograft, being more elastic, less prone to kinking in the curved form, and less thrombogenic in an experimental set-up, represents probably a very useful new generation of xenograft material.

CONCLUSIONS

The results after implantation of human umbilical vein ($n = 5$) were poor because of high frequency of thrombosis, and after implantation of synthetic vascular grafts (PTFE) ($n = 11$) a high incidence of local infections was observed. In most patients therefore a bovine xenograft ($n = 99$) was used. After a follow-up of 1–60 months the calculated failure rate for the first year is 38%. The most common complication was thrombosis, with better results in curved than in straight grafts ($p < 0.05$). Early thromboses were caused by a narrow anastomosis, late thromboses by venous narrowing proximal to the anastomosis. The time delay between construction and first use of the fistula had no influence on the survival rate of the fistulas. Long-term anti-thrombocyte medication showed better results than anticoagulation ($p < 0.05$). A new type of xenograft, more elastic, experimentally less thrombogenic and less prone to kinking, seems to be a promising step forward in the improvement of grafts used for access surgery. From our experience we recommend the use of bovine xenografts for fistula formation whenever the construction of a normal, direct A-V fistula is not possible.

References

1 Chinitz, J. L., Jokojana, T., Bower, R. and Swartz, Ch. (1972). Self-sealing prosthesis for arteriovenous fistula in man. *Trans. Am. Soc. Artif. Intern. Organs*, **23**, 452

2 Forran, R. F., Shore, E. H., Levin, P. N. and Treimann, R. L. (1975). Bovine heterograft for hemodialysis. *West. J. Med.*, **123**, 269

3 Sterling, W. A., Hazel, L. T. and Diethelm, A. G. (1975). Vascular access for hemodialysis by bovine graft arteriovenous fistulas. *Surg. Gynecol. Obstet.*, **141**, 69

4 Zehle, A., Schulz, V., Hottmann, J., Schmitt, N. and Pichelmaier, H. (1979). Arterio-venöse Gefässverbindungen für die Langzeitdialyse. *Chirurgie*, **50**, 345

5 Hollinger, A. and Largiadèr, F. (1973). Das freie Venentransplantat für die Langzeit-Hämodialyse. *Chirurgie*, **44**, 274

6 Geroulanos, S., Von Meiss, U., Walter, P., Uhlschmid, G., Turina, T. and Senning, A. (1982). A new vascular prosthesis for small diameter vessel replacement. *Proceedings of the ASAIO Congress*. (In press)

7 Tellis, V. A., Kohlberg, W. I., Bhat, D. J., Driscott, B. and Veith, F. J. (1979). Expanded polytetrafluoroethylene graft fistula for chronic hemodialysis. *Ann. Surg.*, **189**, 101

8 Rosenberg, N., Thompson, J. E., Keshishian, J. M. and VanderWerf, B. A. (1976). The modified bovine arterial graft. *Arch. Surg.*, **111**, 222

9 Merickel, J. H., Andersen, R. C., Knutson, R., Lipschultz, N. L. and Hitchcock, C. R. (1974). Bovine carotid artery shunts in vascular access surgery. *Arch. Surg.*, **109**, 245

10 Katzman, H. E., Schild, A. F. and VanderWerf, B. A. (1976). Bovine artegraft arterio-venous fistula for hemodialysis in one hundred patients after 'conventional' arteriovenous fistulas failed. *Vasc. Surg.*, **10**, 169

11 Knutson, R,. Wathen, R., Comty, Ch. M. and Shapiro, F. L. (1973). Bovine carotid artery grafts as blood access devices. *Proc. Eur. Dial. Transplant Assoc.*, **10**, 299

12 Burbridge, G. E., Biggers, J. A., Remmers, A. R., Lindley, J. D., Sales, H. E. and Fish, J. C. (1976). Late complications and results of bovine xenografts. *Trans. Am. Soc. Artif. Intern. Organs*, **22**, 418

13 Jokojama, T., Bower, R., Chinitz, J., Schwartz, H. and Schwartz, C. (1974). Experience with hundred bovine arterio grafts for maintenance hemodialysis. *Trans. Am. Soc. Artif. Intern. Organs*, **20**, 328

14 Hirschfeld, J., Molzberger, H. and Von Baejer, H. (1976). Neue arteriovenöse Fistel zur extrakorporalen Hämodialyse unter Verwendung eines Rinderarterien-Heterotransplantates. *Chirurgie*, **49**, 127

15 Kaplan, M. S., Mirahmadi, K. S., Wiener, R. L., Gorman, J. T., Dabirvaziri, N. and Rosen, S. M. (1976). Comparison of 'PTFE' and bovine grafts for blood access in dialysis patients. *Trans. Am. Soc. Artif. Intern. Organs*, **22**, 388

16 Haimov, M., Burrows, L., Baez, A,. Neff, M. and Slifkin, R. (1974). Alternatives for vascular access for hemodialysis: experience with autogenous saphenous vein grafts and bovine heterografts. *Surgery*, **74**, 447

19

Experience with the PTFE graft in the construction of vascular access for haemodialysis

M. HAIMOV AND R. SLIFKIN

The peripheral arteriovenous fistula as originally described by Brescia *et al.* is the vascular access of choice for patients on chronic haemodialysis[1]. For the patient with unsuitable peripheral vessels for a standard peripheral arteriovenous (A-V) fistula, A-V communications have been constructed utilizing a variety of vascular substitutes. This report deals with the experience with 225 PTFE grafts (expanded polytetrafluoroethylene) in the construction of vascular access for maintenance haemodialysis.

MATERIALS AND METHODS

Two hundred and twenty-five PTFE grafts were used in the construction of vascular access for haemodialysis. Fifteen of these grafts were of the non-reinforced type and 210 were of the reinforced type; 210 of these grafts were placed in the upper extremity and ten grafts were placed in the lower extremity. The various configurations of the A-V communication have been described in previous publications[2]. All operations were performed using local anaesthesia on an ambulatory basis. In the forearm the grafts were placed between the radial artery and the antecubical vein or between the brachial artery and brachial vein in a 'U'-shaped fistula as described by May *et al.*[3]. In the upper arm grafts are usually placed between the brachial artery and the brachial or axillary vein in a straight fashion. No systemic anticoagulation or antibiotics were administered.

Table 19.1 PTFE grafts for vascular access

Months	Total	Open	Closed	IP*	CP†
0–3	225	216	9	96	96
3–6	215	211	4	98	94
6–9	191	182	9	95	89
9–12	172	164	8	95	84
12–18	151	145	6	96	80
18–24	141	136	5	96	77
24–30	127	121	6	95	73
30–36	101	96	5	95	69
36–48	86	82	4	95	65
48–60	63	59	4	93	60

* Interval patency
† Cumulative patency

Table 19.2 Grafts for vascular access – cumulative patency

Months	PTFE (225)	Autogenous vein (30)	Bovine heterografts (91)
0–3	96	93	95
3–6	94	86	88
6–9	89	76	82
9–12	84	51	76
12–18	80	33	59
18–24	77	20	42
24–30	73	17	30
30–36	69	10	24
36–48	65	6.6	24

RESULTS

The cumulative patency rates for the 225 PTFE grafts are outlined in Table 19.1. The initial patency rate was 96%; 84% at the end of 1 year; 77% at the end of 2 years; 69% at the end of 3 years; 65% at the end of 4 years and 60% at the end of 5 years. Patency rates were calculated according to the life-table method. In Table 19.2 the cumulative patency for the PTFE graft is compared to similarly calculated patency rates for 30 autogenous saphenous vein grafts and 91 bovine heterografts used for similar purposes and similar configurations during an earlier experience. Full details of this experience have been published[4]. The 1-year patency rate for the PTFE graft was 84% compared to 51% for the autogenous vein graft and 76% for the bovine heterograft. The 2-year patency rate for the PTFE was 77% compared to 20% for the autogenous vein graft and 42% for the bovine heterograft. The 4-year patency rate for the PTFE graft was 65% compared to 6.6% for the autogenous vein graft and 24% for the bovine heterograft. The causes for vascular access failure are outlined in Table 19.3. The main causes for failure were thrombosis (14%); aneurysm (1.3%); ischaemia (1.7%); trauma

(2.6%); primary infection (1.7%); secondary infection (4.4%). Again the causes for failure in the bovine heterograft and autogenous vein series are given for comparison. All percentages are calculated as proportions of the total number of grafts.

Table 19.3 Grafts for vascular access – causes for failure (percentages)

Cause	PTFE*	Bovine heterografts	Autogenous vein
Thrombosis	14	23	97
Graft aneurysm	1.3	10.9	—
Ischaemia	1.7	4.3	—
Trauma	2.6	5.4	3
Primary infection	1.7	4.3	—
Secondary infection	4.4	16.4	—

DISCUSSION

Based on the experience described in this report we have concluded that the PTFE graft is a satisfactory vascular prosthesis when used for the construction of a vascular access for haemodialysis. Patency rates with the PTFE graft when used for that purpose were found to be superior to previously used substitutes, i.e. the autogenous saphenous vein and the bovine heterograft, although inferior to the peripheral A-V fistula which remains the access of choice for patients with renal failure requiring access for haemodialysis. The graft should not be used in any patient in whom a satisfactory peripheral A-V fistula could be constructed. Since the patency expectancy of these grafts is limited it should not be used in patients in whom dialysis is not anticipated in the very near future. The main cause for graft failure was thrombosis caused by rising venous resistance secondary to intimal hyperplasia which occurs at the point of graft vein anastomosis. If this lesion is recognized and diagnosed prior to graft failure some of these grafts can be salvaged by intra-luminal dilatation or surgical revision. The intimal hyperplasia lesions need not be confined to the anastomotic site alone, however, since these lesions may develop at a distance from the anastomotic side and if one confines the revision to the anastomosis alone failure will result. Graft aneurysm was a rare complication and occurred only initially in these series when the non-reinforced graft was used. Ischaemia secondary to arterial 'steal' should be a rare complication if the arterial circulation is carefully evaluated prior to surgery and the anastomosis to the arterial end of the graft is done in such a way to preserve distal pulses and avoid excessive steal. Loss of graft to trauma occurring during the course of haemodialysis is another cause of failure which is partially avoidable. Other causes for graft thrombosis as found in these series were technical, when inadequate-size vessels are used for either the outflow or inflow anastomosis of the graft and on occasions by systemic diseases causing periods of hypotension. Different clinical syndromes were recognized when dealing with graft infections. Some patients developed bacteraemia without local signs of graft sepsis. Occasionally these patients will respond to systemic antibiotics and the access would be saved. If no response is evident within 48 h and no other source for the sepsis is identified the graft should be ligated. In a significant number of patients this is all that is needed and no graft removal will be required. If local signs of infection are present the graft will have to be removed. If the infection has not spread to the arterial anastomosis a small portion of the graft can be spared, thus preserving the continuity of the major artery. If, however, the infection has spread to that area, or a false aneurysm is present, arterial ligation will be required. In none of the patients in whom arterial ligation was required was there an immediate threat to the viability of the extremity. In two patients, however, vascular reconstruction was required following complete healing of the infected area because of persistent ischaemic symptoms. When the three vascular substitutes are compared in terms of patency the PTFE graft appears to be superior. The highest rate of complications occurred in the bovine heterograft series where the high incidence of graft aneurysm formation and septic complications accounted for many of the graft losses. The lowest number of complications was encountered using the autogenous saphenous vein, although this type of arterial substitute yielded the lowest patency rate. Both because of its low long-term patency rate and because of the importance of preserving the autogenous vein for possible use in limb or coronary revascularizations, its use for vascular access does not appear to be justified. The experience with the PTFE graft so far has been found to be satisfactory and it remains our vascular substitute of choice for patients requiring graft A-V fistula for maintenance haemodialysis.

References

1 Brescia, M. T., Cimino, J. E. and Appel, K. (1966). Chronic hemodialysis using venipuncture and surgically created arteriovenous fistula. *N. Engl. J. Med.*, **275**, 1089

2 Haimov, M., Burrows, L., Baez, A., Neff, M. and Slifkin, R. (1974). Alternatives for vascular access. Experience with autogenous vein autografts and bovine heterografts. *Surgery*, **75**, 447

3 May, J., Tiller, D., Johnson, J., Stewart, J. and Sheil, A. G. R. (1969). Saphenous vein arteriovenous fistula in regular dialysis treatment. *N. Engl. J. Med.*, **280**, 770

4 Haimov, M., Burrows, L., Schanzer, H., Neff, M., Baez, A., Kwun, K. and Slifkin, R. (1980). Experience with arterial substitutes in the construction of vascular access for hemodialysis. *J. Cardiovasc. Surg.*, **21**, 149

20

Abstracts of posters on Graft material

Ten years experience on 310 homologous vein grafts for arteriovenous fistula
PH. BONNAUD and N. K. MAN

Three hundred and ten homologous vein grafts were inserted in 248 patients on regular dialysis treatment: 213 times with self-prepared vein grafts (SPG) and 97 times with manufactured homologous vein grafts (MVG). Manufactured vein grafts are selected saphenous stripped veins especially prepared and stored at 4 °C in 2% chloramphenicol solution. They are delivered ready for use in one unit-package container (Vascogref TM). Graft location and configuration included 51 loop and 27 straight on forearm, 4 loop and 78 straight on upper-arm for SPG and 18 loop and 11 straight on forearm, 6 loop and 20 straight on upper-arm for MVG. Ninety-five segmental replacements (59 SPG and 36 MVG) included 40 on previous standard A-V fistula, 38 on SPG and 17 on other xenografts. Thrombosis ratio after 1-year follow-up was 30% for SPG and 10% for MVG. Aneurysm occurred eight times over 69 SPG (11%) and twice over 55 MVG (4%). Regular lumen diameter (average outer diameter: 6–7 mm) and regular wall strength are the advantages of the MVG resulting in lower repair ratio: 11% versus 55% for SPG. The saphenous vein is the graft of choice for short segmental replacement for its flexibility. These data indicate clearly that in our experience better results were obtained with the manufactured vein grafts than those with self-prepared vein grafts for A-V fistula creation and/or repair in patients on regular dialysis treatment.

Secondary vascular access surgery for haemodialysis with PTFE (Gore-tex) graft
J. H. M. TORDOIR, J. M. M. P. H. HERMAN, T. S. KWAN,
F. DIDERICH and J. J. JAKIMOWICZ

A retrospective study has been performed to evaluate the value of PTFE

Gore-tex graft as a secondary access method for haemodialysis. During a period of 4 years in two hospitals, 45 Gore-tex grafts were implanted in 40 dialysis patients. Forty-one of the grafts were placed in the lower arm; 32 of the grafts as a loop and nine grafts straight between the radial artery and the cephalic vein. Four of the grafts were placed in the upper leg.

The complications were: late thrombosis in 20 grafts; on 12 occasions a successful thrombectomy was performed; in six of these cases revision of a venous anastomosis was done.

Local infection occurred in one case. In three patients infected grafts were removed. Pseudoaneurysm formation was encountered in three patients. The cumulative patency rate of the Gore-tex grafts for vascular access in our series is 70.9% after 1 year and 61.8% after 3 years. Because of the results we have obtained, the Gore-tex PTFE graft is currently our vascular substitute of choice for patients requiring graft fistula for the maintenance of haemodialysis.

350 modified bovine carotid arteriovenous fistulas
A. MOUTON, F. FOURNIER and P. BOURQUELOT

The first 350 bovine carotid arteriovenous (A-V) fistulas have been reviewed in March 1982. They have been implanted in the upper extremity for chronic haemodialysis (93%) and chemotherapy (7%) between 25 June 1975 and 31 March 1981; 45% of the patients have already been operated on more than five times for previous angioaccess. The follow-up interval is from 1 to 7 years; 70% of the heterografts are implanted in the arm; 30% heterografts are implanted in the forearm, with the help of an operating microscope. This is particularly efficient for the arterial anastomosis between graft and artery at the wrist. Postoperative infection necessitates removal of the graft. Distal ischaemia is frequent but usually transient. One cardiac failure is observed. Secondary stenosis of the venous anastomosis is the most frequent complication. The necessary investigations to detect (angiography, ultrasonic pulsed Doppler) and to treat (surgery, percutaneous transluminal angioplasty) the stenosis are described. Late patency rate is reported: 90% (1 year), 55% (2 years), 19% (5 years). During 1981, 600 angioaccesses were created: 480 direct A-V fistulas, and 120 bovine graft fistulas.

Dardik biograft for arteriovenous fistula
Ø. BENTDAL, G. SØDAL, H. BONDEVIK, A. JAKOBSEN,
P. FAUCHALD and A. FLATMARK

Dardik biograft has been used for graft fistula in 13 haemodialysis patients because standard A-V fistulas have failed. The Dardik biograft was anastomosed to the brachial artery and to the basilic vein above the elbow with a 50 cm loop on the volar aspect of the forearm. Anticoagulant (salicylate 0.5 g daily) was given to all patients for 6 days. Long-term anticoagulation was given only to one patient with a cardiac valve prosthesis. All patients except one received prophylactic antibiotics for 10 days. Four patients developed graft infection; in one of these patients the graft was infected after kidney transplantation. Two of these patients died, and the deaths may be related to infected graft with septicaemia. The graft was removed in the remaining two patients. The infected grafts remained open for 2, 3, 6 and 10 months respectively. Three of the nine uninfected grafts occluded after 1, 2 and 5 months. Successful thrombectomy and later graft replacement was carried out in two patients, while one remained occluded, and access was established with a Thomas shunt. Four of the remaining six uninfected grafts are still used for haemodialysis for a mean period of 8 months, while one graft functioned for 8 months, when the patient died, and one graft functioned for 5 months until renal transplantation. One of the patients developed a pseudoaneurysm next to the 'factory anastomosis' and was successfully operated.

Bovine and Gore-tex grafts for haemodialysis fistulas
R. VAN SCHILFGAARDE, J. H. VAN BOCKEL, I. SCHICHT and
M. R. LILIEN

Bovine (B) and Gore-tex (G) grafts were used for secondary haemodialysis fistulas in the forearm during two consecutive periods of time. Between January 1975 and January 1979 25 patients received 28 B grafts (follow-up 1–239 weeks, mean 129 weeks) and between March 1979 and September 1981 37 patients received 44 G grafts (follow-up 1–125 weeks, mean 39 weeks). Cumulative patency rates at 1 year and 2 years were 85% (24 patients) and 65% (20 patients) for B, and 58% (19 patients) and 58% (7 patients) for G, respectively. This difference was partly caused by graft loss due to primary thrombosis, which occurred in five G grafts (11%) but in only one B graft (3%). When related to the number of fistulas, thrombosis occurred in 50% of the B grafts and in 43% of the G grafts. When related to the number of weeks during which the fistulas were actually at risk, however, thrombosis occurred in 0.4% of B graft-weeks and in 1.3% of G graft-weeks. In B grafts, 64% of all thrombotic complications could be treated successfully; only 21% of these occurred within the first year. For G grafts, these percentages were 47% and 89%, respectively. Relative differences between B and G grafts in success rate of treatment of other complications like infection (0.5% of B-weeks, 0.9% of G-weeks), false aneurysm (0.4% of B-weeks, 0.3% of G-weeks) and lymphocoele (0.03% of B-weeks, 0.3% of G-weeks) were comparable to those in the presence of thrombosis. We conclude that B grafts showed better patency rates than G grafts at 1 and 2 years. If primary failures due to thrombosis were excluded, patency rates appeared to be in the same order of magnitude for B and G grafts. Treatment of complications appeared to yield slightly better results in B as compared to G grafts.

Comparison of bovine artery and human umbilical vein in vascular access
R. A. DONALDSON, M. G. MCGEOWN and J. F. DOUGLAS

With the advent of suitable graft material extended procedures using autogenous vein for vascular access have been used less frequently. In this series, 16 bovine arterial grafts were used in 10 patients and 21 umbilical vein grafts in 18 patients. Both materials could be used for access immediately after implantation and provided for easy insertion of needles. Of the 16 bovine arterial grafts, three thrombosed within 24 h of insertion but two of these were salvaged by thrombectomy, six thrombosed irretrievably within 90 days, five false aneurysms were encountered, one graft could not be used due to extravasation when needled and two required removal due to thrombosis with infection. Of the 21 umbilical vein grafts one clotted irretrievably within the first 24 h, otherwise thrombosis was not encountered in the first 90 days, two were removed due to infection with sinus formation after successful renal transplantation but no aneurysms occurred. Haemostasis after needling is more easily secured with the umbilical vein grafts.

Comparative study with two vascular grafts for haemodialysis
A. GARCIA-ALFAGEME, C. JUANENA, S. FLÓREZ, P. MARTÍNEZ and J. AGOSTI

We have used as secondary vascular access for haemodialysis, a modified human umbilical cord vein graft in 14 patients (group I), and PTFE expanded graft in 12 (group II). Most of these grafts were inserted in the arm, between the brachial artery and the axillary vein in straight configuration. The mean follow-up is 14 months.

Grafts complication were: *group I:* early failure without recovery of the graft (infection and thrombosis) three cases; late failure without recovery of the graft because of pseudoaneurysm and infection two cases; thrombosis with recovery by surgery, six cases; free of complications, four cases (28%). *Group II:* early failure of the graft (infection), one case; late failure (thrombosis), one case; late thrombosis with graft recovery, three cases; free of complications, seven cases (57%).

Even though these series are small, it seems reasonable to think that PTFE is a more convenient alternative as a vascular access for haemodialysis than biografts.

Histological changes of polytetrafluoroethylene (PTFE) arteriovenous (A-V) fistulas for haemodialysis (HD)

D. FERLUGA, J. DRINOVEC, A. VIZJAK, A. HVALA, J. VARL, M. MALOVRH, R. KVEDER, R. PONIKVAR and A. GUČEK

Histological examination of 10 portions of PTFE and (Gore-tex) fistulas from six HD patients has been performed by light microscopy, four portions also by electron and immunofluorescent microscopy. Grafts have been removed 5–47 (mean 31) months after implantation and 1 week to 23 (mean 7) months after thrombosis. Some parts of removed prostheses of five patients were infected.

Time-correlated morphological examination of PTFE grafts has shown slowly developing neointima. It begins with thin fibrin membrane, and a unicellular thin endothelial layer follows after some weeks. More than 6 months afterwards dense collagen appears; its thickness increases with blood flow and fistula survival. Inner parts of PTFE wall are impregnated with plasma proteins and fibrin up to half of the thickness. Neoadventitia is the most prominent tissue reaction in first weeks after implantation. A continuous layer of foreign body multinucleated cells along the outer surface of graft is formed, a zone of round cell infiltration envelops it and soft fibrous tissue is the most peripheral part. Less than a year later foreign body cells and mononuclear infiltrates are disappearing. Only rare fibroblasts are invading the PTFE wall from the outer surface. Some collagen fibres are seen between plastic fibres. The number of fibroblasts and collagen fibres apparently does not increase with fistula survival. Blood capillaries have not been found in PTFE wall except in fibrous plugs in puncture sites. The most prominent lesion of infected PTFE graft fistula has been sequestration of graft, and complete denudation of outer surface. Infected parts are intensively insudated with fibrin. The tube is thickened and impregnated with basophilic debris and bacteria at some portions. On the sites of sutures in PTFE no tissue reaction has been observed.

Secondary access for chronic intermittent dialysis. Bovine graft A-V fistula

H. H. M. REINAERTS, F. G. M. BUSKENS and S. H. SKOTNICKI

Of the alternatives for secondary access surgery we have used the bovine graft fistula since the end of 1974. In April 1977 we analysed our results and decided to continue with this technique. In this paper we present a second series over a period from 1 January 1977 to 31 December 1981. The series consists of 59 patients with end-stage renal disease, 78 graft fistulas have been created, 53 U-shape and 25 straight grafts. In six patients two fistulas were made, in six patients three were made.

Early complications were seen in 16 patients; nine grafts were lost despite revision. This leaves 88% functioning grafts. Late complications were met in 24 patients, 13 of the fistulas were lost. At the time of analysis 18 graft fistulas at risk were functioning; 10 patients are transplanted successfully, 12 have died.

Bovine graft fistulas are a good alternative in secondary access surgery. The percentage functioning grafts, mean patency rate and actuarial survival time are comparable with series from literature on other grafts. In our material the highest incidence of late complications is between 6 and 9 months. Increased pressure in the venous run-off during dialysis should be considered as the first sign of venous obstruction, which then should be established by shuntography.

The bovine heterograft as dialysis shunt
R. SCHMIDT, S. HORSCH, H. ERASMI and H. PICHLMAIER

At the University Hospital of Cologne between 1974 and 1981 121 bovine heterografts were implanted into 78 patients. Sixty-five grafts were placed as loops, 56 as straight shunts. Shunt thrombosis was the most frequent late complication (67.6%), followed by graft infection (15.3%). Nine of 11 aneurysms observed were due to faulty puncture technique. The cumulative patency rate after 1 year was 59%, and after 2 years 43%, corrective interventions included.

Thrombectomy restored the patency of 80% of the occluded grafts.

Thus, next to the easy and safe puncture, the good response to thrombectomy is one of the advantages of the bovine heterograft.

Access to haemodialysis: comparative evaluation of different grafts
E. DI SALVO, E. MANZO, F. SALZANO DE LUNA, G. NAPPI and M. L. SANTANGELO

Since 1975 in 102 uraemic patients, 130 arteriovenous graft fistulas of the upper limbs have been constructed by interposition of prosthetic materials.

We have used homologous vein graft in 50 cases, autologous vein in three; PTFE in 59; Microvel® in 11; Dardik® in five; and bovine carotid in two placed in a straight line or in a loop-form (70 and 60, respectively). The average age was 35 years (range 12–73). All the patients underwent haemodialysis 3 days weekly with two one-way needles.

The maximum graft survival was 46 months, the average was 14 months for vein, 9 for PTFE and 8.5 for Microvel®.

The complications (early and late thrombosis, infection and aneurysm) occurred in 20% of cases for vein, 35.5% for PTFE and 45.4% for Microvel®.

Our results strongly support a better outcome for vein grafts with a lower rate of complications.

21

Invited comment on papers and posters in Graft material

R. W. G. JOHNSON

Whilst there has always been a general consensus among surgeons that primary access is best affected by internal arteriovenous (A-V) anastomosis at the wrist, there has never been complete agreement about what to do when primary access fails. The choice lies between more proximal direct A-V anastomosis and the use of free grafts which act as conduits which are easy to needle.

Considerable ingenuity has been shown in developing methods to achieve secondary access; as a result two main methods and three types of material have emerged as the principal lines of treatment. Free grafts are either straight or looped, and they are made of autologous or homologous vein, bovine carotid artery or expanded polytetrafluoroethylene (PTFE).

Everyone would like to know which is the best method and what is the material of choice.

On the evidence presented there are three factors that prevent objective comparisons being made; firstly, no group has provided a synchronously conducted prospective randomized trial of the methods or material available.

Secondly, the circumstances under which different authors have used the materials have varied so widely that objective comparison is impossible. In some instances a free graft has been used immediately after failure of the first direct access procedure, whilst other groups have attempted multiple direct access procedures before resorting to a free graft. Thirdly, different methods of assessment have been used ranging from simple percentage patency with time, through estimation of graft life in months to measurement of 'dialysis months'. The latter is the most objective assessment since it indicates patency, use and usability.

Since objective comparison has been ruled out it has been necessary to pool all the information relating to the materials described in order to make some assessment of the consistency of results achieved with the same material from centre to centre. Each material has been assessed for patency, complications and incidence of salvage procedures. Where possible these results have been compared with published results for Cimino–Brescia A-V fistula.

HOMOLOGOUS SAPHENOUS VEIN

This material obtained from stripped varicosities has been extensively used (Table 21.1). Bonnaud and Man in a large personal series obtained excellent results using homologous vein but demonstrated a significant advantage for the commercially prepared vein (Vascogref®). They reported a rather high incidence of true aneurysm which presumably is a reflection of weaknesses in the wall of the varicosities. Nonetheless the patency rate reported is supported by papers from Di Salvo *et al.* and a multicentre study by Berardinelli *et al.* No-one appeared to experience rejection phenomena even when the vein was used fresh, and certainly the material was easy to handle, easy to needle and inexpensive.

Table 21.1 Homologous vein grafts

	Material	*No.*	*Patency* (%)			*Salvage* (%)	*Average function*
			1 year	*2 years*	*3 years*		
Bonnaud and	Saphenous vein	213	70	—	—	55%	>1 year
Man		97	90	—	—	11%	>1 year
Di Salvo *et al.*	Saphenous vein	50	80	—	—	—	14 months
Berardinelli *et al.*	Saphenous vein	190	—	—	—	—	13 months
Donaldson *et al.*	Human umbilical vein	21	90	—	—	—	>90 days
Garcia-Alfageme *et al.*	Human umbilical vein	14	65	—	—	42%	—
Bentdal *et al.*	Human umbilical vein	13	47	—	—	25%	>6 months

BOVINE CAROTID GRAFTS

These have now been extensively used for many years. Experience of almost 700 procedures has been reported here (Table 21.2). Results are again variable reflecting the incidence of high-risk cases (Schmidt *et al.* and Donaldson *et al.*). The largest single series from Mouton *et al.* showed a patency rate of 90% at 1 year followed by accelerated graft loss over the next 2 years. Van Schilfgaarde *et al.* and Reinaerts *et al.* had similar experience with smaller numbers. Decurtins *et al.* had 62% patency at 1 year – using bovine carotid as a last resort!

Table 21.2 Bovine carotid grafts

	No.	*Patency (%)*			*Salvage (%)*	*Average function*
		1 year	*2 years*	*3 years*		
Van Schilfgaarde *et al.*	28	85	65	—	3	>1 year
Mouton *et al.*	350	90	55	19	?	>1 year
Reinaerts *et al.*	78	88	75	—	20	>1 year
Decurtins *et al.*	100	62	—	—	?	>1 year
Schmidt *et al.*	121	59	43	—	68	>1 year
Donaldson *et al.*	16	56	—	—	19	>90 days

HOMOLOGOUS HUMAN UMBILICAL VEIN

Experience with this material was limited and rather variable (Table 21.1). This clearly reflects the desperate nature of many of the situations in which the graft was used (Bentdal *et al.*). Excellent results can be obtained with this material (Donaldson *et al.*) when it is used under ideal circumstances, but it is very expensive, and also rather difficult to handle because of the disparity in thickness between the umbilical vein and the forearm veins. The need for thrombectomy ranged from 25 to 42%; this was well tolerated and most often resulted in significant extension of graft life. The incidence of thrombosis was significantly reduced by giving salicylates (Bentdal *et al.*).

The complications attributable to bovine carotid are usually aneurysm formation, thrombosis, and graft infection. In this series most of the aneurysms reported were false aneurysms unrelated to the graft material. Early thrombosis was usually easily corrected by thrombectomy, but late thrombosis is still a problem occurring between 1 and 3 years. Graft infection has been no more frequent than with any of the other materials.

EXPANDED PTFE

This material is of particular interest since it is the only synthetic material in widespread use for vascular access. The results reported (Table 21.3) have been consistently good. Haimov and Slifkin presented the largest personal

Table 21.3 PTFE grafts

	No.	*Patency (%)*			*Salvage (%)*	*Average function*
		1 year	*2 years*	*3 years*		
Haimov and Slifkin	225	86	76	73	—	>1 year
Tordoir *et al.*	45	70	—	62	44	>1 year
Garcia-Alfageme *et al.*	12	84	—	—	25	?
Van Schilfgaarde *et al.*	44	58	58	—	—	—

series using on occasion some very ingenious sites for access such as a loop based on subclavian artery and subclavian vein – needled on the chest wall. Their patency rates of 86%, 76% and 73% at 1, 2 and 3 years respectively are commendable and are supported in the series presented by Tordoir *et al.* and Garcia-Alfageme *et al.* Only van Schilfgaarde *et al.* reported a rather high early failure rate and they attributed this to technical failures.

The commonest problems associated with PTFE are early thrombosis (44%) (easily corrected by thrombectomy), oedema, skin reaction including ulceration and false aneurysm from poor needling technique.

In summary all three materials presented here can be used effectively and safely as free grafts for secondary access. The rate of early thrombosis, 20–80%, is much higher than with Cimino–Brescia but is also much more easily salvaged by thrombectomy. The result in 1-year patency rates for each material is over 70%, but of course the results do reflect the secondary nature of the access procedure. Long-term graft survival is much worse than with Cimino–Brescia and this must in part reflect the reduced number of needling sites and the higher incidence of false aneurysm.

Most of the complications reported are not criticisms of the material used but rather indications of poor needling technique.

Section V
Haemodynamic sequelae of arteriovenous fistulas

22

Haemodynamics of arteriovenous fistulas

B. A. VANDERWERF, T. WILLIAMS AND L. J. KOEP

When graft arteriovenous (A-V) fistulas are placed for haemodialysis access, assuming that unrestricted venous outflow exists, flow through the A-V fistula doubles in 6 months. The flow through the A-V fistula can go as high as 3000–4000 cc/min.

This chapter describes how this relatively excessive A-V fistula flow is related to the typical complications of A-V fistulas, i.e., thrombosis, infected haematomas, arterial steal, aneurysms, venous hypertension ischaemia and cardiac failure.

THROMBOSIS

Previously, we found that there are two kinds of thrombosis occurring following placement of graft A-V fistulas for haemo-access[2]. If the flow at the time of graft placement is less or equal to 300 cc/min, most patients will thrombose their graft shortly after surgery. This is often related to poor technical aspects of the fistula. When the flow at the time of insertion is 350–800 cc/min, most grafts remained patent for a long time. When, at the time of insertion, the flow is greater than, or equal to 900 cc/min, there is also a high incidence of late thrombosis. Thrombosis secondary to high flow occurs usually 6–12 months after insertion and is often caused by intimal hyperplasia of the outflow veins.

In an attempt to reduce the incidence of thrombosis, the most frequent complication of graft A-V fistulas, we restricted the flow through the graft A-V fistula by creating a narrowing close to the arterial anastomosis. Follow-up flow studies, done at 1 and 6 weeks, and at 6 and 12 months, revealed that the flow through bovine graft fistulas remained the same as it was (600–1000 cc/min) reduced to at the time of surgery. Subsequently, patients who had a bovine graft placed with a controlled narrowing created at the time

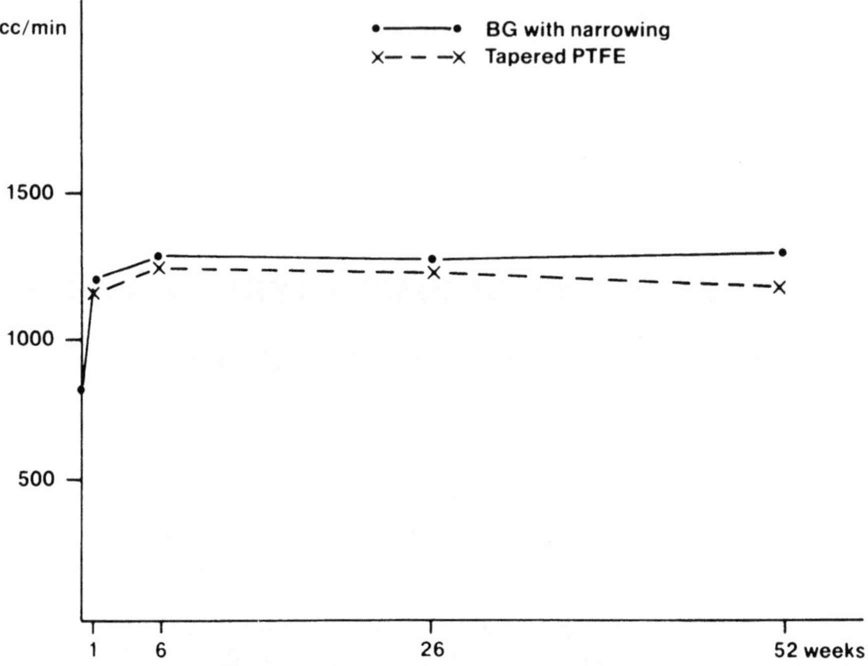

Figure 22.1 Haemodynamics of arteriovenous fistulas

of surgery, using an electromagnetic flowmeter, were compared in a random-ized study with patients who had a Gore-tex graft placed with a standard tapering from 4 to 7 mm close to the arterial anastomosis.

Figure 22.1 shows that the flow studies of these two groups are exactly the same up to 12 months. Although only 10 patients were followed out in each group through 12 months, we did find a reduction of thrombotic incidents. Both bovine and Gore-tex grafts had a thrombotic incidence of once every 40 months of dialysis. This compares favourably with a thrombotic incidence of once every 21 months of dialysis for graft A-V fistulas with unrestricted flow. Follow-up flow studies were done with a technetium dilution technique[3].

INFECTED HAEMATOMAS

Excessive flow A-V fistulas will eventually lead to increased pressure in the graft because intimal hyperplasia narrows the outflow veins. When dialysis needles are removed from high-pressure A-V fistulas there is an increased chance for haematomas, and subsequently more infected haematomas. We believe that the incidence of infected haematomas can be reduced by limiting the flow of graft A-V fistulas.

We have an aggressive policy revising infected grafts. From previous studies[4] we have found that in most cases a successful bovine bypass graft around the area of infection can be performed, making the same access available for immediate and continuing use.

ANEURYSMS

If haematomas do not get infected, they may lead to false aneurysms of graft A-V fistulas. The incidence of aneurysms should be reduced by restricting the flow and pressure of graft A-V fistulas.

ARTERIAL STEAL

Graft A-V fistulas seldom cause arterial steal despite poor circulation in extremities where these grafts are placed. When this occurs it can be related to excessive flow stolen away from the distal part of the extremity. When arterial steal occurs there are several options to cure this. When excessive flow can be reduced significantly, sufficient blood flow to the extremity can be restored. If the A-V fistula flow is not excessive and still causes arterial steal, the fistula may have to be sacrificed to save the extremity. On one such occasion we were able to salvage the fistula and the extremity by converting the graft fistula into an arterial–arterial bypass. CAPD should be considered if new A-V fistulas are too risky for other extremities.

VENOUS HYPERTENSION ISCHAEMIA

Ischaemia distal to an arteriovenous fistula is much more commonly caused by venous hypertension than by arterial steal. If excessive flow causes venous hypertension it is not possible for blood to flow freely through the capillary bed of the distal part of the extremity, and stasis occurs. This causes swelling of the distal part of the extremity and further ischaemic changes. If not properly taken care of, this can eventually lead to loss of the extremity. Angiography will show the extent of the problem and show possibilities for correction. Excessive flow A-V fistulas can cause fibrosis of the outflow veins and sometimes lead to venous hypertension ischaemia.

CARDIAC FAILURE

Excessive fistula flow can cause cardiac failure. When graft fistulas are placed in patients with 'normal' cardiac function, the cardiac output increase is in excess of the flow diverted through the graft fistula (Table 22.1). A combination of different factors, i.e. increased heart rate, decreased afterload and increased preload, is probably responsible for this extra increase of the cardiac output.

When patients present with cardiac failure after their graft fistula placement, there is a relatively simple way to evaluate whether the failure is related to excessive fistula flow. We can measure the cardiac output with the graft open and closed, and if the flow in the fistula is greater than the difference in cardiac output with the graft open and closed, there is direct correlation. Table 22.2 shows an example of such a patient. A frequent mistake is assuming that the flow in the fistula is the same as the difference of the cardiac output with the fistula open and closed.

Table 22.1 Arteriovenous fistulas – effect on cardiac output (CO): Normal cardiac function

	cc/min
CO before fistula	6000
CO after fistula	8500
CO increase	2500
Fistula flow	1500
CO increase more than fistula flow	1000

Table 22.2 Arteriovenous fistulas – effect on cardiac output (CO): Cardiac failure

	cc/min
CO before fistula	4000
CO after fistula	4800
CO increase	800
Fistula flow	2800
CO increase less than fistula flow	2000

In conclusion, we feel that most of the typical complications, i.e. thrombosis, infected haematomas, aneurysms, arterial steal, venous hypertension ischaemia, and cardiac failure are directly related to relatively excessive A-V fistula flows. The flow in the A-V fistula will increase tremendously if not restricted. It is relatively easy to restrict the flow by banding a bovine graft fistula during surgery. With synthetic materials we recommend the use of a graft with a built-in taper, because the electromagnetic flowmeter does not register flow until tissue ingrowth has taken place. A 7 mm diameter graft is easy for needle placement, and if there is a narrowing to 4 mm at the arterial end of the graft the flow will be limited sufficiently.

References

1 VanderWerf, B. A., Kumar, S. S., Pennell, P. and Gottlieb, S. (1978). Cardiac failure from bovine graft arteriovenous fistulas: diagnosis and management. *Am. Soc. Artif. Intern. Organs*, **24**, 474
2 VanderWerf, B. A., Kumar, S. S., Rattazzi, L. C., Perez, G., Katzman, H. E. and Schild, A. F. (1976). Long-term follow-up of bovine graft arteriovenous fistulas. *Proc. Dial. Transplant. Forum*, **6**, 85
3 Gottlieb, S., Garcia, E., Cold, S. B. and VanderWerf, B. A. (1976). Radiotracer method for nonsurgical measurement of blood flow in bovine graft arteriovenous fistulas. *Proc. Dial. Transplant. Forum*, **6**, 107
4 Kumar, S. S., Rattazzi, L. C. and VanderWerf, B. A. (1975). A new treatment of infected bovine graft arteriovenous fistulas. *Proc. Dial. Transplant. Forum.*, **5**, 89

23

Non-invasive Doppler blood flow measurement in the vascular access of haemodialysis patients

B. I. LEVY, J. C. PONSIN, P. BOURQUELOT, E. AMAR AND
J. P. MARTINEAUD

INTRODUCTION

Arteriovenous (A-V) fistulas in haemodialysis patients may result in local and systemic alterations in circulatory haemodynamics. During the last 10 years it has become apparent that patients maintained on chronic haemodialysis programmes died of cardiovascular disease with an incidence greatly in excess of the control group[1]. The chronically increased cardiac work certainly must play a major role in the development of cardiac failure in these patients[2-4]. Most previous descriptions of altered vascular dynamics in A-V fistulas have involved invasive methods to access regional alterations in pressure[5,6] or in blood flow[7,8]. Plethysmography[3], and more recently Doppler ultrasound[9], were used as non-invasive methods to measure A-V fistula blood flow. In fact, plethysmographic results expressed as cm^3/min for each $100\ cm^3$ of tissue are very difficult to measure and interpret in a limb with A-V fistula. Furthermore, we have shown in a previous paper that plethysmographic methods have a poor accuracy in blood flow measurement of the upper limb[10,11]. Previously reported results, obtained using continuous wave Doppler methods, did not give the blood flow rate (cm^3/s) but the blood flow velocity (cm/s). Range gated Doppler velocimetry was undertaken to quantify blood flow rate through the A-V fistula in patients undergoing maintenance hemodialysis.

METHODS

Doppler flowmetry is based on the frequency change ΔF of the emitted wave after its backscattering by moving erythrocytes. ΔF is a function of the emission frequency (F), of the velocity of the red cells (V), and the angle (α) formed by the ultrasonic beam and the direction of the blood displacement. $\Delta F/F = (2V/C)\cos\alpha$ where C is the mean propagation velocity of ultrasounds within tissues (1540 m/s). The method was introduced by Satomura[12] and Franklin[13], who used a continuous emission apparatus with one transmitting and one receiving ultrasonic transducer. In addition to the classical Doppler method, the used apparatus (Echovar Doppler Pulse Alvar R) presents the following characteristics: (i) an adjustable range gated time system; and (ii) a double transducer probe which provides a bidimensional blood velocity measurement and considerably minimizes the error induced by the angle between the ultrasonic beam and the vessel axis[14,15]. A single transducer is alternatively emitter and receiver (Figure 23.1). The ultrasound frequency used is 8 mHz, with emission duration of 0.5 μs pulsed at a repetition frequency of 15 kHz. Between the emitted pulses the transducer operates as a receiver. An electronic gate is adjusted between the pulses, T3 is the time delay, T2 the gate duration. T3 and T2 can be selected in order to analyse the

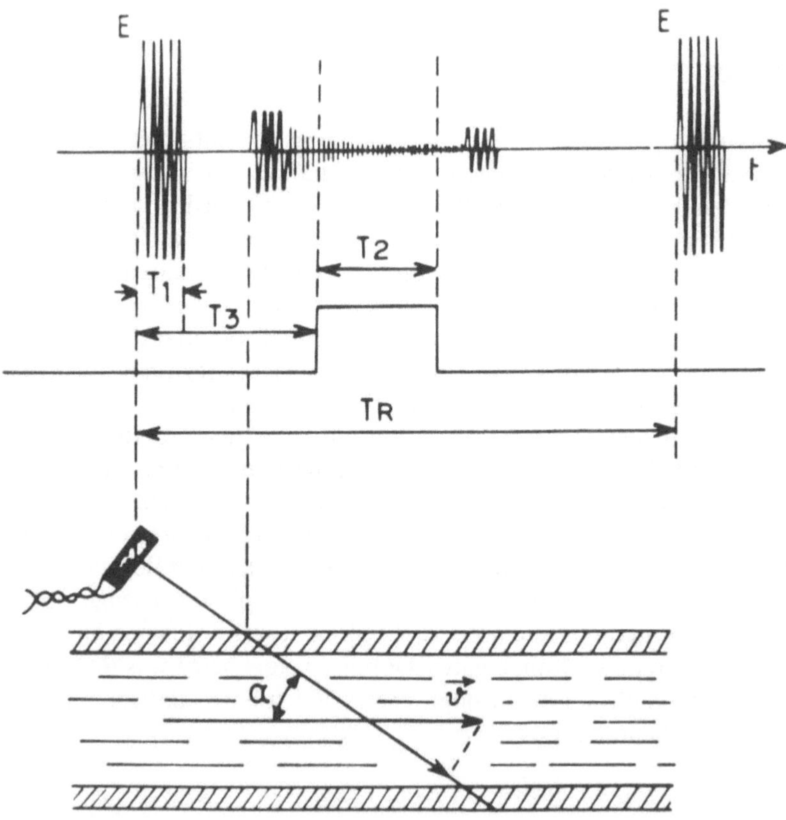

Figure 23.1 Principle of the range gated ultrasonic Doppler flowmeter[14]

Doppler signal in a precisely definite sample volume, at a definite distance from the transducer. With such a system, it is possible to calculate the distance (d) between the red cells and the transducer according to the echocardiographic relation: $d = t \times C/2$. The difference between the measured distances from the transducer to the proximal and to the distal vessel walls is the diameter, D, of the vessel. The time delay T3 and the duration reception T2 represent respectively the deepness and the thickness of the sample volume along the beam axis. The probe includes a double transducer system[16] forming a fixed angle (Figure 23.2). The probe is designed so that the intersection of the beams is located around the distance where the maximal accuracy is needed (5–15 mm). The two transducers were successively activated. A simple calculation then provides the longitudinal velocity within the plane defined by the ultrasonic beam and the vessel axis. From the average velocity of the erythrocytes (V), flow rate can be calculated: $Q = V\pi D^2/4$.

PATIENTS

Two hundred and forty adults (45 ± 13 years), 128 females and 112 males, were studied 0.1 to 14 years (mean: 3.1 ± 2.4) after the A-V fistula was created. The patients were supine, with the hand at the level of the heart, 10 min before the A-V fistula blood flow measurement. Heart rate and arterial blood pressure remained stable during each procedure. We

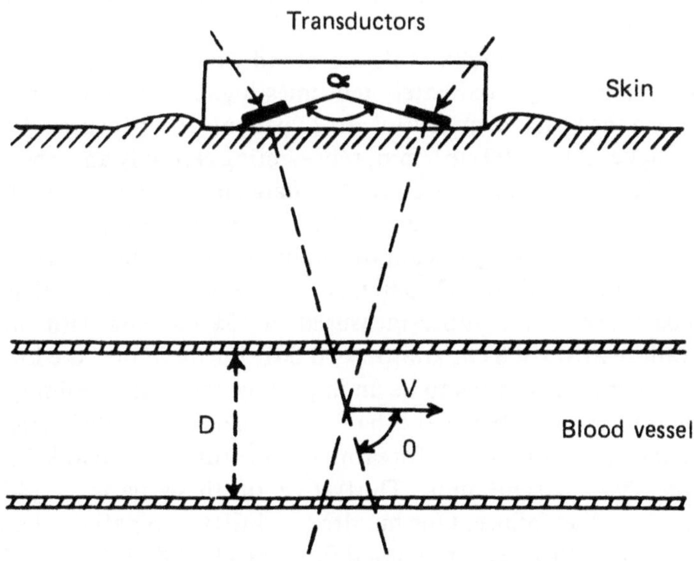

Figure 23.2 Double transductor blood velocity probe

performed an A-V fistula blood flow measurement on 146 patients for systematic investigation, 82 patients for an aetiological investigation of cardiac failure and 12 patients for dialysis difficulties related to low output. Cardiac failure was defined when there were clinical, electrocardiographic, cardiothoracic ratio and echographic evidences. Modified carotid bovine grafts were used in 46 cases, venous grafts were used in 26 patients, 14 heterografts and 12 homografts; 168 patients had standard A-V fistulas. Patients were classified according to the topographic localization of the A-V fistula: 80 patients had a proximal A-V fistula localized in the arm or in the upper third of the forearm, 160 had distal A-V fistula in the forearm or at the wrist level.

Means and standard deviations were calculated according to standard statistical methods; differences in means were assessed by the Student's t test.

RESULTS AND DISCUSSION

Cardiac output can be increased by three major factors in the haemodialysis patients. The first is a decreased total systemic resistance, induced by the A-V fistula, which results in an increased heart rate and stroke volume. The second is a decrease in oxygen transport due to anaemia (mean haematocrit in our patients: $21 \pm 9\%$). The third stimulus to cardiac output is an increased filling of the ventricle (preload increase). All three of these factors may play a role in determining cardiac work and then cardiac failure in the haemodialysis patient. Capelli and Kasparian[2], Drueke et al.[17], and other authors have shown that cardiac index, stroke index and left ventricular work index were generally in the high normal or elevated range in patients receiving haemodialysis.

In our 240 patients, the A-V fistula blood flow was 640 ± 410 cm^3/min. This mean value is approximately ten times higher than the normal blood flow value in the brachial artery[11,18]. In 27 patients the measured AVF blood flow was higher than 2000 cm^3/min, representing certainly an important part of the cardiac output. There are very few data concerning A-V fistula blood flow measurement; our results are in the same range with those reported by Hurwich[3]. There was a significant difference between the A-V fistula blood flow value measured in 82 patients with evidence of cardiac failure (930 ± 460 cm^3/min) and those measured in 158 patients with no sign of cardiac failure (610 ± 308 cm^3/min), $p < 0.001$. Furthermore, the localization of the vascular access seems to be an important factor determining the A-V fistula blood flow. Eighty patients had a proximal A-V fistula localized in the arm or in the upper third of the forearm; the measured A-V fistula blood flow value was 890 ± 320 cm^3/min. Thirty-five of these patients (44%) had evidence of cardiac failure. One hundred and fifty-two patients had a distal vascular access with a measured blood flow of 644 ± 290 cm^3/min; 47 of them (31%) suffered from cardiac failure. A simple electric analogue model

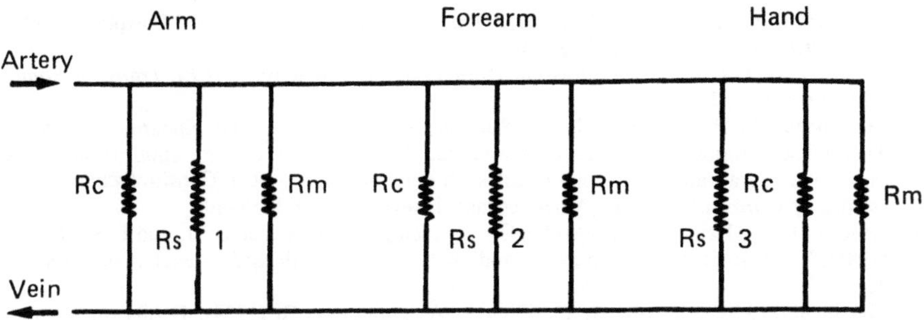

Figure 23.3 Electric analogue model of the upper limb circulation. Rc = cutaneous resistance; Rm = muscular resistance; Rs = arteriovenous fistula (shunt) resistance

(Figure 23.3) can be helpful in understanding these results. Using this model, it is easily demonstrated that the same A-V fistula, with the same diameter, decreases the equivalent resistance of the arm, all the more as the A-V fistula is proximal.

This work demonstrates the incidence of haemodynamic conditions of the A-V fistula; the higher the A-V fistula blood flow rate, the greater is the probability of cardiac failure. Furthermore, this risk increases with time. Range gated Doppler blood flowmetry provides a simple non-invasive and accurate method to monitor the A-V fistula blood flow. Consequently, this important risk factor should be assessed periodically.

References

1 Scharf, S., Wexler, J., Longnecker, R. E. and Blaufox, M. D. (1980). Cardiovascular disease in patients on chronic hemodialysis therapy. *Prog. Cardiovasc. Dis.*, **12**, 343

2 Capelli, J. P. and Kasparian, H. (1977). Cardiac work demands and left ventricular function in end stage renal disease. *Ann. Intern. Med.*, **86**, 261

3 Hurwich, B. J. (1969). Plethysmographic forearm blood flow studies in maintenance hemodialysis patients with radial arteriovenous fistulae. *Nephron*, **6**, 673

4 VanderWerf, B. A., Kumar, S. S. and Pennell, P. (1978). Cardiac failure from bovine graft arteriovenous fistulae, diagnosis and management. *Trans. Am. Soc. Artif. Organs*, **23**, 474

5 Holman, E. and Taylor, G. (1952). Problems in the dynamics of blood flow. Pressure relations at the site of an arteriovenous fistula. *Angiology*, **3**, 415

6 Ingelbrigtsen, R. and Husom, O. (1959). Local blood pressure in congenital arteriovenous fistulae. *Acta Med. Scand.*, **163**, 169

7 Schenk, W. G. Jr, Martin, J. W. and Leslie, M. B. (1960). The regional hemodynamics of chronic experimental arteriovenous fistulas. *Surg. Gynecol. Obstet.*, **110**, 44

8 Anderson, C. B., Etheredge, E. E., Harter, H. R. (1977). Local blood flow characteristics of arteriovenous fistula in the forearm for dialysis. *Surg. Gynecol. Obstet.*, **144**, 531

9 Barnes, R. W. (1978). Non-invasive assessment of arteriovenous fistula. *Angiology*, **29**, 691

10 Levy, B. I., Valladares, W. R., Ghaem, A. and Martineaud, J. P. (1979). Comparison of plethysmographic methods with pulsed Doppler blood flowmetry. *Am. J. Physiol.*, **236**, H899

11 Levy, B. I., Oliva, Y. and Martineaud, J. P. (1981). Hand arterial blood flow responses to local venous congestion. *Am. J. Physiol.*, **240**, H980

12 Satomura, S. (1959). A study of the flow patterns in superficial arteries by ultrasonics. *J. Acoust. Soc. Jpn*, **15**, 151

13 Franklin, D. L., Schlegel, W. and Rushmer, R. F. (1961). Blood flow measured by Doppler frequency shift of backscattered ultrasound. *Science*, **134**, 564

14 Peronneau, P. P. and Leger, F. (1969). Doppler ultrasonic pulsed blood flowmeter. *Proc. 8th Intern. Conf. Med. Biol. Eng.*, **10**

15 Baker, D. W. (1970). Pulsed ultrasonic Doppler blood flow sensing. *IEEE Trans. on Sonics and Ultrasonics*, **3**, 170

16 Peronneau, P. P., Bournat, J. P., Bugnon, A., Barbet, A. and Xhaard, M. (1974). Theoretical and practical aspects of pulsed Doppler flowmetry real time applications to the measure of instantaneous velocity profiles. In Reneman, R. S. (ed.). *Cardiovascular Applications of Ultrasound*, **1**, 66. (Amersterdam: Elsevier–North Holland)

17 Drueke, T., Le Pailleur, C., Sigal Saglier, M., Zingraff, J., Crosnier, J. and DiMatteo, J. (1981). Left ventricular function in hemodialyzed patients with cardiomegaly. *Nephron*, **28**, 80

18 Martineaud, J. P., Ponsin, J. C., Ghaem, A. and Levy, B. (1979). Débits du membre superieur dans differentes circonstances physiologiques. *Hemodynamics of the Limbs*, **1**, 413

24

Haemodynamic consequences of arteriovenous fistulas for dialysis: a prospective study

J. GERSTOFT, J. MORTENSEN, N. B. MOGENSEN AND
A. UHRENHOLDT

INTRODUCTION

Dialysis fistulas have been incriminated in the increased cardiac morbidity in patients on chronic dialysis. The reason for this is the haemodynamic changes observed in animal studies[1] and the observation of high-output cardiac insufficiency in patients with traumatic A-V fistulas[2]. For both observations it is important to know that the A-V fistulas were created between larger vessels than the ones normally used for dialysis fistulas.

In dialysis literature there have been a number of casuistic reports of cardiac insufficiency which disappeared after reduction of fistula flow[3-5]; but in dialysis patients the distinction between overload and cardiac failure is difficult to make. High cardiac output has been observed in patients with A-V fistulas but there are a number of other factors that might contribute to this; i.e. anaemia and overhydration. Reduction in cardiac output after fistula occlusion does not in itself prove a causal relationship between heart failure and fistula flow. It thus seemed to us that the haemodynamic consequences of A-V fistula needed further investigation. To avoid the bias of inhomogeneous groups we decided to investigate the differences in the individual patient model before, and 6 months after, the creation of an A-V fistula.

MATERIAL

Fifteen consecutive patients with slowly progressing chronic uraemia accepted for haemodialysis entered this study. Patients with systemic diseases that might affect cardiac function (diabetes mellitus, collagen diseases, amyloidosis, etc.) were excluded. Three patients dropped out; two because they died a non-cardiac death before the time of follow-up; one because of a severe episode of septicaemia at the time of follow-up.

Of the remaining 12 patients who had entered regular haemodialysis 6 months after the creation of the fistula, two were still on conservative treatment, because the progression of the uraemia had been slow. The medication, which in some patients included cardioactive drugs, was continued unchanged during the observation period.

INVESTIGATIONS

The investigations included the following procedures which were done 2 days before the creation of the fistula and repeated after 6 months.

Physical examination was done by two of the authors. The further decrease in renal function was determined by Cr–EDTA clearance. The maximal working capacity was estimated during exercise cardiography. Echocardiography was done in order to detect pericardial effusion which if found resulted in exclusion from the study. The plasma volume was measured by using radioactive-labelled albumin, and the haematocrit was recorded simultaneously and used for estimation of blood volume.

Right-hand heart catheterization included measurement of pulmonary wedge pressure. During the catheterization exercise was performed, and in the follow-up investigation recordings were made with the fistula open and with the fistula closed, using a blood pressure cuff. Fick's method was used for determination of cardiac output.

The heart volume was measured on chest X-ray under standardized conditions.

RESULTS

No patients had signs of heart failure on the physical examination at entrance or after fistula creation. Echocardiography did not show any pericardial effusion and there had not been any episode with clinical pericarditis. The patients on haemodialysis tolerated the treatment well without episodes of hypotension. Severe hypertension did not occur in any patient and generally there were no problems with overloading.

The results of the investigations are shown in Tables 24.1 and 24.2. The pre- and postfistula results were compared using the Wilcoxon test. Only the increase in blood volume turned out to be significant ($p < 0.001$).

Figure 24.1 shows the correlation between blood volume increase and the fistula flow (measured as cardiac output with a fistula occlusion subtracted

HAEMODYNAMIC CONSEQUENCES OF DIALYSIS FISTULAS

Table 24.1 Status of 12 patients with chronic uraemia 2 days before, and 6 months after, A-V fistula creation

	Before		After	
	$\bar{x}$	SD	$\bar{x}$	SD
Weight (kg)	66	10	67	8
Heart size (ml^3/m^2)	525	164	588	143
Cr–EDTA a clearance (ml/min)	11.1	4.8	7.9	3.6
Working capacity (W)	78	36	82	30
Blood volume (l)	4.3	0.8	5.3*	0.9
Arterial P_0 (mean) (mmHg)	106	8	100	11
β-haemoglobin (mmol/l)	6.1	1.0	6.3	1.1
Haematocrit	28	5	31	6

*$p < 0.001$

Table 24.2 Haemodynamic investigation in 12 patients with chronic uraemia 2 days before, and 6 months after, fistula creation

	Before fistula		6 months after fistula creation		
	Rest	Work	Rest	Work	Fistula occl.
Cardiac output (l/min)	5.9 ± 2.2	9.5 ± 3.5	6.2 ± 2.4	9.9 ± 3.5	5.4 ± 2.4
Heart rate (min^{-1})	75 ± 18	104 ± 15	68 ± 11	96 ± 15	65 ± 10
Stroke volume index (l/m^2)	51 ± 17	51 ± 17	51 ± 15	57 ± 12	46 ± 14
Pulmonary wedge pressure (mmHg)	8 ± 6	22 ± 9	10 ± 5	22 ± 4	13 ± 11
Right atrial pressure (mmHg)	3 ± 2	8 ± 3	4 ± 3	8 ± 2	4 ± 3

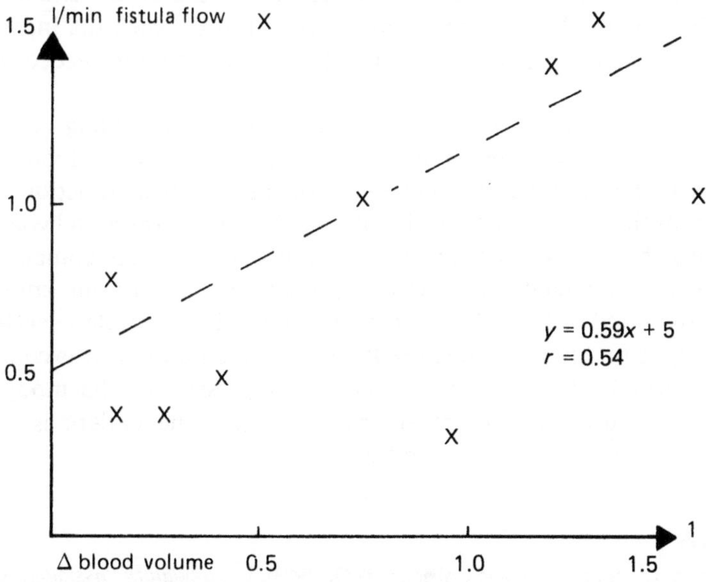

Figure 24.1 Correlation between blood volume increase after A-V fistula creation and fistula flow measure as change in cardiac output after fistula

the cardiac output without fistula occlusion). As can be seen from the figure there are tendencies for a positive correlation, but this appeared to be non-significant using the Spearman test $(0.1 > p > 0.05)$.

DISCUSSION

Between the two points of observation the creation of the A-V fistula was not the only thing that happened to these patients. At least two other things have happened: first most patients have entered dialysis, and second the renal function has deteriorated further. This implies that the results must be viewed as net products of factors that might be working in different directions.

As only two patients stayed out of haemodialysis this study does not tell anything about the isolated effect of haemodialysis on the parameters investigated, as the numbers are too small.

The fact that we did not detect any heart failure or change in pressure in the different parts of the circulation (including the heart) suggests that the haemodynamic status of the patients did not suffer from the A-V fistula. This is in accordance with the unchanged working capacity.

The fistula flow is in accordance with other reports[6]. Our method of measuring the fistula flow is probably not the best, as fistula occlusion itself and pain from the ischaemic arm probably puts a lot of reflexes into work affecting the cardiovascular system, including the cardiac output. The procedure chosen was, however, the only one available to us at the time of investigation. It is possible that the inaccurate measure of the fistula flow is responsible for the lack of significant correlation between the increase in blood volume and the fistula flow. Further investigation is needed on this matter.

The blood volume increase was to be expected according to animal studies[1], but to our knowledge this study is the first showing blood volume increase after fistula creation in patients with impaired renal function. This is important as the kidneys might be involved in increasing the blood volume. It thus seems that the kidneys are of less importance in this compensatory mechanism. Haemodialysis increases haemoglobin[7] but to our knowledge increase in blood volume has not been reported. The isolated effect of haemodialysis on blood volume needs further investigation. It is concluded that the normal sized A-V fistula does not represent any haemodynamic hazard to the uraemic patient entering dialysis. The patient is able to compensate by increasing the blood volume.

References

1 Guyton, A. C., Jones, C. E. and Coleman, T. G. (1973). In *Circulatory Physiology: Cardiac Ouput and its Regulation*, pp. 412–36. (Philadelphia: W. B. Saunders)
2 Pate, J. W., Sherman, R. T., Jackson, T. and Wilson, H. (1965). *J. Trauma*, **5**, 398

3 Bergren, H., Flatmark, A. and Simonsen, S. (1978). *Acta Med. Scand.*, **204**, 191
4 Andersen, C. B., Codd, J. R., Graff, R. A., Groce, M. A., Harter, H. R. and Newton, W. T. (1976). *Arch. Intern. Med.*, **136**, 292
5 George, C. R. P., May, J., Schieb, M., Benson, R. E. and Evans, R. H. (1973). *Med. J. Anaesth.*, **1**, 696
6 Johnson, G. and Bluthe, W. B. (1970). *Ann. Surg.*, **171**, 715
7 Eschlach, J. W., Adamson, J. W. and Cook, J. D. (1970). *Arch. Intern. Med.*, **126**, 812

25

Hyperaemia of the hand in side-to-side arteriovenous fistulas

R. F. M. WOOD AND D. T. REILLY

INTRODUCTION

Hyperaemia of the hand (Figure 25.1) is a recognized complication of side-to-side arteriovenous (A-V) wrist fistulas[1]. The condition is characterized by gradually increasing oedema of the hand and fingers. The thumb and forefinger are usually the most seriously affected digits, becoming erythematous and painful. If remedial action is not taken ischaemic changes of the tips of

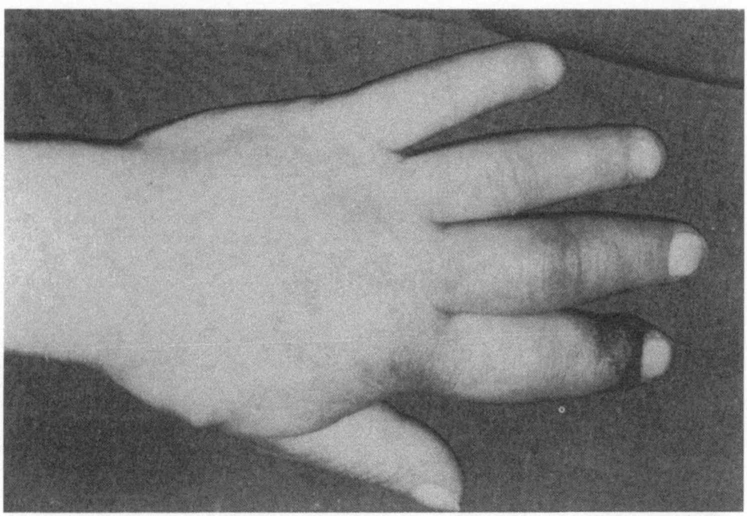

Figure 25.1 Established hyperaemia with marked swelling of the hand and fingers. There are early ischaemic changes of the tip of the index finger

the fingers may develop. Some authorities have recommended that either an end-to-side or end-to-end configuration should be used to avoid the problem[2]. However, many patients, especially those on home dialysis, find the distal segment of cephalic vein extremely useful as a needling site. In this prospective study the incidence of hyperaemia in side-to-side fistulas has been established. Blood flow through the limbs of the fistula was measured at the time of operation in a subgroup of patients to investigate the possibility of identifying those likely to develop hyperaemia. In established cases of hyperaemia, fistula angiography has been undertaken to delineate underlying problems which may be amenable to surgical revision.

PATIENTS AND METHODS

Patients
A total of 136 consecutive patients having side-to-side arteriovenous fistulas were studied prospectively from the time of operation. Details recorded at operation included blood pressure, vessel calibre and size of anastomosis. Postoperative follow-up was carried out regularly at the home dialysis clinic and any patients experiencing fistula problems were admitted for investigation.

Measurement of blood flow
In a subgroup of 23 patients, flow in the proximal and distal limbs of the

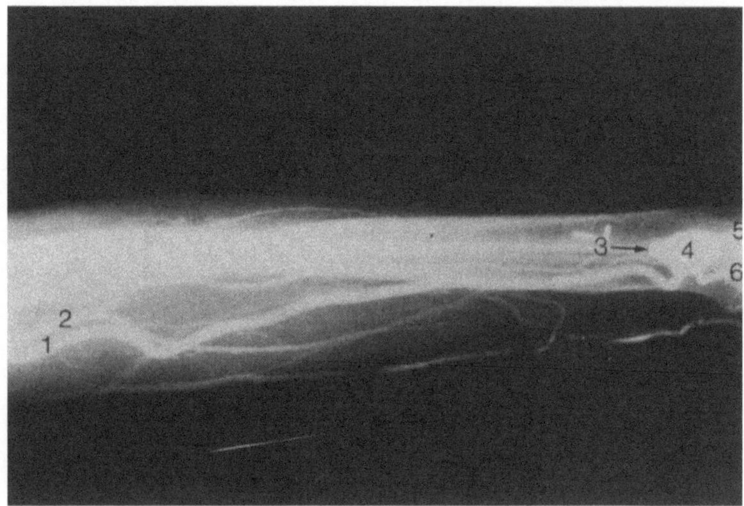

Figure 25.2 Fistula angiography in a case of late hyperaemia: (1) radial artery; (2) ulnar artery; (3) proximal vein stenosis; (4) dilated anastomosis; (5) distal cephalic vein; (6) distal radial artery

fistula was measured at the time of operation. Readings were taken 10 min after construction of the fistula with the vessels fully dilated by topical naftidrofuryl (Praxilene). A model 601D 'Cliniflow' auto-ranging flowmeter (Carolina Medical Electronics) was used with forceps-mounted electromagnetic flow probes of internal circumference 6.8 and 14 mm. The probes were applied constricting the vessel by approximately 10% to ensure good electrical contact. When a stable reading with a good pulsatile wave form was achieved the mean flow in ml/min was recorded.

Fistula angiography
The technique described by Anderson in 1979[3] was used to investigate problem cases. The forearm was positioned on an X-ray table equipped with an automatic cassette changer. A blood pressure cuff was applied above the elbow and a 19-gauge butterfly needle inserted into the distal limb of the fistula, pointing towards the anastomosis. The blood pressure cuff was inflated to 250 mmHg and 20 ml of metrizamide (Amipaque) injected through the butterfly needle. This allowed contrast material to diffuse into all limbs of the fistula. Films were taken at the rate of 2 per second, starting the film sequence ½ s before completing the injection of contrast material. The blood pressure cuff was slowly released after the first two films had been taken.

RESULTS

Incidence and management of hyperaemia
There were six cases of hyperaemia in the series, an incidence of 4.4%. Two patients developed the problem within the first month of the fistula being created. These cases were managed by simple ligation of the distal cephalic vein. In both instances this cured the hyperaemia and the patients continued to dialyse satisfactorily using the proximal limb of the fistula. The remaining four cases of hyperaemia all occurred many months after fistula construction. In the first two of these cases the distal limb of the fistula was divided and ligated but although this solved the hyperaemia it was rapidly followed by failure of the fistula. In the other two cases of late hyperaemia investigation revealed a stenosis of the proximal vein (Figure 25.2). After ligation of the distal vein both fistulas were successfully reconstructed by an end-to-side anastomosis; the cephalic vein above the stenotic segment being joined to the radial artery at a slightly more proximal level in the forearm.

Blood flow studies
The results of the electromagnetic flow measurements in 23 patients are shown in Figure 25.3. The proximal vein flows ranged from 40 to 375 ml/min. In 10 patients there was no measurable flow in the distal vein

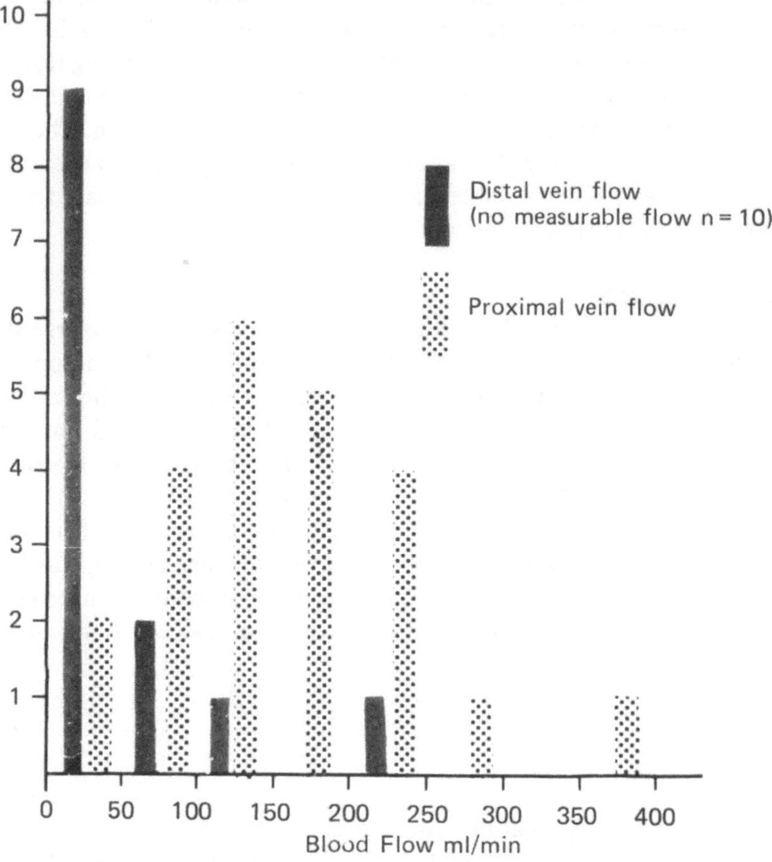

Figure 25.3   Histogram showing the distribution of proximal and distal vein flow in 23 patients having side-to-side fistulas

and in a further nine patients the flow was less than 50 ml/min. There were only four patients in whom the distal flow was greater than 50 ml/min. The distal vein flow exceeded the proximal vein flow in only 2 patients. In the first of these cases the distal vein flow was 210 ml/min with a proximal vein flow of 115 ml/min and the patient dialysed satisfactorily without developing hyperaemia. In the second case the distal vein flow was 60 ml/min with a proximal vein flow of only 40 ml/min. This patient later went on to develop hyperaemia.

DISCUSSION

There is still some controversy over the ideal configuration for an A-V wrist fistula. Side-to-side and end-to-side fistulas have not been compared in a randomized trial but in large series, such as that of Kinneart *et al.* in 1977[4], the long-term patency rate of side-to-side anastomoses was almost 10% greater than for end-to-side procedures. Although intermittent swelling of the hand is mentioned in most series of side-to-side fistulas many authors do not mention hyperaemia as a specific complication. The incidence of six cases in 136 patients (4.4%) in this series compares with the eight cases in 346 patients (2.3%) reported by Giacchino in 1979[5]. Hyperaemia is therefore relatively uncommon and in view of the benefit to the patient of the distal needling site afforded by a side-to-side fistula it remains the procedure of choice.

The measurements of blood flow obtained in this series are equivalent to the values recorded by Anderson *et al.* in 1977[6], in a group of 21 patients with end-to-side fistulas. Excessive distal flow at the time of operation was found in only two out of 23 patients in this study and the individual with a very low proximal flow (40 ml/min) went on to develop hyperaemia. The routine measurement of flow may therefore be helpful in identifying cases likely to develop hyperaemia.

A policy of active investigation of fistula problems can dramatically reduce the need for secondary access procedure such as loop grafts. This is clearly shown in this study where fistula angiography in two late cases of hyperaemia demonstrated a proximal vein stenosis and it was possible both to cure the hyperaemia and successfully reconstruct the fistula.

References

1 Bell, P. R. F. and Calman, K. C. (1974). *Surgical Aspects of Haemodialysis*, pp. 50–51. (Edinburgh: Churchill Livingstone)

2 Bussell, J. A., Abbott, J. A. and Lim, R. C. (1971). A radial steal syndrome with arterio-venous fistula for haemodialysis. *Ann. Intern. Med.*, **75**, 387

3 Anderson, C. B., Gilula, L. A., Sicard, G. A. and Etheredge, E. E. (1979). Venous angiography of subcutaneous hemodialysis fistulas. *Arch. Surg.*, **114**, 1320

4 Kinnaert, P., Vereerstraeten, P., Toussaint, C. and Van Geertruyden, J. (1977). Nine years' experience with internal arteriovenous fistulas for haemodialysis: a study of some factors influencing the results. *Br. J. Surg.*, **64**, 242

5 Giacchino, J. L., Geis, W. P., Buckingham, J. M., Vertuno, L. V. and Bansal, V. K. (1979). Vascular access: long term results, new techniques. *Arch. Surg.*, **114**, 403

6 Anderson, C. B., Etheredge, E. E., Harter, H. R., Graff, R. J., Codd, J. E. and Newton W. T. (1977). Local blood flow characteristics of arteriovenous fistulas in the forearm for dialysis. *Surg. Gynecol. Obstet.*, **144**, 531

26

Abstracts of posters in Haemodynamic sequelae of arteriovenous fistulas

---

Cephalo-basilic anastomosis for venous hypertension
K. OTA, K. TAKAHASHI, R. ARA and T. AGISHI

Use of arteriovenous fistulas has provided undeniable benefit to uraemic patients. Venous hypertension (sore thumb syndrome), however, develops and necessitates recreation of fistulas in some patients. Side-to-side anastomosis, an original type of anastomosis introduced by Brescia and Cimino, is prone to develop this syndrome.

A new operative procedure called cephalo-basilic anastomosis is introduced by us in order to treat this complication, and has been proved to be valid in 14 patients. The operative technique is as follows: dilated limb of the cephalic vein distal to the previous anastomosis is isolated, ligated and severed. A free end of the isolated segment is passed through a subcutaneous tunnel created either ventrally or dorsally. Cephalo-basilic anastomosis is carried out after isolating and ligating the distal part of the basilic vein. Type of anastomosis is selected depending upon the situation of the veins.

Oedema and pain disappeared promptly with concomitant healing of discoloration or a skin ulcer. No recurrence was observed during an observation period of 4 years, except one patient who had his ulnar vein occluded after 14 months.

The advantages of the method are technical simplicity, dramatic effect, no recurrence or damage to the pre-existing fistula.

Cephalo-basilic anastomosis is considered to be a method of choice for sore thumb syndrome.

Venous insufficiency of arteriovenous fistula: symptomatology and treatment

H. D. JAKUBOWSKI, U. RUSCHEWSKI and V. KINDHÄUSER

A total of 826 operations for arteriovenous fistulas were performed in our department between January 1971 and December 1981. In 258 of these cases the operative procedure was necessary for late complications of a fistula, which was established in our own or another hospital. The main causes for reoperation were thrombosis ($n = 129$) and aneurysms ($n = 54$). The problem of venous insufficiency ($n = 35$) has to be stressed, for in many patients the symptoms of this complication are misinterpreted for a long time and treated as an inflammatory process. Principal signs are painful swelling of the hand, phlebectasia on the back of the hand, red or cyanotic discoloration of the skin, and sometimes finger-tip ulcerations. The surgical treatment is simple and effective: in 23 of our 35 patients the venous insufficiency was cured by ligature of the distal venous limb. In 11 patients the symptoms were relieved by anastomosing the distal venous limb end-to-end to an adjacent vein directing the arterialized blood to the proximal venous system. One fistula was closed after successful renal transplantation.

Venous hypertension, a complication of the side-to-side arteriovenous fistula

G. KOOTSTRA and M. J. H. SLOOFF

In several textbooks and leading articles a side-to-side anastomosis between radial artery and cephalic vein is recommended as standard technique for the creation of an arteriovenous (A-V) fistula. We have encountered a late complication in cases where a side-to-side fistula had been constructed. Due to impaired flow – from multiple punctures for dialysis – through to proximal part of the arterialized cephalic vein, the distal collaterals of the vein will be exposed to increased pressure, leading to venous hypertension. This is a clinical entity of which the symptoms equal those in varicose veins: pain, swelling, pigmentation of the skin and eventually trophic ulcers. In radiocephalic A-V fistula the thumb and the first and second finger will be affected. In a case of a side-to-side A-V fistula between ulnar artery and basilic vein we observed venous hypertension of the third and fourth finger, suggesting a segmental venous drainage of the hand. In another case of a known occlusion of the cephalic vein an end-to-side A-V fistula gave venous hypertension too. For prevention of venous hypertension we recommend as standard technique the end-to-side A-V fistula. In case of a pre-existing proximal obstruction of the vein venous hypertension has to be considered as a calculated risk when a standard end-to-side A-V fistula is constructed.

Small inner diameter (3–4 mm) polytetrafluoroethylene (PTFE) grafts for haemodialysis: haemodynamic studies

R. SQUERZANTI, E. De PAOLI VITALI and A. FARINELLI

Arterious venous shunts were implanted into elderly patients undergoing haemodialysis and suffering from diminished heart performance, by grafting a straight bridge, unsuitable for puncture, between a forearm artery and vein (diameter 3–4 mm, $1 = 9.4 \pm 3.2$ cm). Electromagnetic flow measurement, soon after implantation, showed a value of 499 ± 200 ml/min (a value comparable with similar values reported in the literature). All grafts have made veins suitable for dialysis in 2 weeks.

No expansion of the inside diameter of the graft can be reasonably expected owing to the structural features of rigidity. The small inner diameter and the appropriate length of the graft (blood flow-resistant elements) diminish both pressure and flow away from arterial anastomosis.

No worsening effect in the cardiac failure parameters of any of the patients who underwent surgery has so far been found in the 6 months since grafting. In conclusion, PTFE graft (3–4 mm) is recommended in elderly patients especially if suffering from cardiac failure, since these shunts allow only limited blood flow and ensure better survival and fewer complications of A-V fistulas, if compared with PTFE (6–7 mm).

Haemodynamics of arteriovenous fistulas in the human arm

M. J. C. van GEMERT and C. M. A. BRUYNINCKX

A model is used to discuss haemodynamics of arteriovenous fistulas in the human arm. The model assumes that: arteries are rigid tubes with resistance to blood flow; flow and pressure are stationary; veins have no resistance to flow; the blood flow through the arm also flows through the hand; the central aortic pressure is independent of the fistel capacity. This model differs from that discussed by Strandness and Sumner[1] in using zero venous resistance and the blood pressure source located in the central aorta. It is applied to radialis as well as to brachialis fistulas. The results are that, firstly, for a radialis fistula blood flow in the distal arteria radialis is in the fistula direction when $R(rp) R(h) > R(u) R(f)$ where $R(rp)$, $R(h)$, $R(u)$ and $R(f)$ are, respectively, the resistances of the proximal arteria radialis, the hand, the arteria ulnaris, and the fistula. The model confirms that this is the usual situation. Furthermore, finger pressure differences at closed and open radialis fistula appear to be dependent on the resistances of the arm arteries. So, fistula capacity is not uniquely related to finger pressure differences. Secondly, for a brachialis fistula the major haemodynamic changes are caused by the proximal pressure fall between central aorta and fistula. Again there is no unique relation between finger pressure and fistula capacity. Finally, finger ischaemia is shown to be caused by a combination of pressure falls in the proximal arterial system (aorto-brachial) and the distal vascular system. It is emphasized that 'stealing' means stealing of blood pressure instead of blood flow.

Techniques to correct high flow arteriovenous fistulas
A. VEGETO, L. BERARDINELLI, G. STORELLI and R. CANAL

High flow rates in internal angioaccess for haemodialysis can provoke alterations in cardiac parameters. Some surgical techniques adopted at our centre on 12 patients are here proposed: (1) In order to reduce the high flow, a distal arteriovenous (A-V) standard fistula can be usefully transformed into an external A-V shunt. (2) An immediate favourable effect, but without a good long-term result, can be obtained by banding the A-V fistula with a Dacron or homologous venous graft, or a silver clip; the use of textile material increases the risk of infection. (3) A possible alternative method used in four patients is the simple 'capittonage' with multiple continuous sutures of the hypertrophic side of the fistula. This is a good method but it is difficult to determine the resulting diameter of the residual lumen. (4) In our more recent six cases we have resected the excedent portion of the aneurysmatic wall and reconstructed directly the integrity of the vessel with a single continuous suture. This technique has in our hands produced the best functional results.

Reference
1 Strandness, D. E. and Sumner, D. S. (1975). *Hemodynamics for Surgeons*, Chapter 21. (New York: Grune and Stratton)

27

Invited comment on papers and posters in Haemodynamic sequelae of arteriovenous fistula

E. LINDSTEDT

A number of haemodynamic effects are known to occur in patients with congenital and acquired arteriovenous (A-V) fistulas as well as in experimental animals. These effects could be expected to appear even in patients with therapeutic A-V fistulas. Some important changes are:

(1) increased velocity of blood flow;
(2) increased cardiac output;
(3) increased circulating blood volume;
(4) increased oxygen content of venous blood;
(5) high output cardiac failure;
(6) 'steal' of arterial blood pressure;
(7) venous hypertension;
(8) dilation and 'arterialization' of fistula vein;
(9) dilation and 'venization' of fistula artery;
(10) 'endarteritis lenta';
(11) increased skeletal growth.

It is of great importance to recognize and to treat these changes when they are clinically important, and the presentations in this session are directed towards these problems.

Dr Gerstoft and collaborators started a prospective study of the haemodynamic consequences of dialysis fistulas. They found no significant change in cardiac parameters at rest nor, which is important, after exercise. They conclude that no signs of cardiac failure were observed in these patients and their opinion appears to be well founded. They estimated fistula flow as difference between cardiac output with open and closed fistulas. Several authors[1] find these estimations very crude, as a number of technical factors during the examination can affect the cardiac output. They suggest that the increase in blood volume usually found in patients with A-V fistulas makes it easier for the heart to maintain sufficient peripheral circulation. On the other hand, it could increase the risk of high-output cardiac failure. Longitudinal studies of these patients are of great interest, and I hope it will be possible to report the results of follow-up after a year or two for the next Access Conference.

A number of techniques to study A-V fistula flow have been reported but none has proven to be completely satisfactory. Venous occlusion plethysmography has been tried, but failed. We used a dye-dilution technique but, as we do not have a single common path of the blood stream we are not quite sure if the results are true. The most useful method today seems to be Doppler ultrasound techniques as was demonstrated by Dr Lillemor Forsberg in a poster session in Chapter 10. The problem is that we have no absolutely correct method by which we can standardize our investigations.

Levy and collaborators used Doppler blood flow measurement in 240 patients. They used Doppler ultrasound for measuring flow velocity and ultrasound A-scan for determination of vessel diameter. Their results are very interesting, but it is amazing that they found 44% of patients with upper arm fistulas showing clinical signs of cardiac failure. The estimated fistula flows were not very large and would be considered by most cardiologists to produce little consequences for a normal heart. From the discussion it can be concluded that their patients were selected from those having clinical signs of cardiac failure. They have demonstrated well the usefulness of ultrasound techniques to estimate fistula flow in clinical situations with too large or too low fistula flow.

Several presentations in this section deal with the problem of increased venous pressure observed especially in patients with side-to-side anastomoses. Normally the venous pressure in the fistula arm is not very high. Venous pressure was below 15 mmHg, even if the systolic arterial pressure only 2–3 cm proximal to the fistula[2] was 150 mmHg. If the flow on the venous side is unrestricted, most of the pressure gradient seems to be over the fistula itself. If venous flow is obstructed, venous hypertension with the massive oedema, increased skin temperature and possibly ulceration may occur.

Wood and Reilly discussed in their elegant presentation hyperaemia of the hand or, rather, venous hypertension in patients with side-to-side fistulas which occurred in only 4.4% in their prospective study. I support their conclusion that increased distal venous flow thus does not necessarily give problems.

Ota, Takahashi, Ara and Agishi from Tokyo presented a poster called 'Cephalo-basilic anastomosis for venous hypertension'. They suggest that the distal limb of the cephalic vein should be connected to the basilic vein to overcome venous hypertension. Unfortunately, the basilic vein is often, due to its location, difficult to reach for cannulation in many patients. Anyhow, they demonstrate a simple and elegant method to solve the problem of venous hypertension without interfering with the fistula.

Jakubowski, Ruschewski and Kindhäuser from Essen call their poster 'Venous insufficiency of arteriovenous fistula: symptomatology and treatment'. They have experience of a huge number of dialysis patients and have also found venous hypertension to be an important and annoying complication in some cases. They point to the simple treatment with ligation of the distal venous limb which solves the problem in most cases. They also have experience of using the distal venous limb as a bridge to another proximal vein.

Kootstra and Slooff called their poster 'Venous hypertension, a complication of the side-to-side arteriovenous fistula'. In this poster the most impressive case is demonstrated with oedema, cyanotic discoloration and ulcerations of several fingers caused by venous hypertension. They point out that these cases should not be mistaken for arterial steal or infection. I do not support their suggestion that side-to-side fistulas should be avoided, but agree that previous damage to the cephalic vein may lead to venous hypertension if this vein is used for the fistula. I would suggest that the vein used for the fistula should always be checked using vascular dilators or a Fogarty catheter to make sure that the lumen is patent, but also that the venous wall is not damaged from previous thrombophlebitis.

Squerzanti, De Paoli Vitali and Farinelli from Ferrara presented a poster entitled 'Small inner diameter (3–4 mm) polytetrafluoroethylene (PTFE) grafts for haemodialysis: haemodynamic studies'. They report on an elegant technique of preventing excessive flow and growth of the A-V fistula by interposition of a small PTFE prosthesis between the artery and the vein. They found no worsening effect from the fistula on the already poor cardiac function of their patients. In the long run, however, a restriction of the lumen of these small prostheses would be expected due to the formation of pseudo-intima and thrombotic changes at the venous anastomosis.

It is difficult to make haemodynamic studies of A-V fistula both in patients and in experimental animals as so many technical and other factors vary from individual to individual and from time to time. Van Gemert and Bruyninckx from Eindhoven made a most impressive poster presentation 'Haemodynamics of arteriovenous fistulas in the human arm'. They constructed a model to study fistula haemodynamics. They make the assumption that arteries are rigid tubes and veins have no restriction to flow, which is, of course, not always true. They give a good theoretical technique for the study of haemodynamics in and around an A-V fistula but do not consider the progressive changes of arterial resistance due to the development of collaterals, atheromatous changes of the artery and the fistula vein, etc. This model can teach us how haemodynamic changes occur around an A-V fistula and the relative importance of various circulatory parameters. The authors emphasize that 'stealing' means stealing of arterial blood pressure and not primarily of blood flow. Steal of blood pressure does not necessarily mean that clinical symptoms could appear as the body compensates by increasing the capillary bed, thus decreasing the peripheral resistance not only in the fistula and in the collaterals but also in the tissues[3].

Vegeto, Berardinelli, Storelli and Canal from Milan presented a poster called 'Techniques to correct high flow arteriovenous fistulas'. They presented their experiences from converting the fistula to an external shunt or banding the fistula vein with Dacron but they advocate wedge resection of the aneurysmatic venous wall diminishing its diameter by a continuous longitudinal suture, a technique similar to 'end-aneurysmorrhaphy' described by Matas, 1914.

References

1 Lindstedt, E. (1972). Studies in therapeutic arteriovenous fistulae. *Scand. J. Urol. Nephrol.*, Suppl. **14**
2 Göthlin, J., Lindstedt, E. and Olin, T. (1977). A dye-dilution method for the determination of blood flow in Cimino–Brescia arteriovenous fistulae. *Invest. Urol.*, **15**, 167
3 Lindstedt, E. and Westling, H. (1975). Effects of an antebrachial Cimino–Brescia arteriovenous fistula on the local circulation in the hand. *Scand. J. Urol. Nephrol.*, **9**, 119

Section VI
Complications

28

Complications of arteriovenous fistulas and surgical intervention

H. ERASMI, S. HORSCH, R. SCHMIDT AND H. PICHLMAIER

INTRODUCTION

We all know dialysis patients who suffer from a frightening and apparently inexplicable accumulation of arteriovenous (A-V) fistula failures. Numerous procedures to provide vascular access become necessary and eventual rehabilitation is delayed. In order to indicate faults and to prevent unnecessary surgery an analysis of our patients requiring chronic haemodialysis was attempted in this report.

PATIENTS AND METHODS

At the Department of Surgery of the University Hospital of Cologne between 1971 and 1980, 524 subcutaneous A-V fistulas were constructed in 443 patients. Only the results of 299 Cimino and 29 brachial fistulas in 248 patients are reported here. The rest of the patients were not considered because follow-up was not possible. The peripheral A-V fistula as described by Brescia and Cimino[1] is currently the procedure of choice. At the beginning of our observation period the initial A-V fistula was performed as side-to-side anastomosis between radial artery and cephalic vein. After having seen ischaemic complications, the vein distal to the anastomosis was ligated routinely. Since 1980 for haemodynamic reasons we perform only end-to-side anastomosis.

The brachial fistula was our procedure of second choice for a vascular access. It was constructed side-to-side or end-to-side between the brachial artery and the basilic or cephalic vein.

EARLY RESULTS

In 299 Cimino fistulas we observed 42 early thromboses in the first 4 weeks (Table 28.1). In side-to-side anastomosis early thromboses occurred in 14.5%, in side-to-side anastomosis with ligature of the distal vein in 12.2%, and in end-to-side anastomosis in 16.7%. The high percentage of early thromboses in end-to-side anastomoses is due to several factors: operating without magnifying glasses, using veins partially obstructed and damaged by previous venipuncture, and trying the construction of a fistula with thrombectomized veins.

Table 28.1 Early thromboses in ($n = 299$) Cimino fistulas (1 January 1971–31 December 1980). Early thromboses ($n = 42$; 14%)

	n	*Percentage*
Side-to-side anastomosis	23	14.5
Side-to-side anastomosis with ligature of the distal vein	12	12.2
End-to-side anastomosis	7	16.7

Since standardization of our operation technique we observed only nine early thromboses in 82 end-to-side anastomoses between January 1981 and February 1982. This means 10.9% compared with 16.7% in the earlier period.

The aetiology of the early thromboses is listed in Table 28.2. Surgical faults accounted for a third of the fistula failures. In 7.2% the thromboses occurred after the first puncture. In 35.7% narrow and thin veins, arteriosclerosis of the radial artery or damage of the veins caused early thrombosis. In 23.8% the cause of fistula occlusion was unknown.

Table 28.2 Aetiology of early thromboses in ($n = 299$) Cimino fistulas. Aetiology of early thromboses ($n = 42$)

	n	*Percentage*
Unknown	10	23.8
Surgical faults	14	33.3
Traumatic needle puncture	3	7.2
Small capacity of the venous system, obliterated veins	15	35.7

A number of these fistula failures could have been avoided by more careful preoperative examination of the vessels[2]. Palpation of peripheral pulses will provide the information regarding patency and arterial flow. The veins must be examined for size, patency and distribution. Since the preoperative examination was often not thorough and therefore the vessels not suitable, it is clear that only in 23.8% of the cases was fistula patency restored by thrombectomy. In 21.4% a new anastomosis was necessary.

If fistula failure was due to inadequate arterial flow or thin and narrow or obstructed veins a new anastomosis was performed in the contralateral forearm in 33.3%. Brachial fistulas were created in 9.5%, and a graft had to be implanted in 11.9%

LATE RESULTS

In an observation period up to 111 months we encountered 85 late thromboses. The comparison of the different anastomoses shows that end-to-side anastomoses yield a slightly better late result with 12% (Table 28.3). Late thromboses were successfully thrombectomized in 25.9%. In 18.8% construction of a new anastomosis above occlusion was necessary. In 31.8% the replacement of the fistula by a new one on the contralateral side was required. In the remaining patients brachial fistulas were performed or heterografts were implanted.

Table 28.3 Late thromboses in ($n = 299$) Cimino fistulas (1 January 1971–31 December 1980). Late thromboses ($n = 85$; 28.4%)

	n	Percentage
Side-to-side anastomosis	46	54
Side-to-side anastomosis with ligation of the distal vein	29	34
End-to-side anastomosis	10	12

The comparison of early and late thromboses indicates that in the later course surgical technique has less to do with the fistula function than how well the fistula is managed in the dialysis centre. In 36% late thromboses were due to dialysis complications as shown in Table 28.4

Table 28.4 Aetiology of late thromboses ($n = 299$) Cimino fistulas. Aetiology of late thromboses ($n = 85$)

	n	Percentage
Dialysis complications (RR↓, hypovolaemia, pressure, traumatic puncture)	31	36
Aneurysms	15	18
Stenoses	39	46

In 18% late occlusions were caused by an aneurysm and in 46% by stenoses of the venous segment. A short stenosis or a localized aneurysm was corrected by resection and a new end-to-side anastomosis above. If the arterialized segment of the vein was severely stenosed by venipuncture or was largely dilated by aneurysms, salvage of the fistula was not attempted and we proceeded with a new fistula on the contralateral side.

A brachial fistula was only performed if there were no suitable veins in both forearms. In very obese arms with deep-seated veins a graft fistula was constructed. In regard to puncture difficulties in 17.2% and aneurysm formation in 13.6% (compared with 5% in Cimino fistulas) brachial fistulas should be the fistula of second choice[2-4].

Cumulative patency rate for Cimino fistulas – calculated by the life-table-method – was 63% after 1 year, 55% after 2 years, and 46% after 3 years. The mean function was 46.2 months.

CONCLUSION

For patients with renal failure the good function of their dialysis fistula is of vital importance; therefore careful preoperative examination of the upper extremities in regard to suitable vessels is necessary. When performing the initial fistula we should start as peripherally as possible. The fistula of first choice is the end-to-side anastomosis between radial artery and cephalic vein at the level of the wrist. The first fistula should be created long before it is needed for dialysis in order to avoid placing external shunts. In patients with chronic renal failure the vessels for at least one arm should be protected from venipuncture.

The surgical technique should be meticulous and the operation should be carried out by an experienced surgeon.

The late results are much affected by puncture technique and management of the fistulas by the dialysis staff as well as the patients themselves.

References

1 Brescia, M. J., Cimino, J. E., Appel, K. and Jurirch, B. J. (1966). Chronic hemodialysis using venipuncture and a surgically created arteriovenous fistula. *N. Engl. J. Med.*, **275**, 1089
2 Haimov, M. (1981). Vascular access for hemodialysis. *NY State J. Med.*, **81**, 1490
3 Horntrich, J. and Müller, D. (1980). Erfahrungen mit a-v-Fisteln zur Langzeitdialyse unter besonderer Berücksichtigung der Ellenbeugefistel. *Z. Urol. Nephrol.*, **73**, 337
4 Zehle, A., Schulz, V., Kottmann, J., Schmitz, W. and Pichlmaier, H. (1979). Arterio-venöse Gefässverbindungen für die Langzeitdialyse. *Chirurgie*, **50**, 345

29

Non-thrombotic complications of PTFE grafts for haemodialysis

M. J. H. SLOOFF, P. J. H. SMITS, D. H. E. LICHTENDAHL AND
G. K. van der HEM

INTRODUCTION

Thrombosis is the most frequent complication in dialysis grafts. Relatively little attention is paid to the incidence of non-thrombotic complications in these grafts and experience in the treatment of such complications is seldom reported. The aim of this paper is to review our own experience with non-thrombotic complications in a series of 76 PTFE grafts with special regard to their treatment.

MATERIAL AND METHODS

In a 5-year period extending from 1 January 1977 to January 1982, 76 PTFE grafts were implanted for haemodialysis purposes. In the first 3 years Impra grafts (37) were used and from 1 January 1980 only Gore-tex grafts (39).

All 37 Impra grafts were placed in the lower arm, 19 were straight grafts between the radial artery distally and a cubital vein, and 18 were loop grafts between the brachial artery and a cubital vein. Of the 39 Gore-tex grafts 35 were placed in the lower arm, 14 were straight and 21 had a loop configuration. Two straight grafts were placed in the upper arm between the brachial artery at elbow level and the basilic vein near the axilla. Two looped grafts were placed in the thigh between the superficial femoral artery and the femoral vein. All arterial anastomoses were end-graft-to-side artery and all venous anastomoses were end-to-end.

RESULTS

In the 76 PTFE grafts non-thrombotic complications were observed in 30/76 (39%) grafts (Table 29.1).

Table 29.1 Complications in 76 PTFE grafts in relation to graft type and graft configuration

		Impra graft		Gore-tex graft	
		Loop	Straight	Loop	Straight
Bleeding	($n* = 6$)	3	3	0	0
Pseudoaneurysm	($n = 10$)	1	5	3	1
Infection	($n = 7$)	2	1	3	1
Haemodynamic	($n = 4$)	1	0	2	1
Skin erosions	($n = 3$)	2	1	0	0
TOTAL	($n = 30$)	9	10	8	3

*Number of grafts concerned

Bleeding

Bleeding which required surgical intervention was observed in six (Impra) grafts. Bleeding seemed due to puncture lesions, mostly multiple puncture holes in the graft wall too close to one another. In two cases longitudinal tears in the graft wall were present. Only two grafts could be salvaged by suturing the puncture defect in the graft wall. The other four grafts were lost due to massive bleeding, which required ligation of the graft.

Pseudoaneurysm

One or more multiple pseudoaneurysms were observed in 10 (six Impra and four Gore-tex) grafts. Pseudoaneurysm is due to defects in the wall of the grafts caused by punctures. Surgical intervention was undertaken because of imminent rupture and infection. Two grafts were replaced by a new graft because multiple aneurysms were present in the course of the graft. In the remaining eight grafts the affected part of the graft was bypassed by a new graft segment in a parallel subcutaneous tunnel. By doing this the original graft segment with the pseudoaneurysm(s) is isolated and can be excised. When infection was present the wound was left open.

Infection

Infection was seen in seven grafts. Infection was mostly related to secondary operations or due to the neglect of the rules of asepsis. Three grafts were lost due to massive bleeding from the infected arterial anastomoses. In all three cases ligation of the brachial artery at elbow level was required to control the bleeding and all three grafts were removed. In the remaining four grafts infection could be managed by opening the skin over the affected graft segment even in the area of one or both of the anastomoses. Wound debridement is an essential part of the treatment. The wound was left open and cleaned frequently. Secondary healing was awaited. In three cases a skin defect over the graft resulted near the original infected site. In two cases this was closed by means of a bipedical flap and in one case by a bypass graft of the uncovered graft. This latter graft segment was resected after the completion of the bypass.

Haemodynamic changes

Haemodynamic changes occurred due to four grafts. In two cases oedema of the limb was observed. In one case this was caused by a loop graft in the lower arm and in the other case by a loop graft in the thigh. Both cases were treated conservatively by elastic stockings. In two patients with two grafts, one straight graft in the upper arm and one loop graft in the thigh, ischaemia of the limb distal to the arterial anastomosis was observed. The arterial anastomosis was 'banded' and the ischaemic phenomena disappeared. Banding was done under plethysmographic control in such a way that after the narrowing of the arterial anastomosis the peripheral flow as measured by plethysmography was doubled. None of these grafts was lost.

Skin erosions

This type of complication occurred in three grafts. The erosions were all due to a too superficial subcutaneous positioning of the grafts. All erosions were small defects. Although these defects are without consequence, they were treated surgically because patients are often disturbed by them. All defects were closed by means of a bipedical flap. The inner edges of the erosion were excised. A relaxation incision was made and the skin between this relaxation incision and the erosion was undermined and this latter defect was closed. The defect caused by the relaxation incision is left open for secondary healing. In all three cases this surgical intervention was successful.

Overall results

Two types of complications, bleeding and pseudoaneurysms, are due to improper puncture techniques. Table 29.2 shows that in our series these types of complications were more frequent (12/16 grafts) in Impra grafts than in Gore-tex grafts (4/16).

Table 29.2   Complications related to the type of graft used

Graft type		Bleeding	Pseudoaneurysm	
Impra	($n* = 37$)	6	6	12
Gore-tex	($n = 39$)	0	4	4
				16

*Number of grafts concerned

Thirty complications occurred in 30 grafts. Nine of these grafts had to be excised; so only nine (12%) of the original placed 76 grafts were lost. The other 21 grafts with complications could be saved either by surgery (19) or by conservative means. The median survival time of these saved grafts was 12 months.

DISCUSSION

The most frequent complication in access surgery is thrombosis. In the literature this complication and its causes and treatment are discussed extensively. Of the non-thrombotic complications often only the incidence is reported[1-3].

The cause of these mostly infrequent complications or their treatment is not always discussed. The aim of this review is to report our experience with non-thrombotic complications when PTFE grafts are used. Although our own experience is limited several observations can be made. As is shown in Table 29.1, no relation could be found between the incidence of one of the mentioned complications and graft configuration (loop/straight). From Table 29.2 is clear that at least in our series the incidence of bleeding and pseudoaneurysm formation is higher in Impra grafts than in Gore-tex grafts. This observation is confirmed by other authors[4,5].

A possible explanation may be that the Gore-tex graft is reinforced by an extra circular Teflon layer around the proper graft. However our impression is that most of these complications are caused by faulty puncture techniques. All too often the grafts are repeatedly punctured at the same site or the puncture is performed too roughly or under inadequate aseptic circumstances. Proper puncture techniques with frequent changing of the puncture site should prevent these complications[6]. Another important observation is that infection in or around PTFE grafts does not exclude reconstruction and salvage of the graft. The good infection resistance of the PTFE graft is well known[1,5,7].

The operation-related infections are often more massive and therefore more dangerous. In our experience the grafts have often to be removed. However, when the infected site is opened and wound debridement is performed the infection can often be controlled. In some cases these wounds heal secondarily and in other cases reconstructive surgery with a bypass of the affected segment is needed. Banding of the arterial anastomosis of haemo-dialysis grafts for ischaemia of the limb or a steal syndrome was first mentioned by VanderWerf, in 1977[8]. The necessary extent of the narrowing, however, is very difficult to determine. To solve this problem we performed the narrowing of the arterial anastomoses under plethysmographic control. It was decided arbitrarily that the amplitude of the plethysmographic registration on either the finger or toe had to be doubled after the narrowing sutures were placed. Empirically this worked out quite well.

As shown from our experience the surgical treatment of the non-thrombotic complications is worthwhile. Not only are 21/30 grafts with complications saved, but the median survival time of these grafts appeared to be 12 months.

References

1 Butler, H. G., Baker, C. D. and Johnson, J. M. C. (1977). Vascular access for chronic hemodialysis: polytetrafluoroethylene (PTFE) versus bovine heterograft. *Am. J. Surg.*, **134**, 791
2 Tellis, V. A., Kohnberg, W. J., Bhat, D. J., Driscoll, B. and Veith, F. J. (1979). Expanded polytetrafluoroethylene graft fistula for chronic hemodialysis. *Ann. Surg.*, **189**, 101
3 Haimov, M., Burrows, L., Schauzer, H., Neff, M., Baez, A., Kurin, K. and Slifkin, R. (1980). Experience with arterial substitutes in the construction of vascular access for hemodialysis. *J. Cardiovasc. Surg.*, **21**, 149
4 Pasternak, H. M., Paruk, S., Kogan, S. and Levitt, S. (1977). A synthetic vascular conduit (expanded PTFE) for hemodialysis access. *Vasc. Surg.*, **11**, 99
5 Lemaitre, P., Ackman, C. F. D., O'Regan, S., Laplante, M. P. and Kaye, M. (1978). Polytetrafluoroethylene (PTFE) grafts for hemodialysis; 18 months experience. *Clin. Nephrol.*, **10**, 27
6 Merickel, J. H., Andersen, R. C., Knutson, R., Lipschultz, M. L. and Hitchcock, C. R. (1978). Bovine carotid artery shunts in vascular access surgery. *Arch. Surg.*, **109**, 245
7 Slooff, M. J. H. (1981). Secondary access surgery for hemodialysis and chemotherapy. *Neth. J. Surg.*, suppl.
8 VanderWerf, B. A., Ratazzi, L. C., Katzman, H. A. and Schild, A. F. (1977). Prevention and treatment of bovine graft arterio-venous fistula complications. *Dial. Transplant.*, **6**, 27

30

Is angioaccess a limiting factor for haemodialysis of diabetic patients?

J. BOMMER, K. MÖHRING AND E. RITZ

In recent years the number of diabetics on maintenance haemodialysis has increased continuously. According to the figures of the European Transplant Association, in the Federal Republic of Germany, 4.1% of all patients on maintenance haemodialysis and 9.1% of patients admitted during 1980, are diabetics (Dr Wing, London, personal communication). Even higher percentages are reported from the USA[1] where apparently less or no patient selection, particularly with respect to age, is exerted. The increasing prevalence of diabetics in the dialysis population brings into focus specific difficulties because of which medical rehabilitation[3] and survival[3,4] of diabetic patients on maintenance haemodialysis are consistently worse than of non-diabetic patients. Vascular access is one of the main problems consistently commented upon in early reports[5,6]. Angioaccess, in those days, was even regarded as the 'Achilles heel' of haemodialysis in diabetic patients.

Reasons for the poor prognosis of vascular access in the early studies may have included accelerated atherosclerosis, calcification of arterial media and poor venous runoff, particularly in elderly diabetic patients. In addition, the well-known predisposition of diabetics to infection may have contributed to the excessive prevalence of fistula infection.

Since these early reports, considerable improvements in fistula surgery have been made (e.g. changes in anastomosis technique, introduction of PTFE grafts), and patients are dialysed more frequently with improved blood pressure control which avoids hypertensive crises or hypotensive episodes, etc. In view of such advances it appeared of interest to review our experience concerning angioaccess of diabetic patients on maintenance haemodialysis. This issue is of considerable practical importance since alternate modalities of treatment, for example CAPD, are currently available for diabetic patients[7]. Major difficulties with vascular access would be a strong argument in favour of CAPD as the preferred treatment for diabetic patients with uraemia.

PATIENTS AND METHODS

We analysed all patients who were on dialysis between 1 January and 31 December 1980 in the Department of Internal Medicine of the University of Heidelberg. Table 30.1 lists age, sex, underlying disease and percentage of hypertensive patients and duration of haemodialysis in these patients. Fifty-seven patients were non-diabetic, 12 patients were diabetic. Ten patients were uraemic because of diabetic glomerulosclerosis (Kimmelstiel–Wilson), one diabetic patient was uraemic because of polycystic disease and one because of glomerulonephritis. One further patient, in addition to presumed glomerulo-sclerosis and diabetic retinopathy, had pre-existent stable urotuberculosis and urolithiasis. Seven patients were insulin-dependent. Table 30.2 lists the major micro- and macrovascular complications in the diabetic patient population.

Table 30.1

	Diabetic (n = 12)	Non-diabetic (n = 57)
(Kimmelstiel–Wilson) glomerulosclerosis	10	—
Glomerulonephritis	1	33
Pyelonephritis	—	3
Polycystic kidney	1	11
Malignant hypertension	—	3
Miscellaneous	—	7
Age (years)	50.5 ± 11.4	46.5 ± 12.6
Sex	6 m., 6 f.	32 m., 25 f.
Persistent hypertension	3	8
Duration of haemodialysis (months)	29.9 ± 11.3	52.3 ± 35.2

Table 30.2 Microvascular and macrovascular complications in diabetic patients on haemodialysis

Retinopathy	
proliferative	5
background	7
blindness	2 bilateral, 1 unilateral
Polyneuropathy	12
History of myocardial infarction	2
Coronary surgery	1
Angina pectoris	6
Claudicatio intermittens	9
Bypass surgery	1
Amputation of lower limb	3
Amputation of toes	2

Except in cases with preretinal haemorrhage, all patients received on the day of surgery and for 14 days after surgery 500 mg acetylsalicylic acid (Colfarit®) per day. In all except two diabetic patients, the fistula was not cannulated within 6 weeks after fistula surgery. As a prophylactic measure all diabetic patients received 2 g dicloxacillin/day 10–14 days postoperatively.

RESULTS

Type of angioaccess

Table 30.3 shows that a similar proportion of diabetic and non-diabetic patients had Cimino fistulas of the lower arm, Cimino fistulas of the upper arm or polytetrafluoroethylene (PTFE) grafts of the Gore-tex type.

Table 30.3 Fistulas in diabetic patients

	Diabetic ($n = 12$)	Non-diabetic ($n = 57$)
Cimino fistulas		
lower arm	11 (79%)	44 (77%)
upper arm	2 (14%)	6 (11%)
PTFE grafts	1 (7%)	7 (12%)

Surgical revision of fistulas

Table 30.4 demonstrates that in 1980 surgical revision of angioaccess was required in a similar proportion of diabetic and non-diabetic patients.

Table 30.4 Surgical revision of angioaccess in diabetic patients

Diabetic	Non-diabetic
2/12 per year	12/57 per year
1 per 72 months	1 per 57 months

Table 30.5 Infections of angioaccess in diabetic patients

Diabetic	Non-diabetic
1/12 per year	4/57 per year
(7%)	(7%)

Fistula infection

In view of previous reports on the high incidence of angioaccess infection in diabetic patients, it is of note that a similar proportion of diabetic and non-diabetic patients had angioaccess infection (Table 30.5). In diabetics, no

Table 30.6 Angioaccess survival in diabetic patients (18 months post-operative)

	Diabetic ($n = 11$)		Non-diabetic ($n = 57$)	
Functioning	7/11	(64%)	38/57	(69%)
Revision	4/11	(36%)	18/57	(31%)

infections were observed postoperatively. All infections observed in 1980 (Table 30.5) or subsequently occurred beyond the immediate postoperative period, mostly resulting from cannula tract infections at the puncture site or infected haematoma. All infections in diabetics were seen in patients with PTFE grafts.

Postoperative fistula complications

Table 30.6 reviews the proportion of fistulas or grafts of patients who were on dialysis during 1980 which required revision in the first 18 months subsequent to surgical creation of the fistula. There was no obvious difference between non-diabetic and diabetic patients.

DISCUSSION

There are marked differences in recent reports in literature concerning the incidence of angioaccess failure. Shapiro and Comty[3] recently reported an average fistula survival in insulin- and non-insulin-dependent diabetics of 8.5 and 15.7 months respectively. The corresponding survival for bovine grafts was 13.9 and 9.2 months. The number of surgical procedures per year was 2.3 for fistulas and 1.8 for bovine grafts. Although in this report figures for non-diabetic patients were not given, this experience would suggest major difficulties with angioaccess in diabetic patients.

However, other authors reported an experience which is more in line with our own results. El Shahat *et al.*[8] reported the experience of the La Pitié Salpétrière hospital with 56 diabetic patients with a total experience of 1611 patient-months. Approximately 60 out of 82 vascular accesses were classical Cimino–Brescia fistulas. Only in three out of 56 patients could a permanent vascular access not be established, so that primary CAPD treatment was required. Similarly, Levin *et al.*[9] reported that angioaccess function 6, 12 and 18 months postoperatively was similar in diabetic patients and non-diabetic patients both for Cimino fistulas and bovine grafts. An 80% actuarial function rate of Cimino fistulas in diabetic patients after 36 months was also reported by Butt *et al.*[10]. Fifty per cent of fistulas functioned without revision or thrombectomy.

The above-mentioned reports and our own experience permit the following conclusions:

Although undoubtedly angioaccess may be difficult in many diabetic patients, particularly in older individuals, angioaccess is rarely the limiting factor for haemodialysis. With attention to technical detail and fistula care, the incidence of thrombotic and infectious fistula complications is no longer excessive in diabetic patients.

We attribute this more favourable experience to the following factors: timely operation several months ahead of the anticipated beginning of haemodialysis, meticulous blood pressure control, and choice of alternate modalities of angioaccess (upper arm fistulas, PTFE grafts) if difficulties are encountered with classical Brescia–Cimino fistulas.

Acknowledgement

We thank Ms H. Wolff for secretarial help.

References

1 Rao, T. K. S., Hirsch, S., Avram, M. M. and Friedman, E. A. (1980). Prevalence of diabetic nephropathy in Brooklyn. In Friedman, E. A. and l'Esperance, F. A. (eds.). *Diabetic Renal–Retinal Syndrome*, p. 205. (New York: Grune & Stratton)

2 Gutman, R. A., Stead, W. W. and Robinson, R. R. (1981). Physical activity and employment status of patients on maintenance hemodialysis. *N. Engl. J. Med.*, **304**, 309

3 Shapiro, F. L. and Comty, Ch. M. (1980). Hemodialysis in diabetics – 1979 update. In Friedman, E. A. and l'Esperance, F. A. (eds.). *Diabetic Renal–Retinal Syndrome*, p. 333. (New York: Grune & Stratton)

4 Jacobs, C., Broyer, M., Brunner, F. P., Brygner, H., Donckerwolcke, R. A., Kramer, P., Selwood, N. H., Wing, A. J. and Blake, P. H. (1981). Combined report on regular dialysis and transplantation in Europe, XI, 1980. In *Proc. of the Europ. Dial. and Transplant Assoc.*, vol. 18, p. 4. (Tunbridge Wells: Pitman Medical)

5 Ghavamian, M., Gutch, Ch. F., Kopp, K. F. and Kolff, W. J. (1972). The sad truth about hemodialysis in diabetic nephropathy. *J. Am. Med. Assoc.*, **222**, 1386

6 Kassissieh, S. D., Yen, M. C., Lazarus, J. M., Lowrie, E. G., Goldstein, H. H., Takacs, F. J., Hampers, C. L. and Merrill, J. P. (1974). Hemodialysis-related problems in patients with diabetes mellitus. *Kidney Int.*, **6**, 100

7 Katirtzoglou, A., Oreopoulos, D. G., Dombros, N., Blair, G. R., Chisholm, L., Meema, H. E., Ogilvie, R., Vas, S., Leibel, B. and McCreedy, W. (1980). Chronic peritoneal dialysis in diabetics with end-stage renal failure. In Friedman, E. A. and l'Esperance, F. A. (eds.). *Diabetic Renal–Retinal Syndrome*, p. 317. (New York: Grune & Stratton)

8 El Shahat, Y., Rottembourg, J., Jacobs, C. and Legrain, M. (1976). Traitement de l'insuffisance rénale terminale chez les diabétiques insulino-dépendants par les méthodes de dialyse. Un bilan de neuf années d'experience. In Grünfeld, J. -P. (ed.) *Actualités Néphrologiques de L'Hôpital Necker*, p. 222. (Paris: Flammarion Médicine-Sciences)

9 Levin, N. W., Dumler, F., Venkatachalam, K. K., Lakier, J. and Aman, I. (1981). Experience with vascular access survival in diabetic and non-diabetic hemodialysis patients. Abstr. DI-113, p. 421; presented at the 8th International Congress of Nephrology, Athens

10 Butt, K. M. H., Ortega-Gaytan, M., Shirani, K., Hong, J. H., Adamson, R. J., Manis, Th. and Friedman, E. A. (1981). Angioaccess in uremic diabetics. Abstr. In Friedman, E. A. and l'Esperance, F. A. (eds.). *Diabetic Renal–Retinal Syndrome*, pp. 209–210. (New York: Grune & Stratton)

31

Vascular access survival in diabetic and non-diabetic haemodialysis patients

L. C. AMAN, D. W. SMITH, H. K. OH AND N. W. LEVIN

INTRODUCTION

A significant proportion of the 55 000 patients currently haemodialysed in the USA are diabetic, both juvenile and adult onset types[1]. Access site problems faced by haemodialysis patients, including thrombosis, infection and frequent hospitalizations, are compounded in the diabetic haemodialysis population[2]. Construction of an arteriovenous (A-V) fistula is not always possible in diabetics, due to the accelerated arteriosclerosis that occurs in these patients[3-5]. A-V fistulas in diabetics have considerably shorter survival times and higher complication rates than in non-diabetics[2]. Bovine hetero-grafts and polytetrafluoroethylene (PTFE) grafts are alternatives to the A-V fistula but are frequently used as a second or third choice, after problems have already occurred, rather than as a primary access[6-9].

We have previously reported results of a co-operative study[2] that retro-spectively analysed the medical and economic consequences of complications occurring in the use of internal vascular access devices. We have extended this study to analyse in more detail vascular access survival in a diabetic population on haemodialysis.

MATERIALS AND METHODS

Using a standardized reporting procedure, data were obtained from 464 patients on haemodialysis in the participating centres. Permanent internal accesses in patients who had been on chronic haemodialysis (CHD) for a minimum of 3 months were studied: 19% (88) patients were diabetic and 81% (376) were non-diabetic. Table 31.1 shows the distribution of diabetic and non-diabetic patients by race, sex, median age and period of time on dialysis. Table 31.2 shows the distribution of 713 internal accesses in both diabetic and non-diabetic patients.

Table 31.1 Distribution of diabetic and non-diabetic patients

	Diabetic 88 *(19%)*		*Non-diabetic* 376 *(81%)*	
Male	39	(44.3%)	211	(56.1%)
Female	49	(55.7%)	165	(43.9%)
White	23	(26.1%)	174	(46.3%)
Black	65	(73.9%)	202	(53.7%)
Median age	56		50	
Range	20–76		18–85	
Time on CHD	27 months		37 months	
Range	3–74 months		5–143 months	

Percentage distribution is shown in parentheses

Two access survival periods were chosen for analysis: (1) the period until the first complication requiring hospitalization (complication-free survival), and (2) the period until replacement (survival) of the access was necessary[2]. The difference between the two survival times is the extension of survival achieved by surgical techniques.

Table 31.2 Distribution of internal access types

Access type	*Total*	*Patient type*			
		Diabetic		*Non-diabetic*	
A-V fistulas	400	60	(15%)	340	(85%)
Bovine grafts	224	65	(29%)	159	(71%)
PTFE grafts	89	17	(19%)	72	(81%)
Total	713	142	(20%)	571	(80%)

Percentage distribution is shown in parentheses

Survival times were analysed using clinical life-tables with log-rank tests[10] and Cox's multiple variable regression model for censored survival data[11]. Cox's model simultaneously estimates the effect of several risk factors on survival. This permits examination of the main effects of diabetes, sex, age, race and institution, in a single analysis. Furthermore, Cox's model allows examination of the differential effect of other factors on access survival in diabetics and non-diabetics by including the two-factor interactions of diabetes with the other factors of age, sex, race and institution.

RESULTS

Patient data

Graft survival and complication-free graft survival curves are compared in diabetics and non-diabetics with A-V fistulas (Figure 31.1), bovine grafts (Figure 31.2), and PTFE grafts (Figure 31.3). The three types of accesses differed significantly in survival ($p < 0.0001$; log-rank test) in non-diabetics but not in diabetics ($p < 0.43$; log-rank test). Similarly, the complication-free survival of three access types differed significantly in non-diabetics ($p < 0.0001$; log-rank test) but not in diabetics ($p < 0.88$; log-rank test). For A-V fistulas, diabetics differed from non-diabetics in both survival ($p = 0.0001$; log-rank test) and complication-free survival ($p = 0.0002$; log-rank test). For bovine grafts, diabetics were not significantly different from

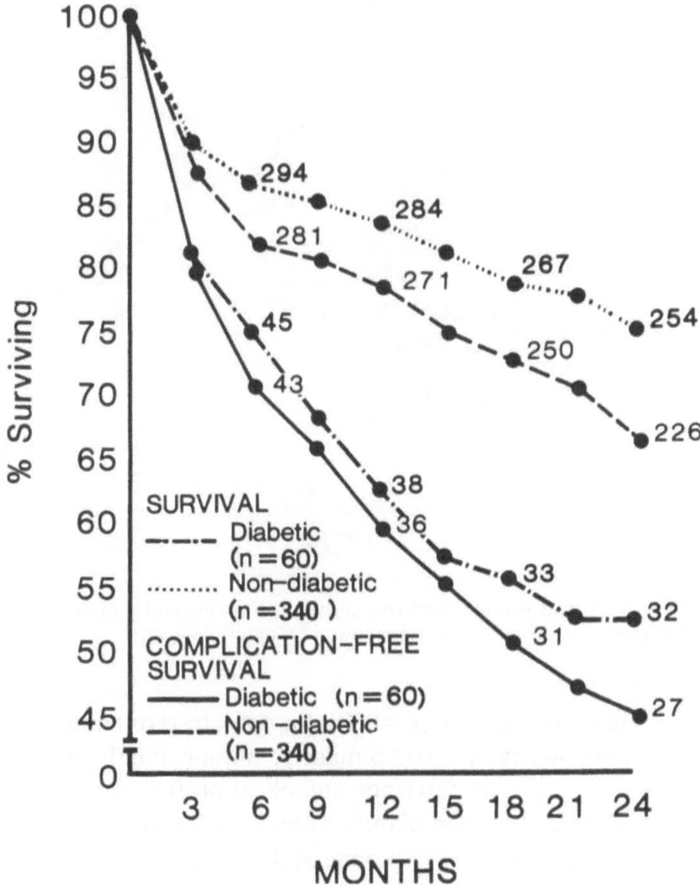

Figure 31.1 Survival and complication-free survival of A-V fistulas in diabetics and non-diabetics (the number of surviving grafts is shown at 6-month intervals)

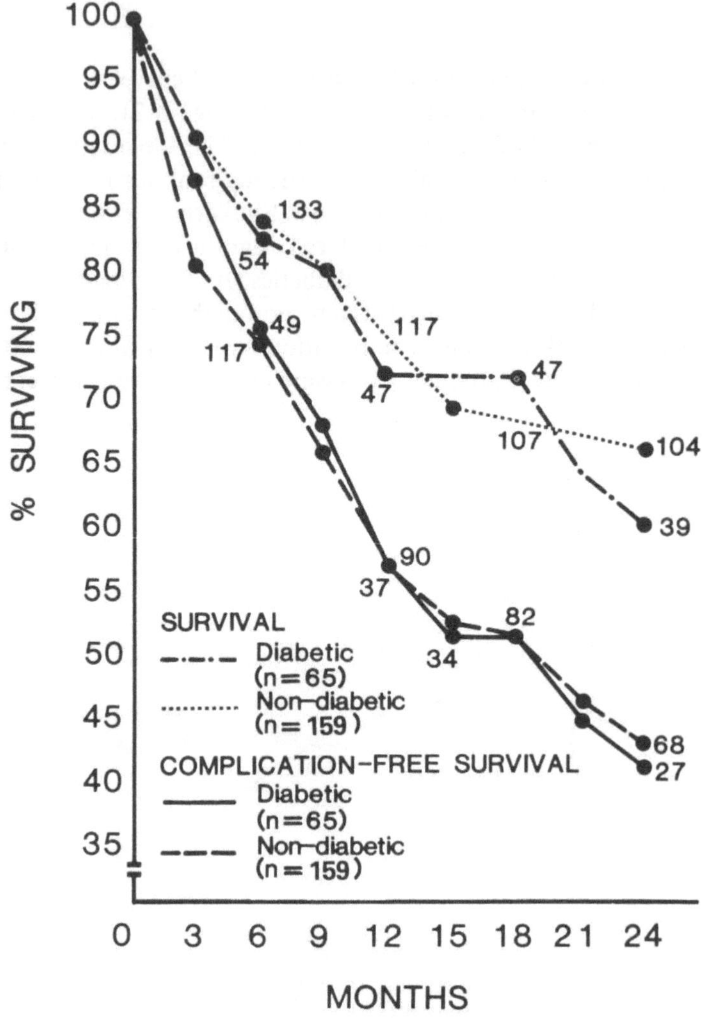

Figure 31.2 Survival and complication-free survival of bovine grafts in diabetics and non-diabetics (the number of surviving grafts is shown at 6-month intervals)

non-diabetics in either survival ($p=0.60$; log-rank test) or complication-free survival ($p=0.90$; log-rank test). Similarly, among PTFE grafts, neither survival ($p=0.09$; log-rank test) nor complication-free survival ($p=0.50$; log-rank test) differed between diabetics and non-diabetics.

For each type of access (A-V, bovine and PTFE), two multiple variable Cox regression models for survival and complication-free survival are shown (Tables 31.3–31.5). The first model for each type of graft includes only the main effects of sex, age, race, diabetes and institution. The second

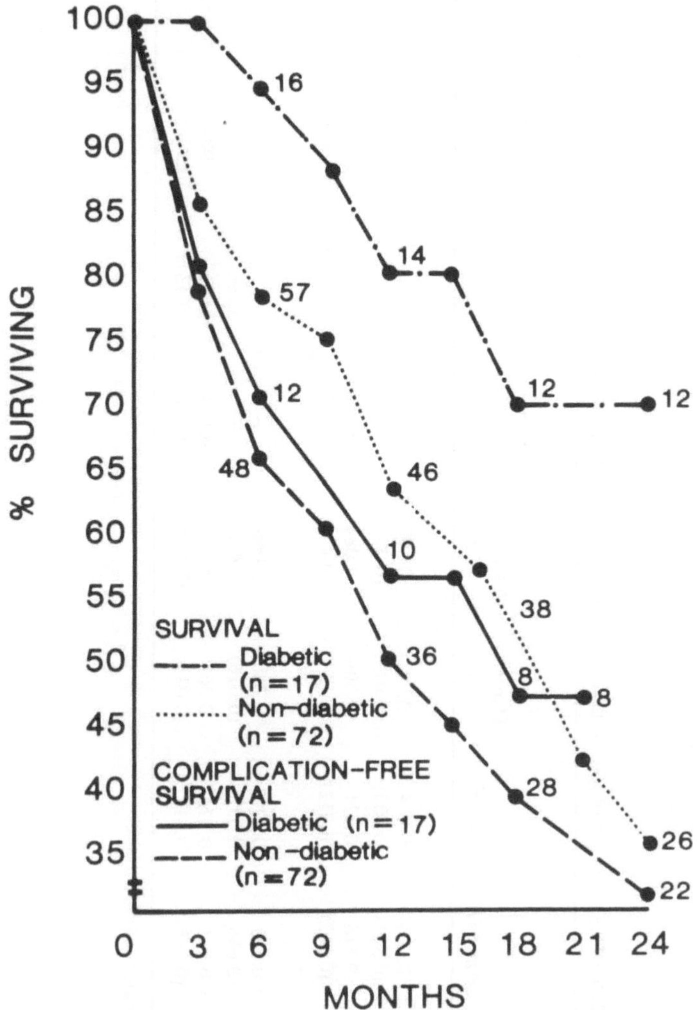

Figure 31.3 Survival and complication-free survival of PTFE grafts in diabetics and non-diabetics (the number of surviving grafts is shown at 6-month intervals)

model adds the interactions of sex, race, diabetes and institution with diabetes, to the first model. Cox's model for the logarithm of the hazard function, which characterizes the survival distribution, is:

$$\log h(t,x) = g(t) + a_1 X_S + a_2 X_A + a_3 X_R + a_4 X_D + a_5 X_I$$

The independent variables, X_S, X_R, X_D and X_I are sex (X_S), race (X_R), diabetes (X_D), institution (X_I), and age (X_A). Independent variables with non-zero coefficients contribute to the hazard (risk of failure) and conse-

Table 31.3 Cox's multiple variable survival analysis for A-V fistulas*

	Sex (S)	Age (A)	Race (R)	Diabetes (D)	Institution (I)	Interaction effects By S	By A	By R	By I
Survival									
Main effects	−0.184	−0.004	−0.274	0.277	0.100	—	—	—	—
	(0.035)	(0.583)	(0.003)	(0.015)	(0.272)	—	—	—	—
Diabetes interactions	−0.216	−0.116	−0.324	0.308	0.084	−0.044	−0.012	−0.062	−0.042
	(0.042)	(0.162)	(0.012)	(0.018)	(0.444)	(0.680)	(0.136)	(0.629)	(0.705)
Complication-free survival									
Main effects	−0.260	−0.003	−0.170	0.248	0.066	—	—	—	—
	(0.001)	(0.666)	(0.032)	(0.016)	(0.418)	—	—	—	—
Diabetes interactions	−0.340	−0.011	−0.172	0.301	0.101	−0.124	−0.012	0.003	0.056
	(0.001)	(0.168)	(0.118)	(0.010)	(0.324)	(0.211)	(0.131)	(0.981)	(0.588)

*Parameter estimates are shown with *p* values in parentheses

Table 31.4 Cox's multiple variable survival analysis for bovine grafts*

	Sex (S)	Age (A)	Race (R)	Diabetes (D)	Institution (I)	Interaction effects			
						By S	By A	By R	By I
Survival									
Main effects	−0.037	0.003	0.087	0.127	−0.216	—	—	—	—
	(0.769)	(0.769)	(0.508)	(0.342)	(0.080)	—	—	—	—
Diabetes interactions	−0.138	0.001	0.165	0.182	−0.136	−0.152	−0.010	0.135	0.201
	(0.367)	(0.953)	(0.290)	(0.271)	(0.314)	(0.320)	(0.248)	(0.385)	(0.138)
Complication-free survival									
Main effects	0.016	0.005	0.146	0.017	0.044	—	—	—	—
	(0.868)	(0.445)	(0.152)	(0.872)	(0.644)	—	—	—	—
Diabetes interactions	−0.055	0.002	0.150	0.003	0.125	−0.126	−0.013	0.003	0.169
	(0.641)	(0.821)	(0.257)	(0.982)	(0.268)	(0.284)	(0.081)	(0.982)	(0.135)

*Parameter estimates are shown with p values in parentheses

Table 31.5   Cox's multiple variable survival analysis for PTFE grafts*

	Sex(S)	Age(A)	Race(R)	Diabetes (D)	Institution (I)
Survival					
Main effects	0.022	0.016	-0.015	-0.520	0.425
	(0.913)	(0.276)	(0.944)	(0.078)	(0.074)
Complication-free survival					
Main effects	0.022	0.016	-0.015	-0.520	0.425
	(0.913)	(0.277)	(0.946)	(0.079)	(0.075)

*Parameter estimates are shown with p values in parentheses

quently affect the survival times. The coefficients (a_I) can be estimated by the method of maximum likelihood. Their estimated standard deviation can be used to test whether the estimates are significantly different from zero, that is whether a variable contributes to the hazard, and to survival. Further details may be found in Kalbfleisch and Prentice[11].

For PTFE grafts the maximum likelihood estimation procedure did not converge to a solution when interactions were included, because the sample sizes were small, so parameter estimates for these models are not reported in Table 31.5. Each table shows the estimated coefficient of age in years, and estimated coefficients of binary dummy variables for categorical variables such as sex and race. Beneath each coefficient is its asymptotic p-value.

The incidences of patient hospitalizations for the management of access complications are shown in Table 31.6. In both diabetics and non-diabetics, thrombosis or poor flow was the most frequent cause for admission. A-V fistulas had the highest incidence, and PTFE grafts the lowest incidence of thrombosis in the diabetic groups. Conversely, bovine grafts had the highest incidence, and A-V fistulas the lowest incidence of thrombosis in the non-diabetic group. Overall, diabetics with PTFE grafts appeared to have the lowest incidence of complications, while those with A-V fistulas had the most complications.

Economic impact

The hospital charges at the time of analysis at one institution (Henry Ford Hospital) for the treatment of access complications of A-V fistulas, bovine and PTFE grafts in diabetic and non-diabetic patients are shown in Table 31.7. These figures include only the costs related to the procedure performed, i.e., semi-private room, local anaesthesia, surgical fees (including materials used) and operating-room fees. Routine laboratory studies, intravenous solutions, antibiotics, and other treatments were excluded. The diabetic group had 0.35 admissions/patient-month at an average cost of $3195.00 per admission. The non-diabetic group had 0.02 admissions/patient-month at an average cost of $4160.00 per admission. The overall annual cost of access

Table 31.6 Access complications requiring hospitalization

Access type	Number of grafts	Aneurysm		Poor flow/ thrombosis		Infection		Other		Total complications	
A-V fistulas	Diabetic (60)	5	(8.3)	35	(58.3)	1	(1.7)	3	(5.0)	44	(73.3)
	Non-diabetic (340)	16	(4.7)	130	(38.2)	21	(6.2)	9	(2.6)	176	(51.8)
Bovine grafts	Diabetic (65)	3	(4.6)	26	(40.0)	9	(13.8)	7	(10.8)	45	(69.2)
	Non-diabetic (159)	17	(10.7)	69	(43.4)	24	(15.1)	7	(4.4)	117	(73.6)
PTFE grafts	Diabetic (17)	0	(0.0)	6	(35.3)	0	(0.0)	0	(0.0)	6	(35.3)
	Non-diabetic (72)	1	(1.4)	29	(40.2)	18	(25.0)	4	(5.6)	52	(72.2)
Total	Diabetic (142)	8	(5.7)	67	(47.2)	10	(7.0)	10	(7.0)	95	(66.9)
	Non-diabetic (571)	34	(6.0)	228	(39.9)	63	(11.0)	20	(3.5)	345	(60.4)

Each entry shows the number of complications with the rate per hundred grafts in parentheses complications for the 187 diabetic and non-diabetic patients is approximately $214 000.00.

The charges were broken down separately for each graft type. In the A-V fistula group 17 diabetics had 0.023 admissions/patient-month at $2204.00 per admission; 40 non-diabetics had 0.009 admissions/patient-month at $3106.00 per admission. In the bovine group 20 diabetics had 0.04 admissions/patient-month at $3886.00 per admission; 42 non-diabetics had 0.034 admissions/patient-month at $4641.00 per admission. Four diabetics with PTFE grafts had 0.073 admission/patient-month at $6327.00 per admission. Six non-diabetics with PTFE grafts had 0.06 admissions/patient-month at $4471.00 per admission.

Table 31.7 Henry Ford Hospital: cost analysis, diabetic vs. non-diabetic patients

Overall (*all three access types*)	Diabetic ($n=43$)	Non-diabetic ($n=144$)
No. patients with complications requiring hospitalization	25	57
No. admissions	46	102
No. days/admission	8.7	8.7
No. patient-months	1279	5120
No. admissions/patient-month	0.035	0.02
Mean cost/admission	$3915.00	$4160.00
Mean cost/patient-month	137.00	83.00
Annual mean cost/patient	1644.00	996.00

DISCUSSION

A-V fistulas in diabetics had significantly lower survival and complication-free survival than in non-diabetics, but surprisingly, such differences were not present for either bovine or PTFE grafts. There is little difference between the survival and complication-free survival curves of A-V fistulas in both diabetics and non-diabetics, indicating that complications occurring in connection with A-V fistulas are difficult to correct and usually result in graft failure. Complication-free survival of bovine and PTFE grafts was shorter than total survival in both the diabetic and non-diabetic groups, indicating that efforts to repair these grafts are effective and more successful than those made to repair A-V fistulas[8].

In six diabetic haemodialysis patients previously reported, all had problems with the internal A-V fistula used as an initial access, requiring revision and/or replacement in all cases[12]. Although this question is controversial, chronic dialysis may contribute to the accelerated arteriosclerosis already present in diabetic patients[13]. This theory suggests that the severe vascular changes that are present in diabetics[4,14] may be a further indication for the use of bovine and/or PTFE grafts as initial accesses in diabetic haemodialysis patients[8,14,15].

The multiple variable survival analyses show that diabetics are at greater risk for both complications and graft failure. The lack of significant interaction with other variables shows that this effect is similar for both sexes, both races, all ages, and different institutions. This confirms the simpler univariate analysis of the same variables[2].

As seen in Table 31.7, diabetics have access complications at a rate nearly double that of non-diabetics. The mean cost/admission is about equal, indicating that when both groups are hospitalized, similar problems are treated. When the charges were broken down further for each access type, the mean cost/admission was generally slightly higher for the non-diabetic group (excluding PTFE grafts), but the number of admissions/patient-month was greater for diabetics, especially those in the A-V fistula group. In the small PTFE graft group, the yearly cost/patient was 30% higher than for the bovine graft group, possibly indicating the bias that in this series PTFE grafts were utilized only after vascular problems had occurred with other access types.

Further clinical trials aiming at prevention of thrombosis as the major access problem, e.g. through antiplatelet drug therapy, are vital to the medical and economic well-being of chronic dialysis patients, especially diabetics. When there is a proven method for the prevention of access site thrombosis, we will no longer need to refer to vascular access as the 'Achilles heel'[16] of the dialysis patient.

Acknowledgements

We are grateful to the following co-operating institutions: BMA of Detroit and Hutzel Hospital, Detroit, Michigan (Franklin D. McDonald, MD, James E. Lawson, DO); Detroit Osteopathic Hospital, Detroit, Michigan (Anthony Malcoun, DO, Michael T. Keefe, DO, Gary L. Slick, DO); Henry Ford Hospital, Detroit, Michigan (Pedro Cortes, MD, Cosme Cruz, MD, Stanley G. Dienst, MD, Francis Dumler, MD, Godofredo Santiago, MD, K. K. Venkatachalam, MD); Mount Carmel Mercy Hospital, Detroit, Michigan (Sidney Baskin, MD); St Clair Renal Center (Joseph Beal, MD); Samaritan Renal Center, Detroit, Michigan (T. Kim, MD, J. Park, MD); Wayne County General Hospital, Westland, Michigan (Gerald A. Rigg, MD); Veteran's Administration Medical Center, Ann Arbor, Michigan (Friedrich K. Port, MD); William Beaumont Hospital, Royal Oak, Michigan (Howard S. Shapiro, MD).

References

1 Friedman, E. A., Delano, R. G. and Butt, K. M. (1978). Pragmatic realities in uremia therapy. *N. Engl. J. Med.*, **298**, 368

2 Aman, L., Levin, N. W. and Smith, D. (1980). Hemodialysis access site morbidity. *Proc. Clin. Dial. Transpl. Forum*, **10**, 277

3 Brescia, M. J., Cimino, J. E., Appel, K. and Hurwich, B. J. (1966). Chronic hemodialysis using a surgically created arteriovenous fistula. *N. Engl. J. Med.*, **275**, 1089

4 Colwell, J. A., Lopes-Virella, M. and Halushka, P. V. (1981). Pathogenesis of atherosclerosis in diabetes mellitus. *Diabetes Care*, **4**, 121

5 Zincke, H. (1976). Critical review of the use of carotid bovine grafts for hemodialysis. *Eur. Surg. Res.*, **8**, 189

6 Baker, L. D., Johnson, J. M. and Goldfarb, D. (1976). Expanded polytetrafluoroethylene (PTFE) subcutaneous arteriovenous conduit: an improved vascular access for chronic hemodialysis. *Trans. Am. Soc. Artif. Intern. Organs*, **22**, 382

7 Elliott, M. P., Gazzaniga, A. B., Thomas, J. M., Haiduc, N. J. and Rosen, S. M. (1977). Use of expanded polytetrafluoroethylene grafts for vascular access in hemodialysis: laboratory and clinical evaluation. *Am. Surg.*, **43**, 455

8 Kaplan, M. S., Mirahmadi, K. S., Winer, R. L., Gorman, J. T., Dabirvaziri, N. and Rosen, S. M. (1976). Comparison of 'PTFE' and bovine grafts for blood access in dialysis patients. *Trans. Am. Soc. Artif. Intern. Organs*, **22**, 388

9 Katzman, H. E., Schild, A. F. and VanderWerf, B. A. (1976). Bovine artegraft arteriovenous fistulas for hemodialysis in one hundred patients after 'conventional' arteriovenous fistulas failed. *Vasc. Surg.*, **10**, 169

10 Peto, R., Pike, M. C., Armitage, P., Breslow, N. E., Cox, D. R., Howard, S. V., Mantel, N., McPherson, K., Peto, J., Smith, P. G. (1976, 1977). Design and analysis of randomized clinical trials requiring prolonged observation of each patient. *Br. J. Cancer*, **34**, 585 (Part I); **35**, 1 (Part II)

11 Kalbfleisch, J. D. and Prentice, R. L. (1980). *The Statistical Analysis of Failure Time Data.* (New York: Wiley)

12 Thayssen, P., Roed-Petersen, K., Nielsen, F. U., Svendsen, V. and Kemp, E. (1977). Treatment of end-stage renal failure in insulin-dependent diabetic patients. *Acta Med. Scand.*, **201**, 469

13 Bagdade, J. D. (1980). *Accelerated Atherosclerosis in Patients on Maintenance Hemodialysis*, pp. 7–20. (Chicago: Year Book Publishers)

14 Giacchino, J. L., Geis, W. P., Buckingham, J. M., Vertuno, L. L. and Bansal, V. K. (1979). Vascular access: long-term results, new techniques. *Arch. Surg.*, **114**, 403

15 Sannella, N. A., Mehigan, J. T., Pennell, J. P., Halpren, B. and Fogarty, T. J. (1976). Initial approach to blood access for the chronic hemodialysis patient − the bovine heterograft. *Trans. Am. Soc. Artif. Intern. Organs*, **22**, 394

16 Kjellstrand, C. M. (1978). The Achilles' heel of the hemodialysis patient. *Arch. Intern. Med.*, **138**, 1063

32

Abstracts of posters in Complications

Analysis of 326 vascular accesses and their complications
M. HABERAL, R. YALIN, A. ÖZENC, Z. ÖNER, H. GÜLAY and
N. BILGIN

From November 1975 to January 1982, 326 vascular accesses have been performed in 258 chronic renal failure patients. Of these patients 161 (62.5%) were male and 97 (37.5%) were female, between the ages of 6 and 65 years. 273 (83.7%) vascular accesses were arteriovenous (A-V) fistulas, 53 graft fistulas were performed. 216 A-V fistulas were performed on the wrist. 179 (82.8%) of these were side-to-side, 44 (20.3%) end-to-side and three (1.3%) end-to-end anastomoses. 54 (19.7%) fistulas were performed on the anticubital area.

27 (50%) of them were side-to-side and 27 (50%) end-to-side anastomoses.

Bleeding 17 (5.2%), early thrombosis 55 (16.9%), late thrombosis 27 (8.2%), infection 25 (7.6%), pseudoaneurysm 15 (4.6%) and reoperation or revision 54 (16.8%). In addition to these complications, one steal syndrome, one left arm disarticulation, and three cyanosis and swelling in the left hand were seen. One graft was removed due to infection and another one due to thrombosis. One of the PTFE grafts has been functioning for 6 months.

The most frequent complication in our series was thrombosis. This, however was mainly due to inherent vascular pathology rather than surgical technique. The vessels of chronic renal patients are of vital importance; therefore they should be used very carefully.

Central venous stenosis following upper arm arteriovenous fistulas
W. P. REED, P. D. LIGHT and J. A. SADLER

The brachial artery to basilic vein fistula with subcutaneous transposition of the vein has provided a useful alternative fistula for patients with inadequate or previously utilized forearm veins. High 1- and 2-year patency rates, with few reported complications, have encouraged use of these fistulas as a first alternative to forearm access. In the past year, three confirmed and two suspected cases of subclavian vein stenosis have appeared as late complications in patients with upper arm fistulas in place for 2–4 years. The most prominent clinical features of this stenosis were uncorrectable fistula thrombosis or the gradual onset of oedema in the involved extremity. It was possible to salvage the fistula and reverse the oedema in one patient by performing a bypass from the cephalad portion of the basilic vein to the jugular vein, but in general central venous stenosis precluded further use of the extremity for vascular access. Although relatively uncommon, the complication of central venous stenosis should caution against moving too rapidly to upper arm fistulas in patients who may require years of dialysis. Every attempt should be made to salvage stenotic or thrombosed forearm fistulas, before using the arm proper.

A study of fistula survival in 25 171 unipuncture haemodialyses
M. DE CLIPPELE, R. VANHOLDER and S. RINGOIR

Fistula survival rate and complication profile occurring in the Brescia–Cimino arteriovenous fistulas of 65 chronic hospital haemodialysis patients, routinely treated with the unipuncture technique, were studied. For that purpose, the history of the fistulas of all patients in our chronic haemodialysis programme between January 1981 and December 1981 is analysed. The average follow-up period per patient was 33.54 ± 3.76 months, covering 25 171 haemodialysis sessions. The fistulas' survival rate averaged 28.31 ± 2.95 months, with 51 fistulas still being patent at the end of the study. Most common complications were thrombosis (13), local infection (18), septicaemia (8), inadequate flow (11) and aneurysm (3). Thirteen fistulas were replaced, the majority because of thrombosis (7). No mortal complications occurred. Twenty-eight fistulas remained in use for more than 3 years, 13 for more than 5 years, four for more than 7 years.

It is concluded that Brescia–Cimino fistulas in chronic unipuncture dialysis have a good survival rate; further studies are necessary to allow a comparison with the bipuncture technique. The unipuncture system used was a pressure–pressure device, the double-headed pump.

Typical stenosis and aneurysms of Cimino fistula by puncture
G. KRÖNUNG

Each puncture of the fistula makes a small separation of the tissue puncture filled by thrombosis. In the case of the often-used 'arterial' and 'venous' area their addition in the longitudinal axis and in the front side of the shunt vessel causes a typical elongation and torsion of the vessel with creation of two aneurysms and a central stenosis. This stenosis often leads to shunt thrombosis by additional turbulence and Bernoulli effect.

Typical cases, and their therapy in rewidening the stenosis by correct puncture and prophylaxis are demonstrated.

Multicentre* study of the vascular access in haemodialysis patients treated with single-needle double-headed blood pump system
J. P. VAN WAELEGHEM and M. M. ELSEVIERS

The survival and complications of 470 vascular accesses (VA) in 291 patients (125 males, 165 females, mean age 47.5 ± 17.1 years) from nine Flemish dialysis centres have been studied. All patients have been routinely dialysed using the single-needle double-headed blood pump system: fourteen per cent of the patients were below 40 years of age, 50% from 40 to 60 and 36% over 60 years. The mean duration of treatment was 42.0 ± 33.9 months. VA survival was calculated (see Table 32.1) using the life-table method.

Patients with a unique puncture site have a significantly lower ($p < 0.001$) incidence of thrombosis, infection and haematoma compared to patients with multiple puncture sites. From this study we conclude: the observed survival rate of the Cimino VA in our patients is comparable to earlier observations in two-needle dialysis, the survival rate of the saphena VA and xenograft being superior in our series. Multiple puncture sites are associated with a higher incidence of VA-associated complications.

Long-term follow-up of 170 Brescia–Cimino fistulas
C. H. RUEGSEGGER, J. P. WAUTERS and R. MOSIMANN

From 1975 to 1981, 170 arteriovenous (A-V) fistulas of the Brescia–Cimino type were created in 146 patients as angioaccess for chronic haemodialysis. The complication rate is relatively important ($55/170 = 33\%$) and necessitated a total of 218 operations (1.5 per patient) to maintain fistula patency. The main cause of complication is obstruction ($34/170 = 20\%$), half of them in the early postoperative period before the fistula was used, half at long-term, i.e. more than 2 months. Emergency desobstruction is useful since 15 out of 33 cases (45%) have been desobstructed, even repeatedly. Emergency desobstruction has saved 35% of the obstructed fistulas during the first year, diminishing to 20% during the fifth year. Peripheral vascular disorders were

*Participating nephrologists: I. Becaus, V. Bosteels, M. Christiaens, M. E. De Broe, J. Hilderson, R. Hombrouckx, L. Jansens, R. Lins, W. Lornoy, M. Segaert, J. Stellaert, H. Thomas and G. A. Verpooten.

Table 32.1 Survival of successive VA and survival and complications of the different types of VA

	1st VA	2nd VA	3rd VA	4th VA	VA overall		Scribner	Cimino	Saphena	Xenograft	
Number	287	110	41	22	470		39	345	38	23	Number
Scribner (%)	9	6	5	18	8		28	10	37	28	Percentage thrombosis
Cimino (%)	86	68	49	23	73		15	12	26	19	Percentage infection
Saphena (%)	3	10	26	27	8		—	3	21	9	Percentage aneurysm
Xenograft (%)	2	15	19	32	11		—	41	42	26	Percentage haematoma
Survival 2 years	74	73	65	55	72		22	80	56	75	2 year survival
Percentage 5 years	59	60	52	36	57		—	65	46	59	5 year survival

observed in five patients (2.9%) mainly as venous hypertension. Eight patients presented with venous stenosis, necessitating widening plasty. Infection rate of the fistulas is low (2.9%), 0.9% as immediate postoperative complication. At long-term 11 cases of carpal tunnel syndrome were observed; in the six operated patients decompression was successful. Life-table analysis of 140 fistulas indicates that 10% of the accesses are lost in the first 2 months, mostly for obstruction. The survival rate of these fistulas is 62% at 5 years. Due to this low long-term complication rate, Brescia–Cimino fistulas still appear the best choice as vascular access when chronic haemodialysis has to be initiated.

Aneurysm incidence in angioaccess for haemodialysis
G. ROMANO, C. SASSAROLI, G. NAPPI and P. DE ROSA

In a period of 7 years 14 aneurysms were observed in patients operated on by angioaccess for haemodialysis. Seven of these involved angioaccess with prosthesis interposition (four true aneurysms on homologous vein graft, two false aneurysms and one true one on PTFE grafts); seven developed at different sites of arteriovenous fistulas (three patients had a false aneurysm at the anastomotic, two patients had a true aneurysm of the host vein, two patients had pulsating haematomas of the humeral artery far away from the vascular access and of traumatic origin).

The pathogenesis of the lesions is analysed in detail (multiple punctures for dialysis, progressive yielding of the vein wall, anastomotic stenosis, infection, etc.).

The goals of a correct therapeutic approach are emphasized: correction of damage, respect for distal vascularization and preservation of the vascular access whenever possible.

131 arteriovenous grafts for haemodialysis vascular access
J. A. C. BUCKELS, M. Y. EZZIBDEH and A. D. BARNES

During a 6-year period (June 1975 to June 1981), 92 haemodialysis patients received 131 arteriovenous grafts – 85 bovine carotid artery; 18 PTFE; 18 umbilical vein: seven Sparks mandril; two autogenous saphenous vein; one velour Dacron. This was the primary access procedure in four patients, and 'second-line' in the remaining 88. The primary graft failure rate was 15.3%, being highest, with the Sparks mandril and umbilical vein grafts which accounted for 11/20 primary failure cases. There were 41 secondary graft failures – 17 due to infection (11.8 months average), and 24 due to thrombosis (8 months average). No difference was seen in the failure rate between loop or straight grafts and arm or leg grafts. Thrombosis was the commonest later complication, though thrombectomy was successful in 37 of 63 cases. Only 35 grafts were complication-free, the remaining patients requiring revision or replacement, many undergoing multiple procedures. (Cases associated with infection underwent an average of 3.4 revisions, compared to 1.6 revisions in non-infected complications.) Overall, 70 patients (76%) had successful grafts – 30 functioning at transplantation; 14 functioning at death, and 26 functioning to date (average patency of 30.6 months). Arteriovenous grafts can provide long-term vascular access, but at significant cost to the patient in terms of high revision rate.

33

Invited comment on papers and posters in Complications

J. BANCEWICZ

I must first stress that my comments on vascular access for haemodialysis are those of an outsider to this field. I have never performed an access procedure for dialysis and it is a minor professional ambition never to do so. The organizers originally asked me to comment on the papers in a symposium on complications because I have previously written about the complications of total parenteral nutrition. It therefore came as a surprise to find that the complications of access for nutrition were not mentioned at all in this symposium and demonstrated only briefly in some of the poster displays belonging to other sessions.

It is significant that this has happened since parenteral nutrition is now a successful and safe form of treatment with a low incidence of major complications. Several years ago, however, it seemed that prolonged access for infusion of hypertonic solutions was a more difficult problem than that of access for dialysis. The advent of silicone intravenous catheters and the Broviac and Hickman catheters for long-term use has revolutionized this field. Complications still exist and the greatest danger is infection, but experience has shown the risk of infection can be minimized by scrupulous attention to aseptic technique. Patients can now enjoy a relatively normal lifestyle if long-term nutritional support is required for 'intestinal failure'. The quality of life in such patients is now better than that of the average dialysis patient.

These comments are not altogether irrelevant in a discussion about the problems of haemodialysis since subclavian vein catheters are now used both for acute haemodialysis and for chronic dialysis in certain problem patients. If these methods are to be successful nephrologists will need to take note of the lessons which have been painfully learnt in the field of parenteral nutrition.

In technical discussions the relatively unbiased comments of an outsider are sometimes helpful and I hope that my remarks will generate some useful thoughts. There are, of course, several reasons why it is important to think about complications. Firstly, it is a basic condition of any form of treatment that the doctor should be aware of the risks. Secondly, he needs to know why complications occur and how they can be avoided. Finally, knowledge of the risks may influence the choice of technique.

In the case of vascular access for dialysis one must obviously consider the site at which an access procedure is done, whether in the upper limb or lower limb, and whether this is distal or proximal. The type of procedure may vary from a standard Brescia arteriovenous (A-V) fistula to more complicated A-V graft procedures involving autogenous vein, heterografts or xenografts, or artificial materials such as PTFE. One must also consider alternative strategies, such as chronic peritoneal dialysis which is now well accepted by many patients, and of course the whole question of central venous catheters will have to be carefully considered over the next few years.

What have we learnt from this symposium? We have heard four excellent papers describing a variety of problems and a few remedies. Dr Erasmi and co-workers have given us an excellent survey of the incidence of complications of A-V fistulas. The main message is that occlusion of the shunt is the most common problem. Early occlusion appears to be related to surgical technique whereas late occlusion depends more on the management of the shunt in the dialysis unit. In the poster display Dr Haberal and his colleagues from Turkey describe an 'Analysis of 326 vascular accesses and their complications' with a very similar list of complications. They suggest that thrombosis is due to inherent vascular pathology rather than surgical technique or puncture technique. I do not think that this is the majority view at this conference. Drs Ruegsegger, Wauters and Mosimann report the 'Long-term follow-up of 170 Brescia–Cimino fistulas' in a poster which presents a similar range of problems but they emphasize the importance of emergency reconstruction of occluded fistulas.

Aneurysms are the topic of a poster by Dr Romano and colleagues from Naples who describe 14 aneurysms following access procedures in the upper limb. It is possible to get an aneurysm at almost any site in an A-V graft. There are a variety of causes, but multiple needle punctures may cause some of the problems and will be discussed later.

Finally, to complete the list of complications, Drs Reed, Light and Sadler have presented an excellent, but disturbing poster on 'Central venous stenosis following upper arm arteriovenous fistulas'. They report a low, but definite incidence of major stenosis of the subclavian vein following brachial artery to basilic vein fistulas. This complication presents as either an uncorrectable fistula thrombosis or the gradual onset of upper limb oedema. Central venous thrombosis generally seems to render a limb useless for further vascular access and is obviously a major and important problem. This should counsel against performing A-V graft fistulas in the upper arm when other options remain open.

During the whole of this conference many have stressed that the Brescia–Cimino fistula at the wrist is the most satisfactory form of access for chronic dialysis. Occlusion of these fistulas is the central problem in dialysis access, and if this problem were solved more complex and troublesome procedures would not be required. It is a tribute to surgical ingenuity and modern technology that A-V graft fistulas can be constructed in difficult situations from a large variety of materials. However, Buckels, Ezzibdeh and Barnes in a study of '131 arteriovenous grafts for haemodialysis vascular access' point out that these procedures have a high complication rate and a limited life. Obviously they have a place, but however interesting and challenging to perform they are stopgap solutions, do not address the main problem, and should not be used when simpler and more effective options are available. Dr Slooff and co-workers' paper on the non-thrombotic complications of PTFE grafts would agree with this and he reports a 39% complication rate.

The two papers from Dr Bommer *et al.* and Miss Aman *et al.* on the subject of access in diabetics provide an intriguing controversy. On the one hand, Dr Bommer reports very satisfactory results with the Brescia fistula in diabetics with no evidence of any increase in the complication rate. Miss Aman, however, reports a much greater incidence of complications with Brescia fistulas and comes to the conclusion that more complicated A-V graft fistulas using prosthetic materials are indicated in diabetic patients. Even as an outsider, however, I am not entirely convinced by her arguments. All that she has demonstrated is that Brescia fistulas in this series do surprisingly badly. This is an interesting and important controversy and the reason for the difference between the two studies should be carefully sought. Clearly, Dr Bommer has demonstrated good results with simple fistulas in diabetics and Reilly, Wood and Bell have described elsewhere in this meeting that the Brescia fistula gives excellent results even when vessels are small. One possible explanation for the poor results in the Detroit series is that different surgeons may have performed the Brescia fistulas to those performing the apparently more challenging prosthetic procedures. Miss Aman's comments would be interesting in this respect. I am sure that most delegates at this conference would agree that surgical technique for the construction of fistulas is extremely important.

What then can be done to minimize the complications of these access procedures? Surgical technique has already been mentioned and micro-surgery, or at least the use of magnifying spectacles, is probably an important aid. Although these papers report similar incidences of shunt thrombosis discussion with a number of surgeons outside this session indicates a wide variation in success rates. Some have extremely good results with Brescia fistulas and virtually never need to use prosthetic materials.

What happens to an A-V fistula after its construction may also influence its fate. Drs De Clippele, Vanholder and Ringoir report 'A study of fistula survival in 25 171 unipuncture haemodialyses' and suggest that puncture technique may be important. I was very interested to see that they report better fistula survival in home dialysis patients than those receiving hospital dialysis. There are obviously many differences between home and hospital dialysis patients, but this experience does show that home patients care for their fistulas extremely well. It has certainly been our experience that home parenteral nutrition patients look after their catheters well and we need to encourage the motivation of our patients and staff.

I was intrigued by Dr Kronung's poster on 'Typical stenosis and aneurysms of Cimino fistula by puncture' in which he describes progressive elongation of the venous limb of the fistula due to repeated punctures at multiple sites. As a result the vein becomes kinked and will eventually be occluded. He makes the challenging suggestion that this kinking can be avoided by proper technique and on occasions may be corrected by remedial puncture in just the right place. Drs Van Waeleghem and Elseviers report a 'Multicentre study of the vascular access in haemodialysis patients treated with single-needle double-headed blood pump system'. Although not a randomized trial, they have at least been able to compare the results between clinics using single-needle and double-needle systems. As far as Brescia fistulas are concerned there did not seem to be much difference between the two methods, but the single-needle method was associated with a significantly lower incidence of thrombosis, infection and haematoma in patients who have more complicated A-V graft fistulas. This observation makes sense and great care is obviously needed with the apparently simple business of needling a graft fistula.

This commentary is certainly not intended as the last word at this symposium. My intention is to encourage thought and discussion. I think it worth repeating, however, that even as an outsider to the field of dialysis, I have been impressed, at this conference, that the central problem of vascular access is that of thrombosis of A-V fistulas and graft fistulas. Some patients manage for many years with a single fistula and occasionally even with a Scribner shunt. Why are the rest different? It is this basic problem that must be addressed and not the question of even more complicated surgical procedures with prosthetic materials if vascular access is to have a low complication rate.

Section VII

Management of complications

34

Complications and surgical treatment after angioaccess

B. M. KEMKES AND F. BORCHARD

The use of the Cimino–Brescia fistula is preferred to obtain vascular access for haemodialysis because of a low rate of occlusion, a lower incidence of complications, and it imposes fewer restrictions on the patient.

MATERIALS AND METHODS

Over a period of 9 years, 703 patients were preferred to long-term angio-access. The conventional arteriovenous (A-V) fistula (Group 1) was attempted in a total of 408 patients (330 times using radial artery, 21 ulnaris artery and 57 brachial artery). Because of puncturing veins occluded due to previous infusions, graft fistulas were used 295 times (Group II). Various synthetic and biological–vascular prostheses have been used. 26 Sparks mandril, 200 bovine grafts (102 Solco®, 98 Johnson®) and 20 human umbilical vein cords (HUVC) (10 Dardik® and 10 Mindich®) and 49 PTFE grafts (Gore-tex®). The longest patency rate in the conventional (A-V fistulas) group is 9 years, in group II it is 7 years. While the complication rate in the conventional A-V fistula was only 11%, the incidence of complications in Group II was 32%. HUVC exhibited the highest failure rate and after 1 year none of the grafts was still functioning.

Due to a failure rate of 41%, we no longer use the Sparks mandril, although one remained patent for 5 years. The Solco® grafts showed a complication rate of 38%, the Artegraft® 18% and the PTFE graft 16%. Nevertheless no patient died due to loss of vascular access.

COMPLICATIONS

The use of different materials created several problems. The most common complication seen was graft thrombosis; 16% in our series within 1 year. The

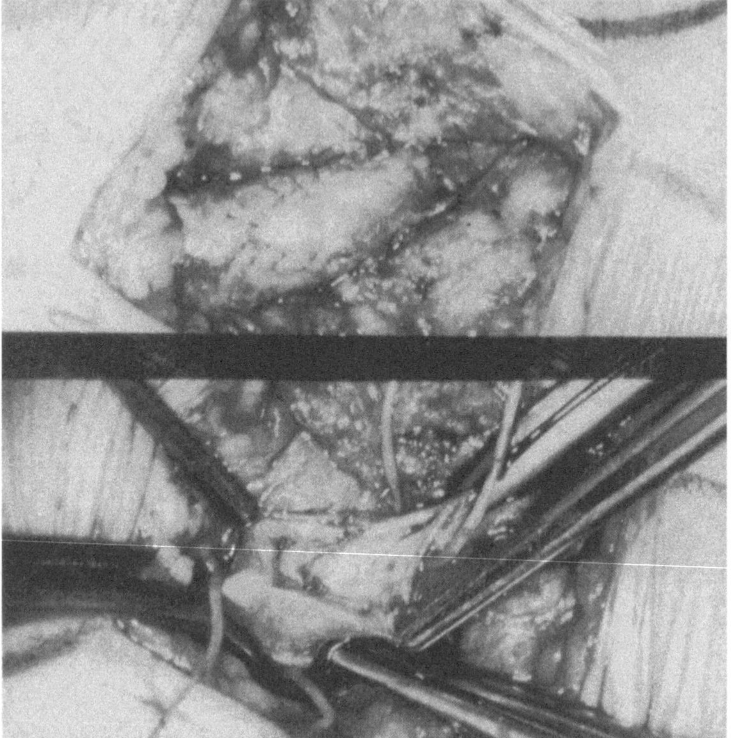

Figure 34.1   Correction of a venous stenotic anastomosis by a patch plasty

function can be re-established easily by means of thrombectomy with a Fogarty catheter within the first 24 h. In PTFE prostheses this is still possible, even after a couple of days. Intimal hyperplasia, as well as pseudodiaphragm formation, usually at the venous anastomosis, was found to be a major cause of graft failure. The latter problem can be corrected with a patch plasty or by a jump graft to a more proximal vein. Another possibility is to construct a new bigger loop around the original[1]. After thrombectomy a longitudinal incision overlapping the lesion in both directions is performed, the stenotic diaphragm removed, and the arteriotomy closed with a venous or heterologous patch (Figure 34.1).

Another reason for thrombosis could be a kinked loop. To avoid this problem, two incisions should be made for positioning the graft in a smooth loop.

We have recognized perigraft seroma formation in 4.6% (Figure 34.2a, b). Seroma aetiology has been ascribed to lymph fistula, graft infection or graft reaction. Erythema and tissue inflammation in the HUVC was very often observed. No treatment methods were found to be effective and the ineffec-

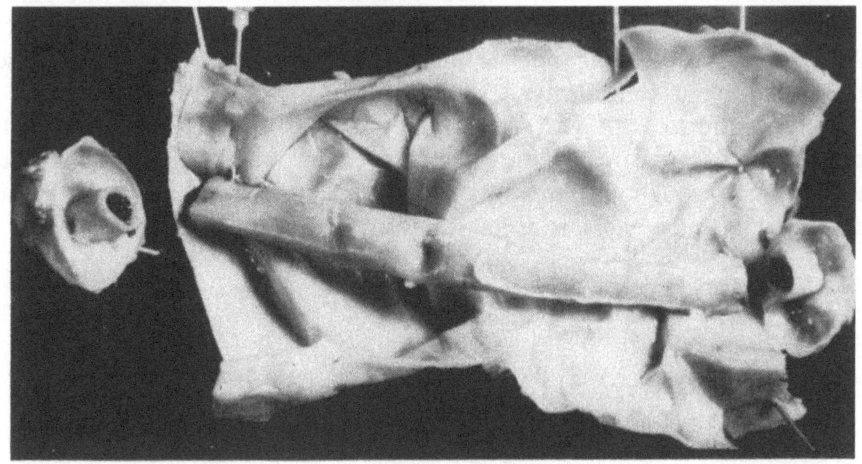

(a)

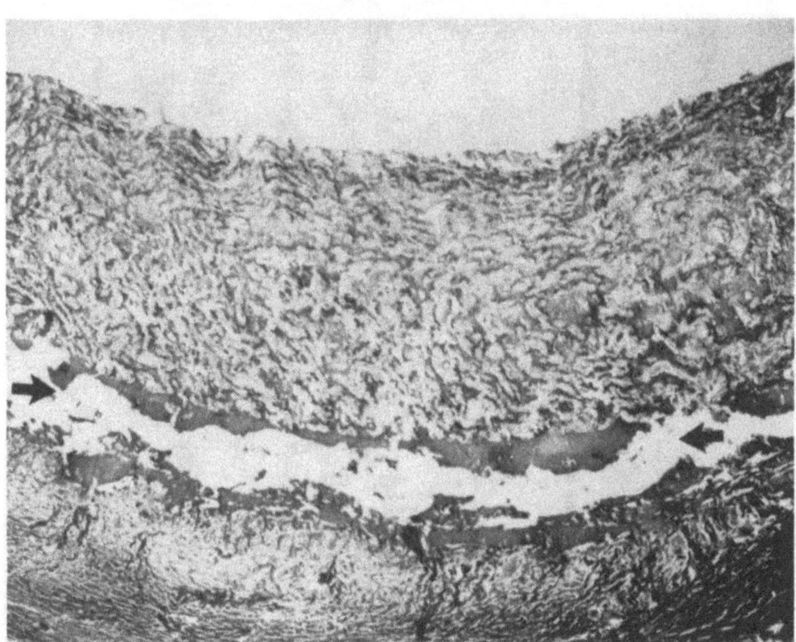

(b)

Figure 34.2 (a) Macroscopical view of a PTFE prosthesis with perigraft seroma. The perigraft accumulation was an erythrocyte-free filtrate either rich or poor in normal serum proteins. (b) Microscopical view of the perigraft seroma (arrow)

tive grafts had to be removed[2]. In cases with small skin ulcerations it is possible to bypass this area with a prosthesis without loss of the graft fistula[1].

Severe ischaemia of the hand in diabetic patients with a high side-to-side A-V fistula were seen between the brachial artery and vein. Symptoms ranged from hand pain, discoloration, venous oedema and swelling of the whole arm to ischaemic neuropathy with marked disability, to gangrene or trophic ulcer. All patients required ligation of the fistula in an effort to relieve these incapacitating arm problems.

Deterioration of the graft substance was also experienced, often with destruction of large areas of the wall in association with multiple thin-walled aneurysms throughout the graft length[3]. A small aneurysm could be corrected by a new end-to-side anastomosis a little bit more proximal[1].

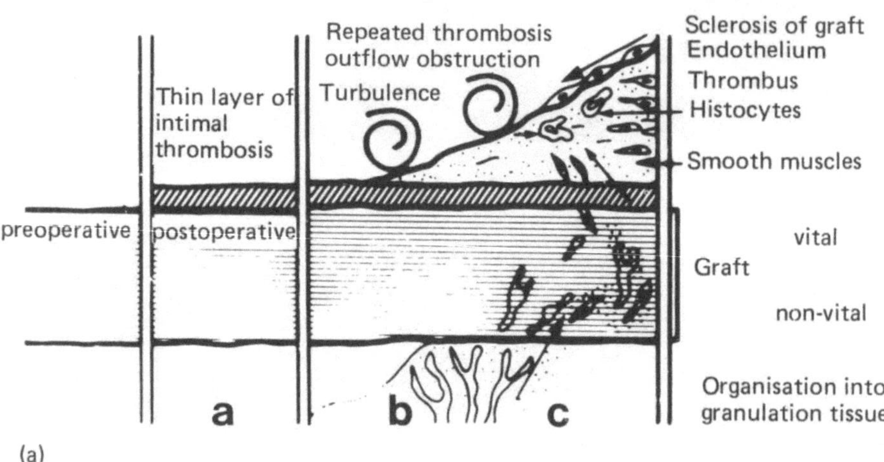

(a)

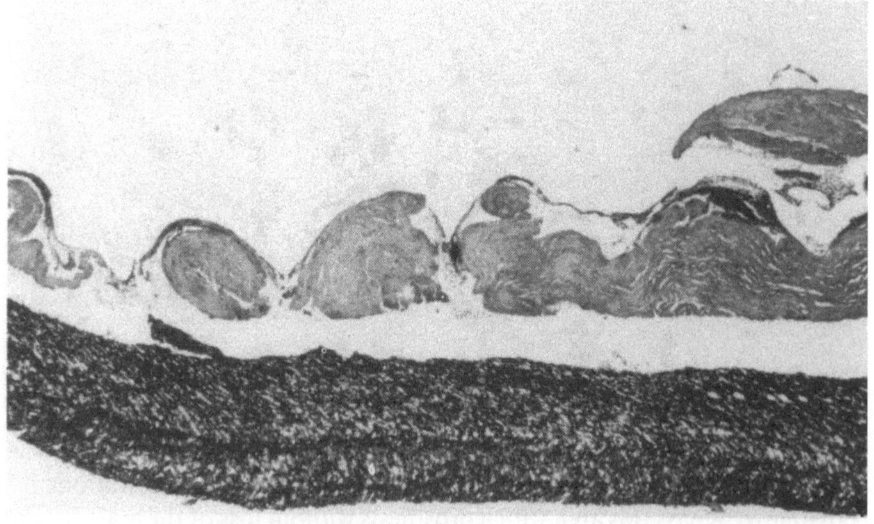

(b)

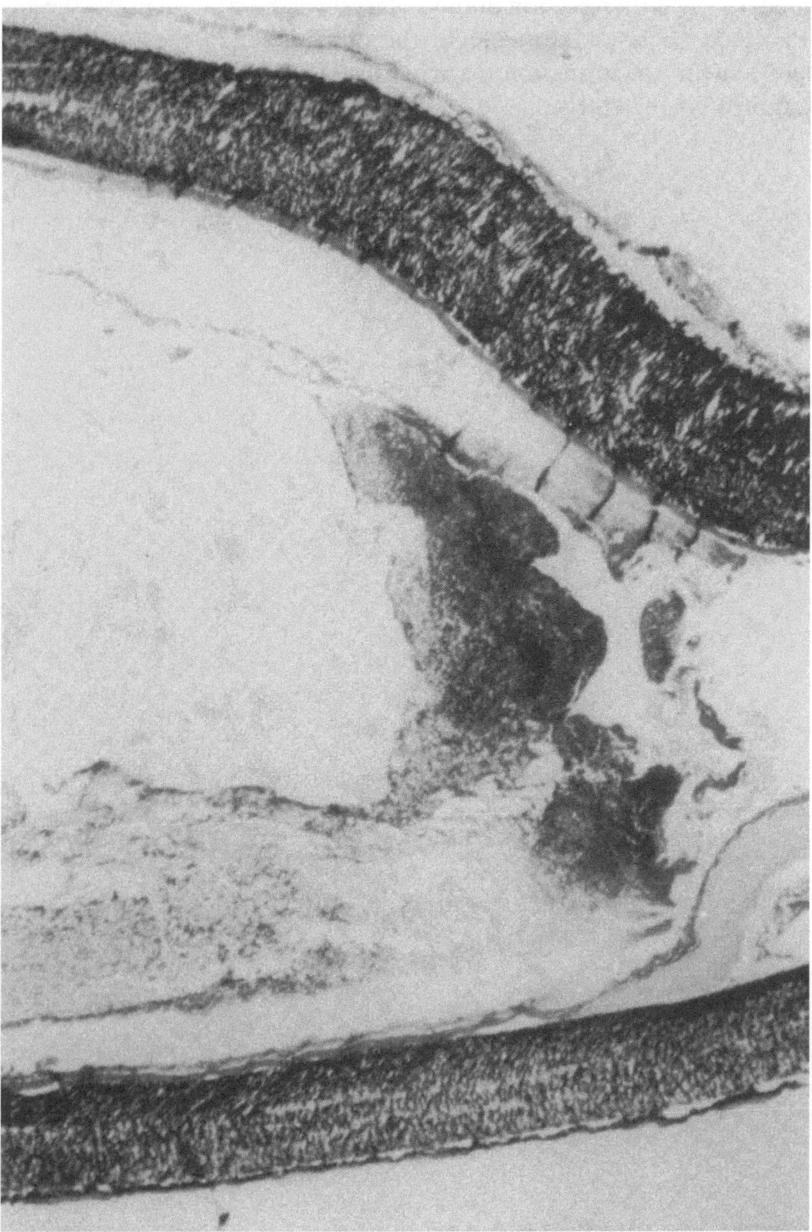

(c)

Figure 34.3 The fate of biological and allogen prostheses: (a) postoperatively you can find a film-like thrombosis; (b) local turbulence causes repeated thrombosis; (c) poor runoff causes an intimal hyperplasia or a pseudodiaphragm with an organized thrombus

Aneurysms in autologous veins were observed between 5 and 8 years of haemodialysis. With resection of the aneurysm and a straight graft, the graft fistula could be re-established. On the other hand in the bovine group (Solco®) aneurysm formation occurred just after 1 year in contrast to the (Johnson®) bovine grafts.

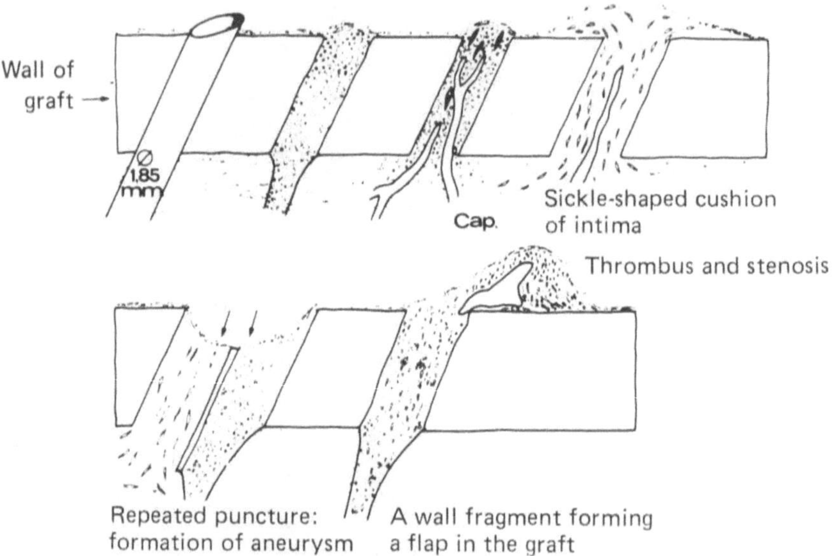

Figure 34.4   Scheme of morphological changes after repeated puncturing of a prosthesis

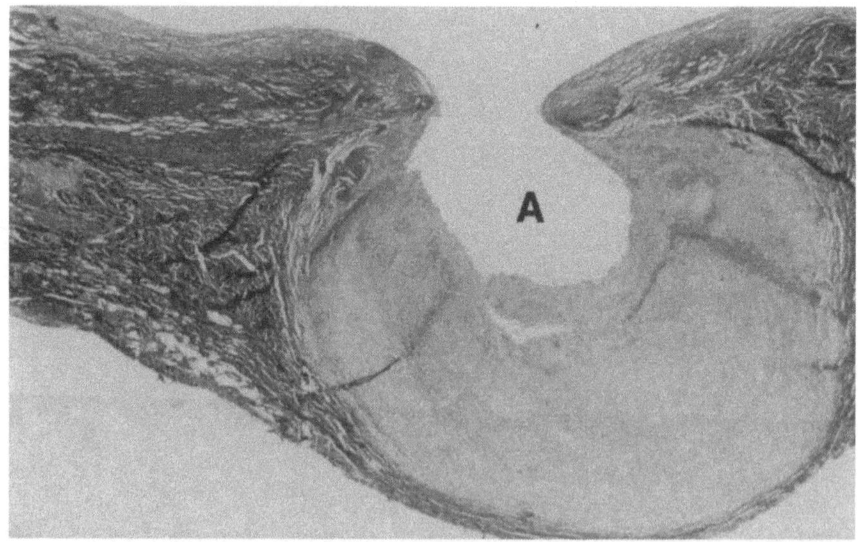

Figure 34.5   Microaneurysm (A) with a parietal thrombus

DISCUSSION

The complications with prostheses could be summarized morphologically in the following scheme (Figure 34.3). Despite the type of the graft material, you can find similar morphological points on both the internal and external layers. The internal layer of all prosthesis, except the autologous vein, shows no viable endothelium. You find only fibrin deposits, covered by endothelial-like cells (Figure 34.4). The presence of subendothelial collagen connective tissue results in the formation of a flat initial thrombosis. Repeated thromboses are usually caused by changes in blood flow rate, for example local turbulences or poor runoff. On the other hand, from the anastomotic site intimal pads are growing in the prostheses. Postoperatively, on the external layer you can find a haemotoma and an enormous number of foreign-body giant cells; after 2 weeks it will be replaced by granulation tissue. Later, capillaries and connective tissue cells are ingrowing. After 3 or 4 years most of these prostheses will be dissolved or show regressive changes like calcification or disintegration of the original matrix. Unfortunately, this disintegration proceeds more quickly than replacement by the patient's own collagen tissue does[4].

A disadvantage of the PTFE prosthesis is the pannus-like proliferation at the anastomotic site as well as the formation of fibrous pads in the area of puncturing (Figure 34.4).

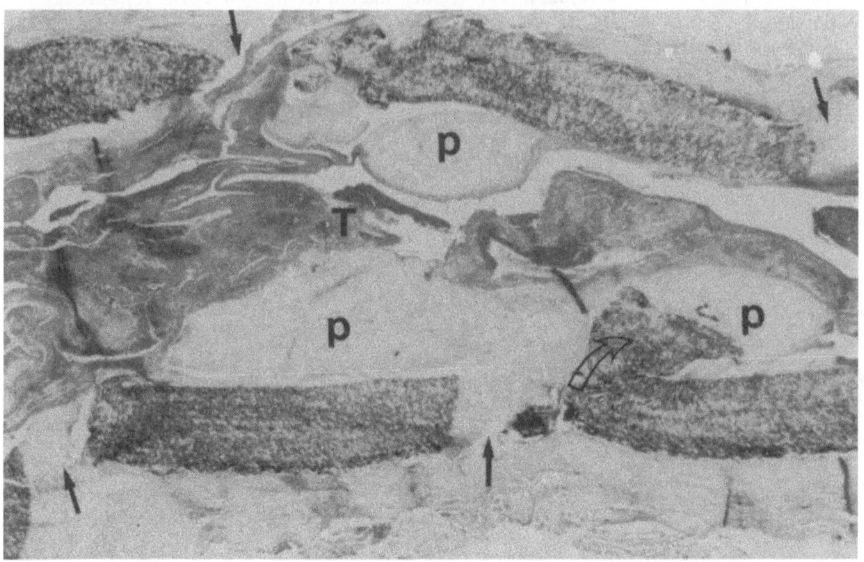

Figure 34.6 Fresh thrombosis (T) of a PTFE prothesis with older fibrous intimal pads (P) in the area of puncturing (arrow). The white arrow shows a flap of PTFE material

After graft puncturing the puncture holes will close with fibrin and a thrombus. Later you can find new deposits of thrombotic material. The other problem is repeated puncturing of the same site. Microaneurysms could occur (Figure 34.5). The third point is producing an intimal flap of PTFE material, which will be covered by new thrombotic deposit (Figure 34.6).

CONCLUSIONS

The continuing appearance of reports of new grafts for access procedures proves that no graft is really satisfactory. Initial reports of new material always sound enthusiastic, but only time reveals the complications and dissatisfactions. Until the ideal access for haemodialysis can be found, it still depends on the surgeon's skill and imagination to make the next angioaccess feasible.

References

1 Kemkes, B. M. (1980). Shuntfibel, Melsungen, Bibliomed.
2 Kemkes, B. M., Reichard, B., Loose, D. A., Borchard, F. and Lenz, W. (1979). Klinische Erfahrungen mit modifizierten homologen Nabelschnurvenen als Gefässprothese zur A-V Fistel. In Ehringer, E., Betz, E., Bollinger, A. and Deutsch, E. (eds.). *Gefässwand, Rezidivprophylaxe, Raynaund-Syndrom*, p. 585. (Baden-Baden, Köln, New York: Witzstrock)
3 Borchard, F., Kemkes, B. M., and Loose, D. A. (1980). Arterienersatz durch biologische Gefässprothesen. Morphologie und klinische Erfahrungen. In Loose, K. E. and Loose, D. A. (eds.). *Gefäss-Patient-Therapie*, p. 191. (Baden-Baden, Köln, New York: Witzstrock)
4 Borchard, F., Loose, D. A. and Kemkes B. M. (1981). Morphologische Befunde an durchstrómten arterio-venösen Fisteln zur Hämodialyse. *Angio*, 3, 135

35

Angiography in the surgical treatment of occluded ePTFE haemodialysis fistulas: a retrospective comparative study in two hospitals

J. H. van BOCKEL, R. J. van DET AND R. van SCHILFGAARDE

INTRODUCTION

An internal arteriovenous (A-V) fistula fashioned at the wrist of the non-dominant arm is the ideal form of angioaccess in patients requiring maintenance haemodialysis[1]. However, this technique is often not feasible, since adequate superficial arm veins are absent in many patients. In these patients an internal A-V access may be created by using venous autografts, modified allografts or xenografts, or prosthetic graft materials.

At the present time, expanded polytetrafluoroethylene (ePTFE) is commonly used with acceptable results[2-4]. Many complications may occur, like infection, (pseudo-)aneurysm and lymphocoele formation, or haemo-dynamic disturbances[5]. But graft occlusion due to thrombosis is the most frequent complication responsible for the loss of a significant number of grafts[6]. The occurrence of thrombosis may be associated with several causative mechanisms, such as hypotensive episodes during dialysis, an obstruction of the inflow or outflow tract, and undue mechanical compression of puncture sites after completion of dialysis. Evidently, mere thrombectomy is often insufficient for successful surgical treatment of occluded grafts. For instance, if an obstruction of the venous outflow tract is the main cause of graft thrombosis, a surgical revision of the venous anastomosis should be added to the thrombectomy.

Conceivably, angiography of the fistula performed immediately following successful thrombectomy of an occluded graft may be helpful in deciding whether any vascular reconstruction should be performed in addition to the thrombectomy. This retrospective study examines this hypothesis by comparing patency rates of ePTFE graft fistulas in two different hospitals, in one of which angiography was applied as a routine in the management of occluded graft fistulas, whereas in the other it was not.

MATERIALS AND METHODS

In the period 1978–1981 a total of 65 ePTFE (Gore-tex) grafts were implanted as a means of secondary vascular access for haemodialysis. At the Municipal Hospital, Leyenburg, The Hague (ZLDH) 21 grafts were implanted in 17 patients, and at the University Hospital, Leiden (AZL) 40 grafts were implanted in 37 patients. The mean follow-up was 61 weeks (ZLDH) and 39 weeks (AZL). All graft fistulas were constructed in a U-loop fashion in the forearm using end-to-side anastomoses, except for four straight grafts between the radial artery and a cubital vein (all four at ZLDH). The surgical technique, postoperative care and treatment of complications except for the attitude to graft occlusion were identical in both hospitals.

Occluded grafts were treated by thrombectomy in both hospitals. However, this thrombectomy was followed by angiography in all instances in the ZLDH patients, whereas this angiography was not performed in the AZL patients. In these latter patients, graft extension with construction of a new venous anastomosis was performed only if a venous outflow tract obstruction was felt to be present by using the Fogarty thrombectomy catheter. In the ZLDH patients, on the other hand, angiography was used to decide whether residual thrombus or stenoses of the inflow or outflow tract were present, and to determine the most appropriate site for an eventual new venous anastomosis.

Angiography was performed as described by Anderson et al.[7]. After placing a blood pressure cuff around the upper arm, all blood flow in the forearm ceases by inflating the cuff to a pressure of about 250 mmHg. Next, a bolus of 20 ml of contrast material is injected into the graft. The contrast material passes through the graft into the venous outflow tract as well as into the artery, since the A-V pressure gradient is eliminated in the presence of an inflated cuff. Serial radiography is performed in at least two projections before and during release of the occluding cuff.

Using this technique angiograms were performed immediately following thrombectomy in 11 ZLDH cases; no complications were observed. Patency rates were determined using the life-table method[8].

RESULTS

The overall incidence of complications did not differ conspicuously in both series.

The incidence of complications such as infection or pseudoaneurysm formation did not differ in both series, neither when related to the number of weeks in use (infection: 0.9% AZL, 0.5% ZLDH; pseudoaneurysm: 0.3% AZL and 0.2% ZLDH) nor when related to the number of graft fistulas (infection: 27% AZL and 28% ZLDH; pseudoaneurysm: 11% AZL and 14% ZLDH).

Thrombosis occurred as often at AZL (1.3%) as at ZLDH (0.8%), when compared to the number of weeks in use. At AZL, 43% of the graft fistulas suffered from a thrombotic episode. At ZLDH this percentage was 71%, which difference is likely to be due to the longer follow-up period at ZLDH. Surgical treatment of thrombosis by means of thrombectomy with or without surgical revision of inflow and outflow tracts was successful in only 60% of the AZL series and in 82% of the ZLDH series. In both series an equal number of venous anastomotic corrections was carried out (AZL: 40%, ZLDH: 45% of the occluded grafts). Restoration of inflow disorders, mostly due to residual thrombus, was judged necessary in three ZLDH cases.

Graft occlusion was a major problem in both hospitals (Figure 35.1) as is shown by a combined cumulative patency rate at 2 years of 30% and 80% in the presence or absence of a thrombotic episode, respectively. These differences in patency were even more remarkable at AZL, but less significant at ZLDH. For the patency rates of graft fistulas with one or more thrombotic episodes at 1 and 2 years at AZL were 23% and at ZLDH 40%, whereas patency rates in graft fistulas not having suffered from a thrombotic episode were 89% (AZL) and 65% (ZLDH), respectively.

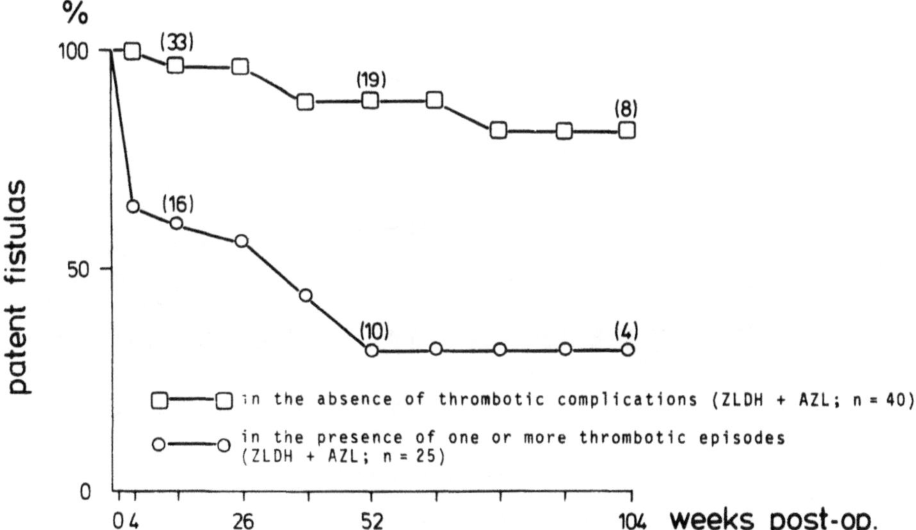

Figure 35.1 Effect of thrombotic complications (including revisions) on the cumulative patency of ePTFE A-V fistulas; combined results in two hospitals (ZLDH + AZL)

Primary failure due to thrombosis (i.e. within 4 weeks postoperatively) occurred in 5/44 (12%) AZL patients, and in 4/21 (19%, all straight grafts) of ZLDH patients. Since angiography was not performed in those patients in which the graft showed primary thrombosis, the effect of angiography in the treatment of occluded graft fistulas can be most clearly shown by excluding those fistulas with primary thrombosis. The favourable effect of routine angiography is evident from the data presented in Figure 35.2, since patency rates at 2 years were 35% if angiography was not applied (AZL) and 67% if it was (ZLDH). These data also demonstrate that the decrease in patency in the AZL series agrees with the number of thrombotic episodes; none of these thrombosed grafts were lost due to complications other than thrombosis.

DISCUSSION

Wide experience with venous angiography in the surgical management of subcutaneous A-V haemodialysis fistulas was first described by Anderson[7]. He observed only one complication in 256 fistulographies, namely the occlusion of an already poorly functioning fistula. Useful information was obtained from 91% of the angiographies performed[9].

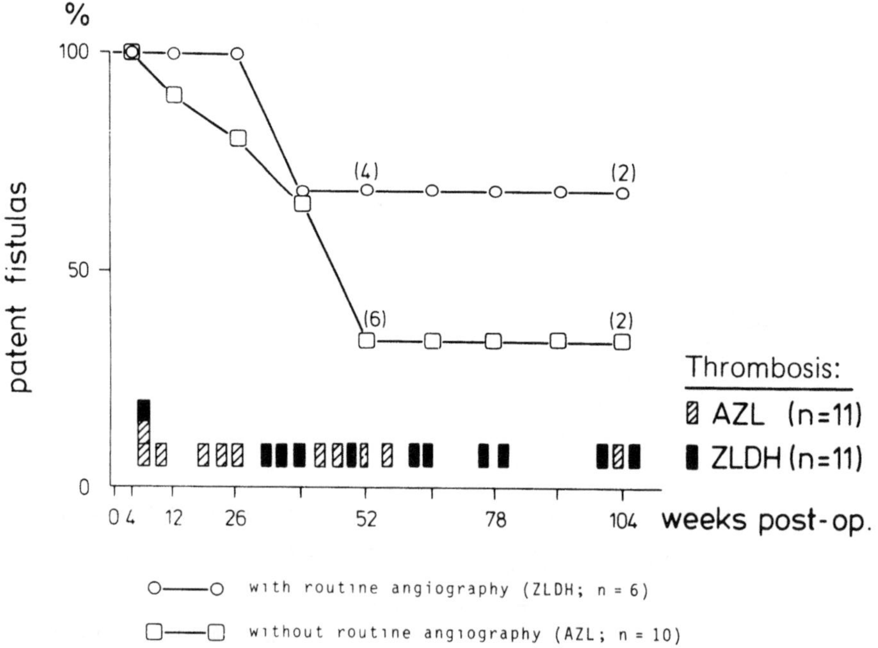

Figure 35.2 Effect of routine angiography on results of surgical treatment of thrombosis in ePTFE A-V fistulas; primary failures have been excluded

This study describes the use of venous angiography performed after surgical intervention by means of thrombectomy in 11 occluded ePTFE graft fistulas. In all instances the graft, together with the anastomotic sites, was adequately visualized, and complications were not observed.

When venous angiography was used routinely in the management of occluded grafts, the 2 years patency rate of graft fistulas having suffered from one or more thrombotic episodes was 67% (ZLDH), whereas it was only 35% if such a routine procedure was not performed (AZL). The number of surgical revisions of venous anastomoses as related to the number of thrombotic episodes in each group (AZL and ZLDH) was the same in both hospitals. In both patient groups the indications for using ePTFE graft for secondary haemodialysis access, the surgical procedures and the post-operative care were identical, and the incidence of late complications such as thrombosis, infection and pseudoaneurysm were in the same order of magnitude. Therefore, both series were judged to be comparable. The only difference was the attitude to the management of late thrombosis and the performance of routine angiography at ZLDH. Apparently the difference in patency in both series, observed in the grafts suffering from one or more thrombotic episodes, was related to the information obtained from the angiography.

On the basis of such angiographic information, secondary surgical procedures can be planned and performed in an adequate fashion. On the one hand the necessity of revising the venous anastomosis may be firmly established, and sometimes the arterial anastomosis may be demonstrated to need surgical correction. In addition, angiography may be helpful in assessing the appropriate site for a new venous anastomosis. On the other hand, superfluous surgical reconstruction of anastomotic sites may be prevented when, after successful thrombectomy, additional abnormalities are demonstrated angiographically to be absent.

Our results corroborate those of Bone[10], who detected 67% significant lesions after thrombectomy in bovine grafts. He, too, stressed the inability to detect outflow obstruction by 'sounding' the outflow with a Fogarty catheter.

CONCLUSION

We conclude that venous angiography performed as a routine after successful thrombectomy of occluded graft fistulas is a valuable means of improving patency rates of ePTFE graft fistulas having suffered from one or more thrombotic episodes. It yields useful information on the basis of which the necessity of an eventual surgical reconstruction of the fistula can be assessed, and this information cannot easily be obtained in any other way. Since the procedure is easy to perform and virtually without risk, we feel that it should be performed routinely, and preferably peroperatively, in all successfully thrombectomized ePTFE graft fistulas. It stands to reason to extend this suggestion, and to apply the technique in the management of any type of occluded haemodialysis graft fistula.

Acknowledgement

The help of M. Lilien in collecting the data is gratefully acknowledged.

References

1 Brescia, M. J., Cimino, J. E., Appel, K. and Hurwich, B. J. (1966). Chronic hemodialysis using venipuncture and a surgically created arterio-venous fistula. *N. Engl. J. Med.*, **275**, 1089

2 Haimov, H., Giron, F. and Jacobson, J. H. (1979). The expanded polytetrafluoroethylene graft. *Arch. Surg.*, **114**, 673

3 Bone, G. E. and Pomajzl, M. J. (1980). Prospective comparison of polytetrafluoroethylene and bovine grafts for hemodialysis. *J. Surg. Res.*, **29**, 223

4 Anderson, C. B., Etheredge, E. E. and Sicard, G. A. (1980). One hundred polytetrafluoroethylene vascular access grafts. *Dial. Transplant.*, **9**, 237

5 Butt, K. M. H., Friedman, E. A. and Kountz, S. L. (1976). Angioaccess. *Curr. Probl. Surg.*, **13**, 44

6 Tellis, V. A., Kohlberg, W. I., Bhat, D. J., Driscoll, B. and Keith, F. J. (1979). Expanded polytetrafluoroethylene graft fistula for chronic hemodialysis. *Ann. Surg.*, **189**, 101

7 Anderson, C. B., Gilula, L. A., Harter, H. R. and Etheredge, E. E. (1978). Venous angiography and the surgical management of subcutaneous hemodialysis fistulas. *Ann. Surg.*, **187**, 194

8 Cutler, S. J. and Ederer, F. (1958). Maximum utilization of the life table method in analyzing survival. *J. Chronic Dis.*, **8**, 699

9 Anderson, C. B., Gilula, L. A., Sicard, G. A. and Etheredge, E. E. (1979). Venous angiography of subcutaneous hemodialysis fistulas. *Arch. Surg.*, **114**, 1320

10 Bone, G. E. and Pomajzl, M. J. (1979). Management of dialysis fistula thrombosis. *Am. J. Surg.*, **138**, 901

36

The management of infected vascular access grafts

J. A. C. BUCKELS, M. Y. EZZIBDEH AND A. D. BARNES

INTRODUCTION

Improvements in both the techniques of and the resources for haemodialysis have led to more patients requiring vascular access for longer periods. An increasing proportion require second-line access when conventional arterio-venous (A-V) and graft fistulas fail. The most serious complication of vascular access grafts is infection, and this chapter reports the management of infected grafts treated at one centre which provides the majority of the second-line access surgery for five haemodialysis units covering a population of 5.5 million.

PATIENTS AND METHODS

During the period June 1975 to June 1981, 93 haemodialysis patients received 136 A-V access grafts (41 male, 52 female: age range 10–57 years, average age 37 years). The indications for graft insertion included primary failure of conventional wrist fistula, small-calibre forearm vessels, obliteration of vessels due to previous infusions or grafts and established fistulas with major cannulation difficulties. In four patients graft placement was the primary access procedure, the remaining 89 patients had previously undergone between one and 10 vascular access operations.

Most grafts were placed in the forearm using a loop configuration based on the antecubital vessels which provided large vessels for anastomoses and a long length (30–35 cm) of graft for cannulation. If this was not possible, thigh or upper arm sites were used. Straight forearm grafts were inserted between enlarged radial arteries and an antecubital vein following wrist fistula which had subsequently produced cannulation difficulties. Thigh grafts were inserted between the common femoral artery (for loop grafts) or distal superficial femoral artery (for straight grafts) and the saphenofemoral junction. Routine anticoagulation was not used and prophylactic systemic antibiotics were not given for initial procedures, though antibiotics were used to cover graft revisions for thrombosis. Details of graft site and configuration are given in Table 36.1, and details of graft materials used are given in Table 36.2.

Table 36.1 Arteriovenous graft site and configuration

		Arm		Leg		
	Total	Loop	Straight	Loop	Straight	Axillo-axillary
Bovine carotid artery	89	71	8	2	7	1
Expanded PTFE	18	1	16	—	1	—
Human umbilical vein	19	14	—	3	2	—
Sparks mandril	7	—	—	—	1	6
Autogenous saphenous vein	2	2	—	—	—	—
Velour Dacron	1	—	—	1	—	—
TOTAL	136	88	24	6	11	7

Table 36.2 Graft material related to infection

Material	Total	No. of infections	Percentage of infections
Bovine carotid artery	89	17	19.1
Human umbilical vein	19	4	21.0
Expanded PTFE	18	1	5.6
Sparks mandril	7	1	14.3
Autogenous saphenous vein	2	—	—
Velour Dacron	1	—	—
TOTAL	136	23	16.9

Bovine carotid artery grafts were most frequently used because of a personal preference for the handling qualities at operation and ease of cannulation. Six of the seven Sparks mandril grafts were inserted axillary artery to contralateral axillary vein early in the series and were soon abandoned due to poor results from this material. This site has been used with other materials and may on occasions be very useful. All patients were fully documented at time of insertion and infective complications were recorded prospectively as they occurred. Graft infection was confirmed by the culture of organisms from pus alongside the graft or from the graft material itself with or without positive blood cultures. All patients with graft infection were treated with systemic antibiotics. Graft infections involving the anastomoses or the entire subcutaneous skin tunnel were treated by graft

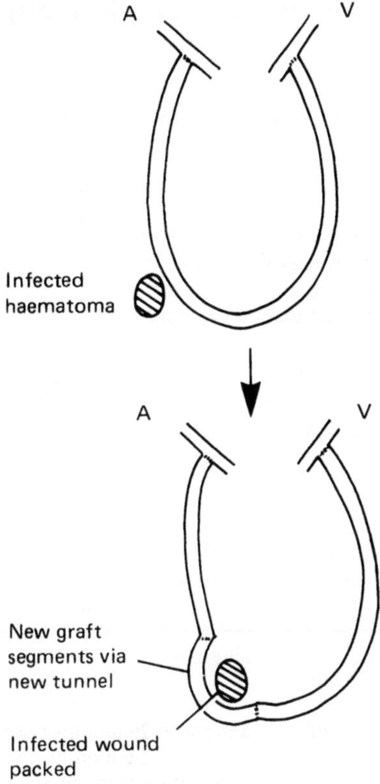

Figure 36.1 Technique of local graft revision

removal and establishment of vascular access at another site. Infections involving a localized area of the graft were treated similarly early in the series, but more recently localized areas of infection have been treated by local excision of the infected segment with insertion of a new graft segment via a new skin tunnel (Figure 36.1). The infected wounds were allowed to heal by secondary intention. All patients have been followed up for at least 6 months.

RESULTS

Graft infection occurred in 23 patients (25% of patients: 12 male, 11 female, average age 39.5 years) which is an overall incidence of 17% of the grafts. There was no difference in infection rate related to graft configuration or graft site. There was a greater incidence of infections related to cannulation puncture than after the primary surgical insertion or revision for thrombosis (Table 36.3). Early graft infection (within 4 weeks of insertion) was seen in seven patients. It involved the arterial anastomosis in two and the skin tunnel in five patients. All these grafts were removed but despite this two patients died from septicaemia.

Table 36.3 Incidence of infection in arteriovenous grafts

	Infections	
	Number	Percentage
Infection after 136 primary procedures	7	5.1
Infection after 85 secondary procedures*	2	2.3
Infection related to cannulation puncture in 116 grafts †	14	12.0
TOTAL INFECTIONS	23	16.9

*85 late thrombectomies
†20 primary failure grafts

Table 36.4 Results in 23 infected arteriovenous grafts

	Outcome
Early infection, 7	all excised
Late infection, 16:	
5 excised	
10 local revision	5 in use at 26 months (average)
	5 failed at 2.6 months (average)
1 aspiration	used until transplant at 26 months

Late graft infection (after 4 weeks from insertion) occurred in 16 patients, related to cannulation puncture in 14 patients and following graft revision for thrombosis in the remaining two patients. Treatment was graft removal in five patients, local graft revision and antibiotics in 10 patients and aspiration and antibiotics in one patient. Of the 10 grafts revised locally, five subsequently failed from recurrent infection at 1–5 months (average 2.6 months) though five continue to be used for haemodialysis at 7–50 months with an average patency of 26 months (Table 36.4). The infected graft treated by aspiration and antibiotics functioned until the patient was successfully transplanted 26 months later. All patients treated by local revision survived. Bacteriological cultures from the infected grafts showed a prominence of the common skin pathogens with 17 infections due to *Staphylococcus aureus*, 2 due to *Micrococcus* and the remaining cases due to *Klebsiella* sp., *Streptococcus faecalis*, alpha-haemolytic *Streptococcus* and *Peptostreptococcus*. At present, of the 23 patients who developed graft infection 10 are maintained on haemodialysis, eight have had successful renal transplants, three died on haemodialysis from non-infective causes and two died from graft infection-related septicaemia.

DISCUSSION

Infection of any vascular graft is a grave complication which may lead to septicaemia and secondary haemorrhage. Usually the accepted treatment is graft excision. Graft infection in the haemodialysis patient carries the additional consequence of loss of vascular access for life-supporting therapy, which has led to our present policy of local graft revision whenever possible.

The high infection rate associated with vascular access sites is partially due to immunodeficiency in the chronic renal failure patient. Moreover, haemodialysis patients have a higher carriage rate for *Staph. aureus*, estimated at over 60%, compared with 10% in a control population[1]. Contamination by skin bacteria during the operation probably accounts for the early infections seen in this series.

Infection following secondary procedures has been more common and Bhat *et al.*[2] report an incidence of 17%. In this series the incidence was lower at 2.3%, possibly because of the routine administration of the antistaphylococcal agent flucloxacillin to patients undergoing thrombectomy or revision. Serious cannulation sepsis, however, has been a major problem. This occurs as a result of infections of subcutaneous haematomas following haemodialysis needle puncture. Minor cannulation sepsis, although common, has not been evaluated in this population as most patients underwent dialysis at home or at other dialysis centres and minor septic episodes were treated with antibiotics by local physicians. Only infections which persisted or led to major graft haemorrhage and were referred for surgical assessment are included in these series. Cannulation sepsis in expanded PTFE grafts has been treated successfully with local incision and drainage and parenteral antibiotics[2]. Our initial attempts to reproduce these results with bovine carotid artery grafts failed due to recurrent haemorrhage from exposed graft, and our early practice with serious cannulation sepsis was graft removal and establishment of vascular access at an alternative site. More recently we have employed the technique of local revision described by Kumar *et al.*[3]. Though many surgeons have been unable to salvage infected bovine grafts[4,5] local revision has been successful on occasions[3,6,7]. In this series the 10 grafts undergoing local revision comprised seven bovine, two umbilical vein and one PTFE. A successful outcome was obtained in three bovine, one umbilical vein and the one PTFE, being a salvage rate of 50% with an encouraging long-term average patency of 26 months.

We conclude that early graft infection involving either an anastomosis or the skin tunnel requires graft excision and is accompanied by significant mortality. Locally infected grafts may be treated by local graft revision which provides long-term patency in 50% of patients without mortality.

References

1 Appel, G. B. (1978). Vascular access infections with long term haemodialysis. *Arch. Intern. Med.*, **138**, 1610

2 Bhat, D. J., Tellis, V. A., Kohlberg, W. I., Driscoll, B. and Veith, F. J. (1980). Management of sepsis involving expanded polytetrafluoroethylene grafts for haemodialysis access. *Surgery*, **87**, 445
3 Kumar, S., Rattazzi, L. and VanderWerf, B. (1976). A new treatment for infected bovine graft (BG) arteriovenous fistulas (AVF). *Clin. Dial. Transplant. Forum* (Abstr.), 22
4 Tellis, V. A., Kohlberg, W. I., Bhat, D. J., Driscoll, B. and Veith, F. J. (1979). Expanded polytetrafluoroethylene graft fistula for chronic haemodialysis. *Ann. Surg.*, **189**, 101
5 Guillou, P. J., Levenson, S. H. and Kester, R. C. (1980). The complications of arteriovenous grafts for vascular access. *Br. J. Surg.*, **67**, 517
6 Butler, H. G., Baker, L. D. and Johnson, J. M. (1977). Vascular access for chronic haemodialysis: polytetrafluoroethylene (PTFE) versus bovine heterograft. *Am. J. Surg.*, **134**, 79
7 Rolley, R. T., Sterioff, S. and Williams, G. M. (1976). Arteriovenous fistulas for dialysis using modified bovine artery. *Surg. Gynecol. Obstet.*, **142**, 700

37

Abstracts of posters in Management of complications

Short-term follow-up of percutaneous transluminal angioplasty of stenoses located on fistulas used for haemodialysis
J. C. GAUX, P. BOURQUELOT, B. GUIDET, M. SEUROT,
A. RAYNAUD and D. BLANCHARD

Forty-five stenoses behind arteriovenous (A-V) fistulas in 35 (haemodialysed patients were treated with percutaneous transluminal angioplasty (PTA). Immediate stenoses dilatation results in relation to A-V fistula type were haemodynamically significant in 34 cases (76%), with poorer results on bovine heterograft stenoses (13 cases = 62%). Dilatation results in relation to the site of the lesion showed haemodynamically efficient angioplasty on stenoses next to anastomosis (93%) but a poor result on distal lesion (15 cases = 40%). We observed nine cases of thrombosis but four recovered after treatment, three after local fibrinolytic perfusion, one after surgical thrombectomy. Follow-up over period of 1–10 months (mean 4.8 months) including angiography and appreciation of the dialysis quality were performed in 28 patients who had a successful dilatation. PTA appears to be a technically feasible and clinically effective method of treating stenoses lying on the venous limb fistula in patients on chronic haemodialysis.

Effects of smoking on arteriovenous fistula patency
P. J. A. GRIFFIN, F. DAVIES and G. A. COLES

The adverse effects of smoking on disease in general and vascular disease in particular, are now well established[1]. Recently it has been our impression that amongst our haemodialysis population the number of smokers requiring new fistulas or fistula revision was higher than non-smokers. This hypothesis has been tested by questioning our haemodialysis population on their smoking habits and fistula patency. We have found 37% of smokers required new fistulas or fistula revision while only 6% of non-smokers did so (see Table 37.1).

Table 37.1

	One fistula	More than one fistula	
Smokers	17	10	
Non-smokers	27	1 }	} $p<0.002$
Ex-smokers	23	2 }	

This number of fistula failures in smokers is highly significant; we thus feel all haemodialysis patients should be strongly advised to refrain from smoking.

Reference

1 *Med. J. Australia.* (1975) **2** Suppl., 3–4. List of illnesses associated with smoking

Vascular access for chronic haemodialysis: a 10-year survey with 136 patients
PH. MORINIÈRE, J. P. VERMYNCK, D. ABET, P. RINGOT,
J. BURNAY, J. F. DE FREMONT, B. COEVOET, J. PIETRI and
A. FOURNIER

Brescia arteriovenous (A-V) fistula was performed as first vascular access in 133 patients (mean ($\pm$SD) age 48$\pm$14 years, mean dialysis duration 40$\pm$28 months). It was definitively successful in 73 patients (54%), failed immediately in 25 (18%) or after 1–72 months in 35 (28%). An *in situ* repair of the first A-V fistula performed in 10 cases was successful in all. A second A-V fistula was performed in 31 patients with definitive success in 14 (50%), immediate failure in 4 (13%) and failure after 1–24 months in 13. A graft was performed as first procedure in 3 patients and as second procedure in 19 patients, with definitive success in 7 patients (32%) immediate failure in 3 and after 1–72 months in 12. A second graft was made in 32 and three grafts or more were made in 19 patients so that a total of 92 grafts was made. Autologous or homologous saphenous veins were used in 80 cases. Calf carotid was used in five cases, Gore-tex® in four and Dardik® in five cases. Twenty-six patients died during the period: in nine cases the death was indirectly related to under-dialysis (cachexia, pericarditis) or secondary to complications of anaesthesia or catheterisms. Two of these deaths came from the 73 patients group with successful first A-V fistula and seven from the 60 patients group with unsuccessful first A-V fistula ($\chi^2 = 5.6$; $p<0.02$). The following non-fatal complications were observed: septicaemia (10), local infections with loss of vascular access (10), vascular ruptures (7), distal steal syndromes (4) with finger necrosis leading to amputation (2) and transfer to peritoneal dialysis either transitorily (7) or definitively (3) with three peritonitis. Except one septicaemia and one focal infection, all these complications were observed exclusively in the group with the first unsuccessful A-V fistulas.

Conclusions:

(1) The quality of the first A-V fistula is a primary determinant of morbidity and mortality of the patients on chronic haemodialysis.

(2) After an unsuccessful first A-V fistula *in situ* correction or creation of a second A-V fistula is a preferable procedure to graft since they are more likely to be definitively successful (60% *vs.* 32%).

Percutaneous transluminal angioplasty in failing arteriovenous fistula
S. K. S. SO, W. R. CASTANEDA-ZUNIGA, D. HUNTER,
D. E. R. SUTHERLAND and K. AMPLATZ

Three patients with failing Brescia arteriovenous fistulas due to one or more proximal stenotic venous segments underwent Gruntzig balloon angio-dilatation with uniform success. One patient was started on haemodialysis immediately after the procedure and underwent a subsequent pre-transplant splenectomy in 4 days. All three patients are still on haemodialysis with functioning fistulas. Balloon dilatation was performed on an outpatient basis at the time of venous cine-fistulography eliminating the need for a second procedure. By using the distal vein of the fistula or by direct puncture of the distal part of the fistula, both the proximal arterial and venous vessels were easily accessible for catheterization and angiodilatation. There were no complications, and the procedure was rapid and well tolerated by the patients. No hospitalization was required, and the patients did not require elaborate anticoagulation therapy short of the empirical use of one or two tablets of aspirin per day. Our 100% success rate shows that percutaneous transluminal angiodilatation via the distal vein or distal part of the fistula at the time of venous fistulography can be a rapid and effective method of managing failing arteriovenous fistulas.

The frequency of thrombosis in patients with central venous catheters is high
G. WICKBOM, T. ANDERSSON, M. BRODIN and E. LINDBERG

Thrombosis of the upper central veins associated with central venous catheters (CVC) has previously been reported in 0–15%. Phlebography has usually been done via peripheral arm veins. There are reasons to believe that the incidence of thrombosis is considerably higher.

Sixty-seven patients with CVC via internal jugular vein or subclavian vein have been examined by contrast injection through the CVC during catheter extraction. The examination was documented on 35 mm X-ray film via image intensifier. The catheters were indwelling 5 to 72 days. The tip of the catheter was positioned in the superior vena cava (SVC). Fifty-two patients had silicon rubber catheters and 15 had a Teflon catheter. Heparin 5000 i.u. $\times$ 2–3 s.c. was given to 31 patients, five had acetylsalicylic acid 1 g, two had Rheomacrodex and 30 did not receive any anticoagulant therapy. Nine patients were free of thrombosis (13%). Fifty-eight patients (87%) had developed varying degrees of intravenous aggregations, from fibrin sleeve formation around the catheter to total occlusion of the SVC in six patients (9%). Anticoagulant prophylaxis did not seem to have any effect. No difference was noticed between the different catheter materials, catheterization time or underlying disease. Cultures from the catheter tip and skin puncture site did not show any significant growth of bacteria. We feel that use of CVC must be utterly restricted; a better anticoagulant prophylaxis is mandatory. Total parenteral nutrition via peripheral vein, as well as enteral nutrition, must be used whenever possible.

The relation between spontaneous and induced platelet aggregation and arteriovenous fistula thrombosis in chronic haemodialysis patients
J. VLACHOYANNIS, V. BELWE and W. SCHOEPPE

In addition to vascular changes, enhanced platelet aggregation has been discussed as a cause of arteriovenous (A-V) fistula thrombosis in chronic haemodialysis patients.

Spontaneous and ADP- as well as collagen-induced aggregation was studied in two groups of chronic haemodialysis patients. In the first group of 10 patients (I), recurrent fistula thrombosis occurred, whereas in the second group of 10 patients (II) no fistula problems were encountered. The evaluations were carried out prior to haemodialysis with plasma containing 200 000 platelets/μl after the method of Born. In group I, 36 fistulas of various types had been employed which remained patent for an average of 7.6±0.2 months ($\bar{x}$±SEM). In group II, the fistulas stayed open for an average of 27.7±2.4 months.

Using ADP-induced aggregation at a concentration of 10^{-5} mol/l, group I displayed a T50%-value 36±0.1 s. *vs.* 34.8±6.8, respectively. For collagen-induced aggregation at a concentration of 5 γ/ml, α^2/TR values were 78.6±3.0 and 79.4±1.8, respectively. The differences were not significant at these and other concentrations.

These results demonstrate that there is no correlation between the rate of A-V fistula thrombosis and spontaneous as well as ADP- and collagen-induced platelet aggregation in chronic haemodialysis patients. The preventive administration of antiplatelet agents in haemodialysis patients thus does not appear to be justified.

The place for secondary access procedures in a new dialysis population
D. T. REILLY, R. F. M. WOOD and P. R. F. BELL

A radiocephalic fistula is accepted to be the best form of access procedure for haemodialysis; most reviews of patency rates are biased because of previous access operations. In an attempt to define the need for more exotic procedures than simple wrist fistulas, 157 unselected consecutive patients accepted onto the dialysis programme were studied prospectively over a 5-year period. Only three patients were unable to have a primary wrist fistula. Eighty per cent of fistulas were patent at 1 year, and 65% were patent 4 years after construction, when 78% of patients were dialysing on either a first or second wrist fistula. In the 51 patients who had access problems, 107 procedures became necessary to re-establish satisfactory access; 42 were salvage procedures and 65 new fistula operations of which only four were loop grafts. Failure was twice as common when vein diameter was 2 mm or less but 14% of the successful fistulas were constructed using 2 mm diameter veins. It is concluded that the majority of patients are suitable for primary wrist fistula despite small vessels, and the place for grafts is strictly limited.

The subclavian vein: ultimate refuge for haemodialysis?
J. R. BEUKHOF, A. M. TEGZESS, G. GO, E. VAN GOGH,
B. K. BEGEMAN and G. K. VAN DER HEM

Since October 1979, 15 intensive care patients (ICP) were dialysed via the subclavian vein (SV) using non-tunnelled argon cannulas; 22 chronic dialysis patients (CP) were dialysed by means of 35 tunnelled Uldall catheters; ($n=236$ dialyses, CP + ICP). In order to determine the merits and demerits of this method several aspects were studied.

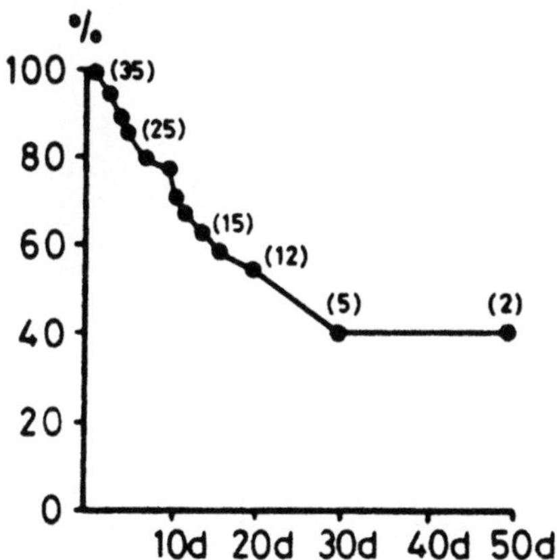

Figure 37.1 Actuarial catheter survival

Lethal complications did not occur (ICP + CP). Long-term complications could be observed in the 22 CP; six complications did not lead to removal of the catheter (reversible oedema, two; bleeding, two; tension pneumothorax, one; small pneumothorax, one, 15 complications however, required removal/replacement (sepsis, two; tunnel infection, one; luxation, two; external leak, one; obstruction, nine). Actuarial cannula survival is given in Figure 37.1. Efficiency of dialysis via SV (E′SV) can be defined as the ratio of effective versus *in vitro* dialyser clearance; E′SV-can be calculated from urea concentrations and generation rate, dialysis time, body weight and distribution volume. E′SV for single cannula (SC) dialysis was 0.47 ± 0.13 ($x \pm 1$ SD), much lower than E′ for other routes (0.77 ± 0.21) ($p < 0.01$, Wilcoxon). This is probably due to the large recirculation (14.3–24.5%). E′SV (SC) was especially low in patients with heart failure and could be improved approximately 100% by returning the blood into a peripheral vein.

Conclusions:

(1) Dialysis via the SV can be a life-saving procedure;
(2) Because of the low E′SV (SC) the venous blood should be infused into a peripheral vein whenever possible;
(3) Overall cannula survival was disappointing, but can be improved by tunnelling, by flushing $\geq 1 \times /24$ h and by restriction of its use to dialysis only.

38

Invited comment on papers and posters in Management of complications

R. HORSCH

Failure and complications of arteriovenous (A-V) fistulas had been attributed to many factors inducing accelerated thrombosis, such as haemodialysis alterations, material interaction and surgical problems.

Thrombosis represents the most frequent complication of A-V fistulas. Particularly demoralizing to the patient, the dialysis personnel and the surgeon are repetitive episodes of fistula occlusion. These necessitate multiple operative procedures for thrombectomy or construction of new fistulas.

Table 38.1   Causes of thrombosis in A-V fistulas

(a)	**Surgical causes** Inadequate surgical technique Inadequate arterial flow Outflow obstruction due to neointimal fibroplasia Aneurysm formation
(b)	**Inadequate handling by dialysis personnel** Improper puncture technique Early cannulation of new immature fistulas Excessive compression of puncture sites after decannulation and over-zealous banding
(c)	**Risk factors inducing vascular diseases or** **complications** Prolonged systemic hypotension Uraemic hypercoagulopathy Hyperlipaemic state Smoking

In the pathogenesis of fistula thrombosis one can differentiate between early and late thrombosis, or they can be classified according to cause (Table

"

38.1a). For example surgical causes include inadequate surgical techniques which can result in insufficient arterial flow or outflow obstruction. This, however, in grafts is generally due to neointimal fibroplasia. Aneurysm formation of the anastomotic site may also result from inadequate surgical techniques.

Careless handling by the dialysis personnel is in our opinion the most frequent cause for fistula thrombosis. This can be the puncture technique, the early cannulation of new or immature fistulas or the excessive compression and over-zealous banding after decannulation (Table 38.1b). For this reason home dialysis patients have in our experience fewer fistula complications than patients dialysed in the hospital.

Further causes of thrombosis include factors inducing vascular diseases or complications. These include prolonged systemic hypotension, sometimes caused by excessive dialysis, the uraemic hypercoagulopathy and a hyper-lipaemic state, and perhaps smoking (Table 38.1c).

As J. H. van Bockel *et al.* demonstrated in the management of fistula thrombosis angiography is very helpful since thrombosis is often associated with anatomical problems that need repair. This was the reason why, in patients referred to angiography, the patency rates were higher than in the group treated by thrombectomy alone.

In the literature similar results were reported by Bone *et al.*[1]. It is therefore evident that the intraoperative fistulography with immediate revision of an identified defect is still more effective than the angiographic examination after emergency thrombectomy.

The paper of B. M. Kemkes and F. Borchard clearly underlined the following facts: the superiority in patency of autologous graft fistulas, the use of Sparks mandril is obsolete, and bovine grafts have higher complication rates than PTFE grafts. With respect to bovine grafts one should, however, consider that in most retrospective studies the patency rates of these grafts are perhaps so discouraging since these grafts were used a long time prior to PTFE grafts and the knowledge as to how to put them in was not so precise at that time. The author demonstrated further that surgical treatment of occluded or ruined fistulas is possible and worthwhile even in nearly hopeless situations.

Every method to avoid repetitive surgery for thrombectomy, allowing an undisturbed dialysis, is a blessing for both patient and doctor. It seems that percutaneous transluminal angioplasty (PTA) is becoming an accepted therapeutic method for stenotic arterial disease. Not only are arteriosclerotic lesions of coronary, renal and peripheral arteries treated effectively by PTA but also stenoses located on A-V fistulas, as has been shown by the poster of So *et al.* Apart from some case reports no greater series of patients with A-V fistula stenoses treated with PTA are described in the literature.

So allow me to make some critical remarks from the surgeon's view. Any new procedure must be compared with existing and acknowledged effective modes of treatment. In this case the appropriate comparison is surgical angioplasty. It would seem helpful to review the problem of fistula stenosis from the standpoint of what surgical angioplasty or revision has to offer. The central questions would appear to be: is PTA as effective as surgical angioplasty or revision? Is the morbidity of PTA comparable or better? How durable are PTA results? These questions cannot be precisely answered at this time; further experience with this method of therapy is necessary to demonstrate long-term results.

Infections in primary autologous A-V fistulas are rare, and as Kaiser *et al.*[4] demonstrated they generally respond to antibiotic therapy. Infected graft-fistulas are more frequent and often resist every form of antibiotic therapy. I agree with Buckles *et al.* that localized infected portions of the graft can be excised and a bypass operation should be performed. On the other hand it is known that bacteria are not only limited to the infected region of the graft (if it is not completely incorporated) but are also found in areas which outwardly appear inconspicuous. If graft infection persists, one should also consider that the patient cannot undergo kidney transplantation perhaps for a longer time.

Griffin *et al.* found that 37% of smokers had complications with their fistula while only 6% of the non-smokers did so. While the authors considered the renal disease and hypertension they did not examine haematocrit or lipid metabolism, platelet function or arteriosclerosis. All these factors are also well-known risks inducing vascular diseases or complications. On the other hand it seems that smoking influences prostaglandin metabolism, especially the release of thromboxane. Thromboxane has an aggregating action and works against prostacyclin that is produced within the endothelial cells of the vessels and has antiaggregating action. The question therefore is: why have smokers more complications; are the complications due to changes of the vessels or do they have altered platelet function, for example?

Spontaneous and induced platelet aggregation was studied by Vlachoyannis *et al.* The results caused the authors to conclude that the preventive administration of antiplatelet agents without correcting the underlying cause is not justified. Dr Vlachoyannis' results and conclusions are not in agreement with studies of Schulz[2], Oblath[3] or Harter[4]. These authors were able to demonstrate impressively the effect of antiplatelet aggregating agents for the prophylaxis of A-V fistula thrombosis.

Thrombosis is not only a problem of patients with A-V fistulas but also of intensive care patients. Wickbom and his group found varying degrees of intravenous aggregation following central venous catheterization. Only 13% of the patients examined were free of thrombosis. The reported method of examination is much more sensitive than phlebography via the peripheral arm veins. I was surprised that the authors managed to get satisfactory exposures with the low volume of X-ray contrast medium which can be injected through a thin catheter per time.

Nevertheless cannulation of the subclavian vein can be the ultimate refuge of haemodialysis as Dr Beukhof *et al.* demonstrated. Complications such as obstruction, bleeding and sepsis, however, often required removal or replacement of the catheter. Therefore in my opinion and experience the best vascular access in acute renal failure is still the Scribner shunt. With experience it can be placed in about ½ h. The method has a high efficiency and a low complication rate.

A-V fistula complications can be minimized by great experience in the field of access surgery as Reilly *et al.* demonstrated. One-year patency rates of 80% and 4-year patency rates of 65% of primary wrist fistulas are outstanding results. That only four from 65 patients required further grafts demonstrated that grafts are sometimes implanted uncritically and without real indication.

Therefore at the end of the symposium about graft-fistula complications let me give some recommendations to reduce factors causing complications of graft-fistulas:

(1) minimize angles and abrupt changes in calibre; taper a graft if necessary;
(2) use microsurgical technique;
(3) prescribe an antiplatelet agent;
(4) administer an antibiotic selectively;
(5) perform an antiseptic and proper puncture technique;
(6) avoid unilocular puncture technique; alternate puncture sites.

References

1 Bone, G. E. and Pomazyl, R. N. (1979). Management of dialysis fistula thrombosis. *Am. J. Surg.*, **138**, 901

2 Schulz, V., Zehle, A., Kindler, J. *et al.* (1981). Dipyridamol-Azetylsalizylsäure zur Prophylaxe von Shunt-Thrombosen bei chronischen Dialysepatienten. *Nieren- und Hochdruckkrankheiten*, **1**, 49

3 Oblath, R. W., Buckley, F. O., Green, R. M. *et al.* (1978). Prevention of platelet aggregation and adherence to prosthetic vascular grafts by aspirin and dipyridamole. *Surgery*, **84**, 37

4 Harter, H. R., Burch, J. W., Majerus, P. W. *et al.* (1979). Prevention of thrombosis in patients on hemodialysis by low-dose aspirin. *N. Engl. J. Med.*, **301**, 577

5 Humphries, A. L., Nesbit, R. R., Caruana, R. J. *et al.* (1981). Thirty-six recommendations for vascular access operations. *Am. Surg.*, **47**, 145

6 Kaiser, A. B., Clayson, K. R. and Mulherin, J. L. (1978). Antibiotic prophylaxis in vascular surgery. *Ann. Surg.*, **88**, 283

Section VIII
Access for total parenteral nutrition

39

Vascular access for total parenteral nutrition (TPN)

B. J. ROWLANDS, D. J. HOELZER AND T. C. FLYNN

INTRODUCTION

Over the past decade, total parenteral nutrition (TPN) has become an important aspect of the clinical management of many hospitalized patients, and more recently for patients in the home. A reduction or total lack of oral intake, together with an increase in resting metabolic expenditure due to surgery, trauma or infection leads to an erosion of tissue stores of carbohydrate, fat and protein to satisfy energy demands. It is well documented that this catabolic response to starvation and stress is associated with an increase in morbidity and mortality, but appropriate nutritional support either enterally or intravenously will enhance the patient's ability to respond to the increased metabolic stress and will favour a successful outcome of the illness. In patients who are unable to digest and absorb sufficient nutrients via the gastrointestinal tract, amino acids, carbohydrate, fat, vitamins and minerals may be delivered through a central venous catheter, placed and maintained under sterile conditions. Although TPN has gained wide acceptance as an important modality of treatment in a wide variety of clinical conditions there are still numerous reports appearing in the literature which document the metabolic, infectious, technical, mechanical and thrombotic complications of the procedure. This chapter will review the methods of placement and management of central venous catheters for TPN in adults and children, both in the hospital and at home, which enable nutrient solutions to be administered safely over a prolonged period.

PLACEMENT OF A CENTRAL VENOUS LINE

There are several basic principles that need to be observed if the complications of central venous catheter placement and TPN are to be avoided. They are:

(1) The safe placement of the catheter under sterile conditions so that the tip of the catheter lies within the lumen of a large central vein, preferably the superior vena cava.

(2) Obsessional catheter care ensuring that all dressing and tube changes are carried out under sterile conditions.

(3) Preparation and storage of all solutions for infusion under optimal conditions to ensure that the chances of contamination of nutrient infusions is minimized.

(4) Accurate patient monitoring to ensure that metabolic, infective, thrombotic or mechanical problems do not arise and that nutrients are utilized for optimal tissue repair and recovery.

Hypertonic nutrient solutions containing amino acids, carbohydrate, vitamins and minerals are usually infused into a large central vein with high blood flow to avoid the problem of thrombophlebitis that occurs commonly when peripheral veins are used. The most commonly used route of access is via the subclavian veins using an infraclavicular approach which has the advantage that complications are few, the catheter is easy to maintain and the patient is free to move all four limbs at will without fear of dislodging or kinking the catheter. Following placement of the catheter a chest X-ray is taken to confirm the position of the catheter tip and hypertonic solutions are only infused if it is located optimally in the superior vena cava. Subclavian vein catheterization was first described by Aubaniac in 1952[1] and several articles contain excellent descriptions of the technique for TPN catheter placement[2,3]. It may be performed under sterile conditions in the operating room or at the patient's bedside, provided the patient can be maintained comfortably in the Trendelenburg position throughout the procedure. This, together with adequate hydration, ensures maximum distension of the central veins and prevents air embolism during insertion. The patient lies on a small roll placed longitudinally in the middle of the back which allows the shoulders to fall backwards. With the arms in neutral position at the side and the head slightly extended the subclavian vein is situated between the inner third of the clavicle and first rib. With meticulous attention to proper positioning of the patient, the catheter may easily be introduced from either side. The skin of the neck, shoulder and upper chest is shaved and prepared using povidone–iodine solution and is draped with sterile towels. Local anaesthetic is infiltrated below the clavicle into the skin, subcutaneous tissues and periosteum. Using strict aseptic technique with sterile gloves and instruments, a 2 inch long, 14-gauge needle attached to a 5 ml syringe is used to locate the subclavian vein by passing it horizontally from the anaesthetized area under the clavicle towards the posterior aspect of the suprasternal notch. When negative pressure exerted continuously on the syringe produces a 'flashback' of blood, the vein has been entered and the patient is asked to perform a Valsalva manoeuvre while the syringe is detached and a 16-gauge 8 inch long polythene catheter is introduced through the needle into the venous system. When the catheter has been fully introduced, the needle and catheter are withdrawn as a unit and the catheter is secured to the skin with a 3–0 silk suture and a guard is placed over the needle. Never withdraw the catheter through the needle tip as this may lead to transection and embolization of the catheter tip. The catheter is then connected to the i.v. bottle and tubing and its position within the central veins confirmed by the back flow of blood when the bottle is lowered below the level of the heart. The position of the tip of the catheter is confirmed radiologically and then the procedure is completed by applying povidone–iodine ointment to the catheter exit site and covering it with a sterile dressing. Finally, adequate function and position of the catheter are confirmed by the unimpeded flow of fluid from the i.v. bottle into the central veins.

Other techniques such as the supraclavicular cannulation of the subclavian vein[4], and the use of the internal jugular vein[5] have also been used for TPN catheters, and long catheters have been introduced into the central veins via the brachial, cephalic and long saphenous veins, but all these techniques appear to have a higher incidence of technical failure and infectious and thrombophlebitic complications.

Several different types of catheters are available commercially for use in delivery of TPN, including catheters made out of Teflon, Silastic, polyethylene and rubber, and those that employ a catheter-over-needle or split-needle techniques of insertion rather than the catheter-through-needle technique described above. The developments in techniques and materials are designed to reduce complications, ease insertion and maintenance, and allow the catheter to be used over a prolonged period. The development of the Broviac–Scribner and Hickman catheters have been important for the safe delivery of prolonged parenteral nutrition[6]. These catheters are Silastic, are flexible and less thrombogenic than polyethylene and have a Dacron cuff which lies subcutaneously, and acts as a barrier to the passage of bacteria from the skin puncture wound to the site of insertion into the vein. These catheters may be inserted into the subclavian vein using a technique that employs a guide wire and split-needle introducer and are tunnelled across the chest wall in the subcutaneous tissue to the skin exit site over the lower chest or upper abdomen[7]. This allows easier catheter care and management for the patient receiving ambulatory home hyperalimentation[8].

CATHETER CARE

The lowest incidence of catheter- and TPN-related complications have been reported from those units that employ strict protocols for the insertion of catheters, and the management and monitoring of patients receiving TPN[9]. This is best carried out by a team of specially trained nurses who have responsibility for the day-to-day management of these patients' nutritional support and perform all procedures related to catheter care. Dressing changes of the catheter exit site should be carried out three times per week or whenever their is soilage of the dressing using a strict aseptic technique. Some units employ a new transparent dressing which needs less attention and allows direct observation of the catheter exit site, but there is no proven advantage of this method. The i.v. tubing should be changed daily. The TPN catheter should not be used for blood sampling, central venous pressure measurement or for the infusion of blood products and intravenous medications. All these procedures require unnecessary manipulation of the line and increase the potential for infectious and thrombotic complications. It is vitally important to distinguish between the central venous line that is placed for the delivery of TPN and that which is used for monitoring or fluid resuscitation, as the former requires a much stricter management protocol. Suspected catheter sepsis should be managed by culturing the intravenous nutrients and tubing and by drawing blood cultures through the catheter. The catheter should be removed if the fever persists, if blood cultures are positive or if the patient shows signs of systemic sepsis for which there is no other obvious cause. Using these techniques, a subclavian catheter may be maintained for prolonged periods without complications although recently we have adopted a policy of routinely changing these catheters over a guide wire when they have been in place for 60 days.

COMPLICATIONS OF VASCULAR ACCESS FOR TPN

Metabolic, infectious, technical, mechanical, thrombotic and embolic complications may all arise during the insertion of central venous catheters and the administration of TPN. The metabolic complications usually arise from the use of inappropriate TPN regimen with insufficient monitoring of the patients and most are potentially avoidable[10]. The technical and mechanical complications arise either at the time of insertion of the catheter or during subsequent use of the catheter for the administration of TPN (Table 39.1). Infectious complications arise due to contaminated solutions, improper use of the line, catheter sepsis or increased susceptibility of the patient (Table 39.2). Thrombotic and embolic complications are given in Table 39.3.

A number of studies have reviewed the incidence of catheter-associated complications in patients receiving TPN. Ryan *et al.* (1974) showed that an infection rate of 3% occurred when a strict aseptic protocol was followed compared to a 20% incidence when breaks of protocol were observed[11]. They also noticed a 4% incidence of venous thrombosis. Copeland *et al.* reported a

Table 39.1 Technical and mechanical complications of TPN

At insertion

Pneumothorax	Subclavian artery laceration
Haemothorax	Subclavian vein laceration
	Brachial plexus injury
Misplaced catheter	Phrenic nerve injury
Catheter embolism	Thoracic duct injury
Air embolism	Tracheal injury

During use

Pump malfunction	Hydrothorax
Kinking of tubing or catheter	Hydromediastinum
Air embolism	Subcutaneous emphysema

Table 39.2 Infectious complications of TPN

Contaminated solutions	Poor preparation
	Defective bottles
	In-use contamination
	Additives
Improper use of catheter	Frequent disconnection
	In-line filters, stopcocks
	Manometer for CVP measurement
	Piggy-back infusions
	Environmental contamination
Catheter sepsis	Bacteraemia
	Septicaemia
	Septic thrombophlebitis
	Septic embolism
Patient related	Any condition causing an increased susceptibility to infection, e.g. diabetes, malignancy, chronic malnutrition, extremes of age

Table 39.3 Thrombotic and embolic complications of TPN

Venous thrombosis
Pulmonary embolism
Air embolism
Catheter embolism

2% incidence of infection in a group of patients who were at high risk due to malignant disease and treatment with chemotherapy[9]. Padberg *et al.* (1981) reviewed the risks associated with central venous catheterization for TPN over 3291 patient days of therapy and found a 2.8% incidence of infection, 4.8% incidence of pleural and mediastinal complications, 11.8% incidence of misplaced catheter tips on initial insertion, and a 4.8% incidence of venous thrombosis[12]. All studies have concluded that compliance to a strict management protocol by an experienced team is important for safe effective use of central venous catheters and parenteral nutrition therapy.

VASCULAR ACCESS IN INFANTS AND CHILDREN

Vascular access for total parenteral nutrition in infants and children continues to be a technically difficult and often tedious problem. During the 1970s the use of peripherally administered total parenteral nutrition became widespread, adequate calorie intakes being achieved through the use of fat emulsions[13]. The complications of peripheral parenteral nutrition in children are now well documented and several authors have questioned the safety and efficacy of this route of nutritional support[14]. Traditionally, central venous catheterization in children has been accomplished by a 'cut down' of the veins of the head and neck (cephalic, jugular and facial veins). These central lines can be inserted at the bedside under local anaesthesia and are usually tunnelled away from the site of the venous entry with exiting of the catheter behind the patient's ear. The catheter may also be tunnelled onto the anterior chest wall for greater ease of dressing care and cosmetic reasons. As in the adult, central venous lines may be introduced into the inferior vena cava by cannulating the distal saphenous vein in the ilio-inguinal area, and this approach compares favourably with other methods[15].

Central venous access through infraclavicular venous cannulization has recently become more widely accepted although early experiences with this technique were associated with numerous complications[16,17]. More recently, several authors utilizing a different catheter system have reported lengthy experience with subclavian catheterization and have achieved excellent results[18,19]. However, the system still has problems which several centres are currently seeking to resolve[20]. Recently the development of a 'peel-away sheath' for the placement of Broviac and Hickman catheters has been used in children which has the major advantage that the subclavian vein can be cannulated multiple times[21]. Currently at the University of Texas Medical School at Houston, the route of vascular access for TPN in children is determined by caloric need and by the duration of anticipated total parenteral support. For children requiring less than a month of therapy, subclavian catheterization is employed, and in those patients needing prolonged support Broviac, Hickman and Scribner paediatric catheters are introduced.

References

1 Aubaniac, R. (1952). L'injection intraveineuse sous claviculaire: avantages et technique. *Presse Méd.*, **60**, 1456
2 Duke, J. H. and Dudrick, S. J. (1975). Parenteral feeding. In Ballinger, W. F. *et al.* (eds.) *Manual of Surgical Nutrition.* pp. 285–317. (Philadelphia: W. B. Saunders)
3 Steiger, E. and Grundfest, S. (1980). Intravenous hyperalimentation: Vascular access and administration. In Dietel, M. (ed.) *Nutrition in Clinical Surgery.* pp. 53–64. (Baltimore: Williams and Wilkins)
4 Yoffa, D. (1963). Supraclavicular subclavian venipuncture and catheterisation. *Lancet*, **2**, 614

5 Benotti, P. N., Bothe, A., Miller, J. D. *et al.* (1977). Safe cannulation of the internal jugular vein for long term hyperalimentation. *Surg. Gynecol. Obstet.*, **144**, 574

6 Broviac, J. W., Cole, J. J. and Scribner, B. N. (1973). A silicone rubber atrial catheter for prolonged parenteral alimentation. *Surg. Gynecol. Obstet.*, **136**, 602

7 Stellato, T. A., Gauderer, M. W. and Cohen, A. M. (1981). Direct central vein puncture for silicone rubber catheter insertion. *Surgery*, **90**, 896

8 Dudrick, S. J., Englert, D. M., Barroso, A. O. *et al.* (1981). Update on ambulatory home hyperalimentation. *Nutr. Supp. Serv.*, **1**, 18

9 Copeland, E. M., MacFadyen, B. V., McGown, C. *et al.* (1974). The use of hyperalimentation in patients with potential sepsis. *Surg. Gynecol. Obstet.*, **138**, 377

10 Rowlands, B. J. and Dudrick, S. J. (1981). Nutritional support of the infected patient. In Powanda, M. C. and Canonico, P. G. (eds.) *Infection: The Physiological and Metabolic Responses of the Host.* pp. 359–397. (Amsterdam: Elsevier)

11 Ryan, J. A., Abel, W. M., Abbott, W. M. *et al.* (1974). Catheter complications in total parenteral nutrition. *N. Engl. J. Med.*, **290**, 757

12 Padburg, F. T., Ruggiero, J., Blackburn, G. L. *et al.* (1981). Central venous catheterization for parenteral nutrition. *Ann. Surg.*, **193**, 264

13 Coran, A. G. (1974). Total intravenous feeding of infants and children without the use of central venous catheter. *Ann. Surg.*, **179**, 445

14 Ziegler, M., Jakobowski, D., Hoelzer, D. *et al.* (1980). Route of parenteral nutrition: Proposed criteria revision. *J. Pediatr. Surg.*, **15**, 472

15 Fonkalsrud, E. W., Berquist, W., Burke, M. *et al.* (1982). Long term hyperalimentation in children through saphenous central venous catheterization. *Am. J. Surg.*, **143**, 209

16 Morgan, W. W. and Harkins, G. A. (1972). Percutaneous introduction of long-term indwelling venous catheters in infants. *J. Pediatr. Surg.*, **7**, 538

17 Groff, D. B. and Ahmed, N. (1974). Subclavian vein catheterization in the infant. *J. Pediatr. Surg.*, **9**, 171

18 Filston, H. C. and Grant, J. P. (1979). A safer system for percutaneous subclavian venous catheterization in newborn infants. *J. Pediatr. Surg.*, **14**, 564

19 Eichelberger, M. R., Rous, P. G., Hoelzer, D. J. *et al.* (1981). Percutaneous subclavian venous catheters in neonates and children. *J. Pediatr. Surg.*, **16**, 547

20 Hoelzer, D. J., Musemeche, C. A. and Brooks, B. F. (1982). Evolution of the ideal central venous catheter. In *Controversies in Pediatric Surgery.* University of Texas Press, (In press)

21 Gauderer, M. W., Stellato, T. A. and Izant, R. J. (1982). Subclavian puncture for the placement of the Broviac Silastic catheter in children. *J. Pediatr. Surg.* (In press)

40

Stenosis of the subclavian vein after percutaneous catheterization

J. ZINGRAFF, A. DANA, Z. FEDJELLI, T. DRUËKE AND
P. BOURQUELOT

Catheterization of the subclavian vein, a nowadays widely used technique in intensive care units[3-5], is more and more promoted as a transient vascular access in patients treated by chronic haemodialysis[6-8].

Thrombosis of the catheter is considered as a minor complication almost always successfully treated by changing the catheter with the help of a guide wire without the need of a second venous puncture. Thrombosis of the subclavian vein is seldom mentioned and seems clinically very exceptional. However, this contrasts strikingly with the high incidence of subclavian occlusion found during autopsy in a series of intensive care patients reported by Erben *et al.*[1].

In patients with end-stage renal disease who need a lifelong treatment by chronic haemodialysis, vascular access is of major importance. When waiting for a functioning permanent access the subclavian catheter seems an attractive alternative to a Scribner shunt or to repeated puncture of the femoral vein. However, a possible stenosis of the subclavian vein after removal of the catheter may compromise subsequent vascular procedures in the homolateral arm.

Hence, we believe that it might be of great interest to check systematically by serial radiography the post-catheter integrity of the subclavian vein.

PATIENTS AND METHODS

Fifteen patients have been selected for this study: 7 males, 8 females. Their mean age was 47 years (range: 24–72 years). Four of them were already on haemodialysis when referred to our hospital for thrombosis of their fistula.

The other 11 patients started treatment by dialysis without being previously prepared to it. Catheters were left in place during a mean time of 27 days (range 1–100). Six times, the catheter was removed in febrile patients; in four of these patients, *Staphylococcus epidermidis* was found on blood cultures and on the removed catheter. In the two other patients, the fever was unrelated to the catheter: septicaemia with a urinary bacteria in one, infected bronchopathy in the other. In all the other patients the catheter was removed because of the correct functioning of the permanent vascular access or, in one case, because of the onset of a peritoneal dialysis programme. Three times, the catheter had to be changed with the help of a guide wire, twice for thrombosis and once for kinking of the catheter.

None of the patients had clinical signs of subclavian thrombosis. At least, one week after catheter removal, the subclavian vein was visualized by means of an i.v. shot of 40 to 60 ml of Télébrix 38 in the homolateral cubital fossa.

RESULTS

In four of the 15 patients of this study, a stenosis of the subclavian vein could be evidenced: complete in two cases, partial in the two others. Moreover, the suspicion of a slight stenosis exists in one other patient.

In this small series the influence of the duration of the catheter on the incidence of venous stenosis is not easily evaluated. In the four-above-described cases, the catheter was left in place 1, 25, 48 and 100 days respectively (mean 43.5 days versus 21 days in the 11 other cases). In one case, the catheter was removed the first day after being introduced because of a septicaemia. In another patient, the catheter was replaced because of poor blood flow. The second catheter was removed after a total duration of subclavian catheterization of 100 days. In the two other patients, catheter functioning was uneventful.

COMMENTS

In patients with end-stage renal disease, the delay to realize a functional permanent vascular access may take several weeks. During this period, a temporary access should not cut off the vascular tree of the patient. For this reason, a Scribner's shunt must be avoided. The alternative means is the percutaneous puncture of a large vein: the femoral, jugular or subclavian vein. Subclavian catheters may be left *in situ* for a long period with a minimal discomfort for the patient and is preferred to the repeated puncture of the femoral vein as well by the patients as by the medical staff. Hence, many authors consider the subclavian way the method of choice for temporary vascular access[6–9].

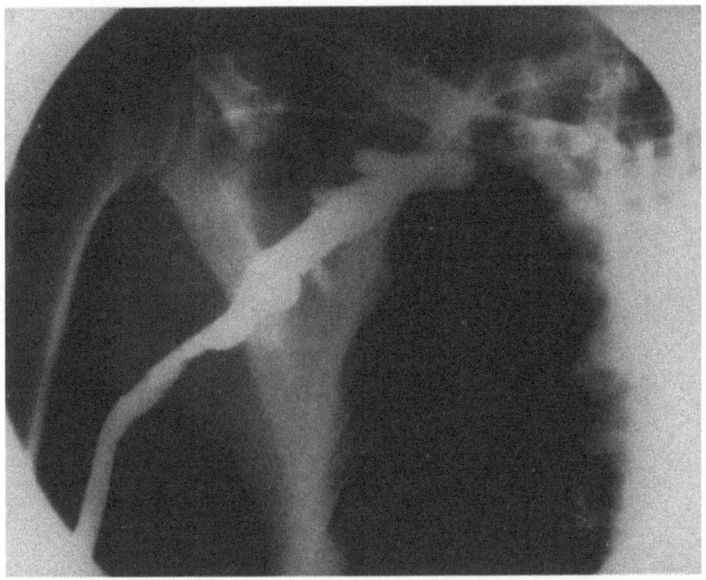

Figure 40.1 Complete obstruction of the right subclavian vein in a 56-year-old man. The catheter functioned quite satisfactorily during 48 days without any complication

However, to appreciate the long-term innocuity of this technique, a careful evaluation of the risk of postcatheter obstruction seems indicated, specially in chronic dialysis patients. Clinical signs of thrombophlebitis fail mostly, in contrast to the high incidence (25–30%) of post-catheter lesions revealed when one systematically looked for it either by autopsy[1] or by angiography as demonstrated in this preliminary study. The risk of subclavian stenosis should be counterbalanced against the advantages of the method.

References

1 Erben, J., Kvasnicka, J., Bastecky, J. *et al.* (1979). Long-term experience with the technique of sub-clavian and femoral vein cannulation in hemodialysis. *Artific. Org.*, **3**, 241

2 Henzel, J. H. and de Weese, M. S. (1971). Morbid and mortal complications associated with prolonged central venous cannulation. *Am. J. Surg.*, **121**, 600

3 Herbst, C. A. (1978). Indications, management and complications of percutaneous sub-clavian catheters. *Arch. Surg.*, **113**, 1421

4 Linos, D. A., Mucha, P., van Heerden, J. A. (1980). Sub-clavian vein. A golden route. *Mayo Clin. Proc.*, **55**, 315

5 Schwarzbeck, A., Brittinger, W. D., Strauch, M. (1978). Percutaneous cannulation of sub-clavian vein for acute haemodialysis. *Proc. Eur. Dial. Trans. Assoc.*, **15**, 575

6 Simons, O., Khazine, F., Haas, T. *et al.* (1980). Repetitive hemodialysis by temporary venous subclavian cannulation. *Kidney Int.*, **18**, 801 (Abstract)

7 Smith, S. B., Wombolt, D. G., Hurwitz, *et al.* (1979). Experience with subclavian vein for vascular access. *Clin. Exp. Dial. Apheresis*, **5**, 293

8 Uldall, P. R., Dyck, R. F., Woods, F., *et al.* (1979). A subclavian cannula for temporary vascular access for hemodialysis or plasmapheresis. *Dial. Transpl.*, **8**, 963

9 Verbanck, J., Vanholder, R. and Ringoir, S. (1981). A 4-year study of subclavian vein access for single needle hemodialysis. XVIIIth Congress of the EDTA, Paris 1981, Abstracts, p. 91

41

The use of arteriovenous fistulas for long-term parenteral nutrition

L. G. J. ENGELS, S. H. SKOTNICKI, F. G. M. BUSKENS AND
J. H. M. van TONGEREN

At present parenteral nutrition is an established mode of nutritional support in many pathological conditions. Long-term parenteral nutrition (LTPN) at home also has become an accepted entity, especially in short bowel syndrome patients. Vascular access of LTPN is generally achieved with indwelling central venous catheters[1-11]. Because of suspected recurrent thrombosis arteriovenous (A-V) fistulas are not recommended to administer LTPN in patients with chronic intestinal disease[2]. We present data of seven patients on LTPN via A-V fistulas.

PATIENTS AND METHODS

There were four female and three male patients, aged 17–67 years (mean 40.7 years) at the start of LTPN at home. The indications for LTPN were: a short bowel syndrome in four patients, a high-output end jejunostomy in two patients and scleroderma of the small bowel with repetitive paralytic ileus and severe malabsorption while on enteral nutrition in one patient. The length of the jejunal–ileal remnant in the short bowel syndrome patients varied from 0 to 50 cm (mean 25 cm). In both high-output end jejunostomy patients with Crohn's disease the remaining jejunum measured 100 cm. The causes of the short bowel syndrome were small bowel volvulus in two patients, strangulation ileus in one and mesenteric infarction in another patient.

Eight access procedures were used in these seven patients. Two patients had a Cimino fistula, in the other patients six bovine graft fistulas were created. Two bovine grafts were located at a thigh because of poor arm vessels, the other fistulas were situated at a forearm. In this study we grouped the Cimino and the bovine graft fistulas and named them A-V fistulas. In general one of the family members inserted and removed a small butterfly needle in the A-V fistula. To prevent thrombosis all patients received coumarin anticoagulant therapy.

RESULTS

The A-V fistulas used were functioning during a mean period of 14.3 months (range 5–54). Early thrombosis, defined as A-V fistula obliterations within 24 h postoperatively[12], occurred in one bovine graft which could be successfully managed by immediate thrombectomy. The course of LTPN via Cimino fistulas in two patients was uneventful during 14 and 9 months respectively. Late bovine graft thrombosis (beyond 24 h postoperatively[12]) took place on six occasions after an average use of 18.9 months (range 2.5–51). Thrombectomy was successful in three graft thromboses but unsuccessful in one case. Thrombectomy was not carried out for a graft obliteration developed during a non-graft derived serious septic shock and for another graft thrombosis due to extravasation of the parenteral nutrition solutions. The latter graft was situated too deep subcutaneously, and this caused frequent problems when inserting the needle.

DISCUSSION

A-V fistulas are rarely applied to administer LTPN. From the literature[7,13–20] we have gathered data on experiences with A-V fistulas in LTPN. Altogether 30 A-V fistulas were used in 25 patients. On three, the data were insufficient, leaving 27 A-V fistulas for an evaluation; these are summarized in Table 41.1. As in our patients A-V fistula thrombosis was the major complication. Mean patency of all A-V fistulas was 25.5 months (range 1–86). Obviously the best results were obtained with Cimino fistulas. Nearly similar results were achieved when using saphenous vein loops and bovine grafts.

Table 41.1 Arteriovenous fistulas in LTPN; literature data[7,13–20]

Number and type of A-V fistulas	Mean usefulness (months)	A-V fistula thrombosis (number)
7 Cimino	38.6	1
9 Saphenous vein loops	24.5	4
7 Bovine grafts	29.2	6
4 PTFE*	3	2

*PTFE = polytetrafluoroethylene

Except for venous thrombosis, complications of central venous catheters in LTPN include catheter sepsis, blockage and migration. These complications occur more frequently than is generally believed. In all but one[9] of some recent published studies[4-11] dealing with 675 central venous catheters in 381 patients the mean catheter survival time did not exceed 10 months. Moreover, when putting together the catheter complications mentioned in these series[4-11] the percentage of catheter sepsis amounted to 16.4. Unacceptable catheter migration occurred in 18.6% of all catheters, venous thrombosis in 8.7% and catheter blockage in 8.6%.

CONCLUSIONS

When considering LTPN our experiences and literature data indicate that A-V fistulas are valuable alternatives for central venous catheters. Except for A-V fistula thrombosis other complications are seldom seen. At present the best results are obtained when using Cimino fistulas. To prevent A-V fistula thrombosis anticoagulant therapy is recommended.

References

1 Broviac, J. W., Cole, J. J. and Scribner, B. H. (1973). A silicone rubber atrial catheter for prolonged parenteral nutrition. *Surg. Gynecol. Obstet.*, **136**, 602
2 Riella, M. C. and Scribner, B. H. (1976). Five years experience with a right atrial catheter for prolonged parenteral nutrition at home. *Surg. Gynecol. Obstet.*, **143**, 205
3 Jeejeebhoy, K. N., Langer, B., Tsallas, G. *et al.* (1976). Total parenteral nutrition at home: studies in patients surviving 4 months to 5 years. *Gastroenterology*, **71**, 943
4 Rault, R. M. and Scribner, B. H. (1977). Parenteral nutrition in the home. In Glass, G. B. J. (ed.). *Progress in Gastroenterology*. Vol. III, chap. 19. (New York: Grune & Stratton)
5 Strobel, C. T., Byrne, W. J., Fonkalsrud, E. W. *et al.* (1978). Home parenteral nutrition: results in 34 pediatric patients. *Ann. Surg.*, **188**, 394
6 Dudrick, S. J., Englert, D. M., Van Buren, C. T. *et al.* (1979). New concepts of ambulatory home hyperalimentation. *J. PEN.*, **3**, 72
7 Byrne, W. J., Ament, M. E., Burke, M. *et al.* (1979). Home parenteral nutrition. *Surg. Gynecol. Obstet.*, **149**, 593
8 Grundfest, S., Steiger, E., Sattler, L. *et al.* (1979). The current status of home total parenteral nutrition. *Artif. Organs*, **30**, 156
9 Fleming, C. R., Beart, Jr, R. W., Berkner, S. *et al.* (1980). Home parenteral nutrition for management of the severely malnourished patient. *Gastroenterology*, **79**, 11
10 Greig, P. D., Jeejeebhoy, K. N., Langer, B. *et al.* (1981). A decade of home parenteral nutrition. *Gastroenterology*, **80**, 1164
11 Ladefoged, K., Efsen, F., Krogh, Christoffersen, J. *et al.* (1981). Long-term parenteral nutrition: II. Catheter-related complications. *Scand. J. Gastroenterol.*, **16**, 913
12 Slooff, M. J. H. (1981). Secondary access surgery for hemodialysis and chemotherapy. *Thesis*, Groningen, The Netherlands
13 Jamieson, A. and Dirnfeld, V. (1972). Long-term parenteral nutrition by means of an arteriovenous (A-V) fistula. *Vasc. Surg.*, **6**, 251
14 McGill, D. B. (1974). Long-term parenteral nutrition. *Gastroenterology*, **67**, 195
15 Zincke, H., Hirsche, B. L., Armamoo, D. G. *et al.* (1974). The use of bovine carotid grafts for hemodialysis and hyperalimentation. *Surg. Gynecol. Obstet.*, **139**, 350
16 Heizer, W. D. and Orringer, E. P. (1977). Parenteral nutrition at home for five years via arteriovenous fistulas. *Gastroenterology*, **72**, 527

17 Buselmeier, Th. J., Kjellstrand, C. M., Sutherland, D. E. R. *et al.* (1977). Peripheral blood access for hyperalimentation. Use of expanding polytetrafluoroethylene arteriovenous conduit. *J. Am. Med. Assoc.*, **238**, 2399
18 Guba, Jr, A. M., Collins, Jr, G. J., Rich, N. M. *et al.* (1979). Nondialysis uses for vascular access procedures. *Ann. Surg.*, **190**, 72
19 Fry, P. D. and Allardyce, D. B. (1979). Polytetrafluoroethylene grafts for vascular access for hyperalimentation. *Can. J. Surg.*, **22**, 154
20 Baird, R. M., Rae, A. I. and Chan-Yan, C. (1980). Long-term parenteral nutrition with arteriovenous fistulas. *Am. J. Surg.*, **139**, 637

42

Exchange of central venous catheters via a guidewire

F. BOZZETTI, G. TERNO, G. BONFANTI, D. SCARPA,
M. AMMATUNA AND A. PUPA

Maintenance of a long-term intravenous nutritional support is frequently associated with catheter-related complications including contamination or sepsis, break of the line and additional cumulative risk for repeated percutaneous cannulations. Exchange of the catheter over a guidewire has been increasingly used all over the world[1-5] with the purpose of reducing the risk of a new percutaneous cannulation or of effectively treating the catheter sepsis. However, demonstration of the efficacy of a routine exchange of the catheter for prevention of sepsis and the evaluation of its safety and efficacy in the treatment of sepsis are still lacking. The present study analyses the safety of a weekly exchange via a guidewire of central venous catheters and its efficacy in the treatment or prevention of catheter sepsis by comparing a series of 64 prospectively studied patients to a series of historical controls[6].

PATIENTS AND METHODS

From September 1980 to February 1982, 64 patients admitted to the Istituto Nazionale Tumori of Milan and candidates for intravenous nutritional support entered in a protocol which included the weekly exchange of the catheter via a guidewire as well as central and peripheral blood culture. If a patient developed a symptomatology that suggested a possible catheter-related infection, the catheter was promptly exchanged and cultures were immediately taken. A total of 218 catheters were positioned in 64 patients.

The catheter exchange is generally performed at the bedside, while the patient is lying in a Trendelenburg position. A strict aseptic technique is essential to avoid any contamination of the newly placed catheter. The ipsilateral chest, shoulder and neck are prepared with ether or acetone and scrubbed with a povidone–iodine solution. The physician wears a mask and sterile gloves to prepare the field of the infraclavicular region. No local anaesthesia is necessary. The indwelling catheter is disconnected from the i.v. tubing, and an appropriate guidewire is then measured for the appropriate length from the catheter to approximately 4 cm below the sternal notch. With increased usage, guidewires of adequate length similar to those of the subclavian catheters are now available. The guidewire is gently introduced with the flexible end first through the lumen of the catheter up to a previously measured length so that the entire catheter is filled with the guidewire. The old catheter is removed and the tip is retained for aerobic and anaerobic bacteria and fungi culture. The new catheter is then threaded over the guidewire and passed through the previous subcutaneous tunnel into the intravascular space. The guidewire is then removed and the catheter hub kept covered until proper blood flow has been established and i.v. tubing connected to prevent occurrence of air emboli. The catheter is then secured to the skin with a sterile air-occlusive dressing.

The rate of colonization and sepsis was finally compared to the figures of 112 historical controls, recently published[6], and the outcome of contaminated catheters and septic patients was analysed.

RESULTS

The population of micro-organisms cultured from the catheter tip is shown in Table 42.1. In the present series the overall colonization rate of catheters was 14.6%, and the sepsis rate (positivity of the tip of the catheter and blood for the same micro-organism) was 2.2%. These values compare favourably ($p = 0.01$) with the previously reported 25.0% and 7.6% in historical controls.

Table 42.1　Micro-organisms cultured on the tip of 218 catheters

Type of micro-organism	No. of positive cultures	
Bacteria	14	
Staphylococcus albus		6
Diphtheroides		4
S. aureus		3
S. aureus + Proteus		1
Fungi	16	
Candida		16
Mixed	2	
S. albus + Candida		1
Acinetobacter + Candida		1
TOTAL	32	(14.6%)

However, if we correlated the incidence of sepsis to the patients, we did not find any significant difference between treated patients and historical controls. In fact, the present sepsis rate was 6.2% for *Candida* and 1.5% for bacteria, which are not very different from the 3.5% for *Candida* and 4.4% for bacteria of historical controls.

With reference to the efficacy of the technique of catheter exchange via a guidewire, we can observe that by this approach three-quarters of the contaminated catheters became negative after the first exchange, and all were negative at the fourth exchange (Table 42.2). All the five cases of sepsis resolved spontaneously with the catheter exchange (Table 42.3).

Table 42.2 Outcome of 22 catheters with microbial contamination (positive catheter but negative peripheral blood culture)

Micro-organism population (no.)	I Exchange	II Exchange	III Exchange	IV Exchange
Candida (9)	6	2	1	0
Candida + *Acinetobacter* (1)	0	0	0	0
Staphylococcus albus (5)	0	0	0	0
Diphtheroides (4)	0	0	0	0
S. aureus (3)	0	0	0	0
TOTAL (22)	27.2*	9.0*	4.5*	0*

*Percentage positive

Table 42.3 Outcome of five septic patients (catheter tips positive for the same micro-organism cultured from the peripheral blood)

Micro-organism population (no.)	I Exchange	
	Percentage of patients with sepsis	Percentage of patients with residual contamination
Candida (4)	0	3
Staphylococcus albus (1)	0	0
TOTAL (5)	0	60*

Candida

DISCUSSION

Preliminary analysis of these results shows that the routine weekly exchange of catheter via guidewire has no appreciable efficacy in reducing the overall colonization and sepsis rate. However, it appears that this technique carries no risk of cross-contamination and, as a matter of fact, both colonization and sepsis were drastically reduced when positive catheters were exchanged. Therefore, while the role of routine exchange in preventing sepsis must be further evaluated on a larger number of patients, its role in contaminated catheters or in septic patients must be emphasized.

Our data clearly show that when a patient with a central venous catheter develops unexplained fever, exchange via a guidewire is a safe and potentially curative approach. Therefore, if a patient is in total parenteral nutrition, nutritional support need not be discontinued.

Since venous catheters are thrombogenic a small but definite risk for thromboembolism does exist, and, in fact, a reversible episode occurred in our experience. The risk for thromboembolism can be minimized if a phlebogram is done prior to the exchange. Alternatively, one should preferably use silastic catheters, which are much less thrombogenic than the polyvinyl ones. The actual incidence of thromboembolism with uncontrolled exchange of silastic catheters can be approximately estimated at 0.1% level.

References

1 Fried, D. A. and Berk, J. L. (1980). Simple, rapid method for insertion of a Swan–Ganz catheter using an existing central venous or Swan–Ganz catheter. *Am. J. Surg.*, **139**, 454
2 Grave, A. H., Carpenter, C. M. and Schiller, W. R. (1981). Management of central venous catheters using a wire introducer. *Am. J. Surg.*, **142**, 752
3 Montaque, R. N. and Steiger, E. (1981). The safety of changing subclavian catheters over guidewires. *JPEN*, **5**, 575
4 Ruggiero, P. R. and Aisenstein, T. J. (1981). Central venous catheter exchange: indications and technique. *Nutr. Supp. Serv.*, **1**, 16
5 Shoum, S., Kahn, R. C., Carlon, G. C. and Howland, W. S. (1981). A guidewire technique for replacement of Swan–Ganz catheters. *Anesth. Analg.*, **55**, 455
6 Bozzetti, F., Terno, G., Camerini, E., Baticci, F., Scarpa, D. and Pupa, A. (1982). Pathogenesis and predictability of central venous catheter sepsis. *Surgery*, **91**, 383

43

Abstracts of posters in Access for total parenteral nutrition

---

Clinical results of 502 cases of caval catheterization through the internal jugular vein

C. U. CASCIANI, A. ARULLANI, G. CAPPELLO, R. DE VITTORI, L. MESCHINI and E. SPERA

Out of 628 cases of central venous catheterization for total parenteral nutrition on surgical patients, 502 were performed through the internal jugular vein. In all cases catheterization of the internal jugular vein was performed with percutaneous puncture from the anterior margin of the sternocleidomastoid muscle. Puncture of the vein was impossible in 14% of the cases in which the catheterization of the controlateral internal jugular vein or the subclavian route was attempted. If we exclude failure of the catheterization which accounted for 13.6% of cases, the technical complication rate was surprisingly low (Table 43.1).

Table 43.1

Complications	Incidence %
Puncture impossible	13.6
False position	0.4
Arterial puncture	0.4
Hydropericardium	0.4
Phlebitis	0.2

The advantages of internal jugular vein catheterization in respect to the more widely used subclavian route are discussed. Furthermore the authors report two cases of hydropericardium which occurred in two patients. The diagnosis of this new complication of central venous catheterization which can be confused with metabolic complications or other cardiac disorders is described. The physiopathology of hydropericardium and its possible connection with right atrium wall perforation are discussed.

Intravenous access for total parenteral nutrition
M. F. SMITH and M. J. LINDOP

This paper describes the technique of silicone catheter insertion with subcutaneous tunnelling. 120 insertions in 89 patients are reviewed in which the sepsis rate was 8%, the number of lines lasting long enough for completion of treatment was 88% and pneumothorax occurred in only one patient. Other complications reviewed include kinked, obstructed, misplaced and perforated catheters and also two cases of catheter occlusion by mineral growth. Methods are discussed for overcoming problems during insertion, including choice of vein, failure of the catheter to pass into the superior vena cava, location of the great veins and damage to the catheter during insertion and tunnelling. A video tape is available demonstrating the current technique.

Subcutaneous tunnelling of central venous catheter for home and in-hospital parenteral hyperalimentation – a prospective study
R. SCHMIDT, J. M. MÜLLER, S. HORSCH, H. ERASMI and
H. PICHLMAIER

Despite the statement of several authors that subcutaneous tunnelling of central venous catheters (CVC) will reduce the incidence of septicaemia in parenteral nutrition (PN) no prospective or comparative trial was able to support this opinion.

As a first step for comparative trial we studied prospectively the complication rate associated with subcutaneous tunnelling catheter.

In 160 cancer patients 182 subcutaneous tunnelled catheters were inserted for pre- and postoperative PN.

Complications due to the insertion of CVCs were puncture of the subclavian artery in two cases and the pneumothorax in one case. Eight patients developed a catheter-related sepsis. The incidence of septicaemia was therefore 1.79 cases per 1000 days of PN.

In 89 patients a Broviac®-type catheter using mainly the peel-away introducer technique described by Hickmann was inserted for home PN. One patient developed a superior vena cava thrombosis after 5 months. The incidence of catheter-related septicaemia was 0.9 cases per 1000 days of PN.

On the basis of these results we planned a comparative study which we are now doing.

Thrombosis around central venous catheters

R. PEETERS, F. VAN ELST, L. HENDRICKX, I. DE LEEUW and
A. HUBENS

In a prospective trial, 35 consecutive central venous catheters were studied by trans-catheter phlebography during their removal after completion of parenteral nutrition (only four catheters were not used for total parenteral nutrition. The mean catheter lifetime was 26.5 days (range 5–92 days). Five of the catheters were PVC, placed by percutaneous function, 31 were silicone catheters, one placed by punction, 30 by cephalic vein surgical cut-down and tunnellization.

Around 29 catheters developed some form of thrombosis (83%); six catheters were negative.

There were 21 simple sleeves, four sleeves with teardrop-like thrombi and four cases of full thrombosis of the superior caval vein.

In this positive group, we encountered three cases of pulmonary embolism, and two clinically evident cases of caval vein thrombosis. Three phlebographies were repeated after 24 h and in two cases the thrombosis was still evident.

Thrombotic occlusion of superior vena cava following total parenteral nutrition – more common than earlier recognized?

E. LINDBERG, T. ANDERSSON and G. WICKBOM

Very little is written about symptoms of thrombosis of superior vena cava (SVC). Moreover, there is controversy about the treatment of choice and also about the frequency. During the last 2 years approximately 750 central venous catheters (CVC) were inserted in our institution. In nine of the patients occluding thrombosis of SVC was diagnosed by phlebography. Five patients were female, four male, age 29–64. Reason for CVC was total parenteral nutrition or postoperative bleeding. Seven had silicon and two had Teflon catheters. Four patients had their first CVC, two had their second and three had previously had several catheters. Catheters had been in place for 2–31 days. Two patients had had heparin 5000 i.u. × 3 s.c. as antithrombotic prophylaxis. Symptoms of thrombosis of SVC varied widely. One patient had no symptoms before the catheter was withdrawn. Three had moderate chest discomfort and fever. Three patients also had swelling of the neck and face. Only two patients had severe cyanosis and obvious venous stasis; one of these also developed extensive pulmonary embolization. Seven patients were treated with streptokinase, one with heparin infusion. One patient received no treatment. All are now free of symptoms. Thrombosis of SVC in association with CVC was diagnosed at a frequency of 1–2%. In a controlled study of 67 patients in our institution 9% had SVC thrombosis. Symptoms are often mild and non-specific; in many cases it may occur unnoticed. Acute thrombosis of SVC is more likely to give severe symptoms; slowly progressing occlusion may allow collaterals to open up. It is a serious condition and the risk for pulmonary embolization is high. Immediate thrombolytic treatment is recommended. When repeated catheterization is considered an upper venogram may be valuable.

Surgical cannulation of the external jugular vein for total parenteral nutrition in 112 patients
J. L. GOUZI, B. PRADERE, Y. PARENT and E. BLOOM

The preferred technique was denudation of the external jugular vein at the base of the neck, insertion of a silicone catheter in the superior vena cava, subcutaneous tunnel in the front of the chest. One hundred and twenty-six catheters were placed in 112 critically ill patients who suffered with: peritonitis and/or digestive fistula (83), or severe pancreatitis (29). Sixty-six per cent were septic at the time of catheter insertion. Total parenteral nutrition was performed during an average of 31.5 days per patient. There was no immediate complication of catheterization.

A septic state occurred in 39 patients with 43 catheters. The relations with catheterization showed:

(1)   proved catheter sepsis   10.3%
(2)   questionable catheter sepsis   10.3%
(3)   removed catheters but no infectant 13.5%.

Peripheral versus central venous access for postoperative total parenteral nutrition
M. GEORGIEFF, L. W. STORZ and H. LUTZ

The insertion of a central venous catheter (CVC) for postoperative total parenteral nutrition (TPN) bears the overall incidence of 4–12% complications[1]. Furthermore the short-term PO intravenous nutrition support (INS) for a 3–6 day period after elective surgery has developed to a specific, adapted therapy. In our study we intended to evaluate the technical complications and the metabolic response of CVC access for hypercaloric TPN compared with peripheral venous access for hypocaloric TPN. Group I (GI) 40 patients who had to undergo gastric operation received preoperatively a CVC that was inserted from the vena basilica up to the subclavian vein. They were fed by TPN PO for 5 days. Group II (GII) 24 patients – gastric operation – received their nutrients by peripheral venous access for the same period. In GI three patients or 7.5% developed a thrombophlebitis, five patients developed a phlebitis; all eight patients received a new CVC.

Two patients needed a CVC change due to technical problems, an overall CVC change in this GII of 25%. In GII 15 patients or 62.5% developed a location infiltration and required a change of the cannula. GII showed a significantly better metabolic response to the hypocaloric infusion therapy compared with GI on hypercaloric TPN. On PO day 5 GII had a significantly higher total protein, albumin and transferrin and significantly lower liver specific enzyme changes.

These results indicate that patients after elective surgery do not necessarily need hypercaloric TPN. Nutritional requirements are more adequate and more safely met by peripheral venous hypocaloric TPN.

Reference

1 Grant, I. (1980). *Handbook of TPN*. (Philadelphia: W. B. Saunders)

Factors influencing catheter sepsis
M. F. VON MEYENFELDT, P. C. M. DE JONG, J. STAPERT, P. B. SOETERS and R. WESDORP

In an effort to diminish the incidence of the most frequent complications of total parenteral nutrition (TPN), catheter sepsis, the following studies were undertaken. Technical problems regarding the tunnelling of catheters were studied in 70 catheters, inserted for TPN. There was no difference between conventionally inserted ($n = 28$) and tunnelled ($n = 42$) catheters regarding technical insertion problems, pneumothorax and sepsis. The tunnelled catheters remained in place for a significantly longer period of time. A possibly diminishing effect of a 10 cm subcutaneous tunnel on the incidence of catheter sepsis, presumably by creation of a longer anatomical distance between puncture site and vein, was studied in a prospective randomized trial, involving 150 catheters. Eighty-one catheters were inserted according to the conventional technique; 69 catheters were tunnelled. Catheter sepsis was defined as an episode of clinical sepsis for which no other cause can be identified, and which resolves upon catheter removal. No differences between the two techniques were recorded, suggesting the tunnelling of PVC subclavian catheters as not useful in diminishing the incidence of catheter sepsis. Since systemic candidiasis is one of the more lethal complications of TPN, the influence of caloric source and intake on *Candida* pathogenesis was evaluated in an animal study, employing a hyperalimented rat model of systemic candidiasis. From this study it is concluded that the central catheter may contribute, in malnutrition, to the persistence of *Candida* in the tissues. Infusion of lipid or high concentrations of glucose may enhance *Candida* proliferation.

44

Invited comment on papers and posters in Access for total parenteral nutrition

R. I. C. WESDORP

It is a great honour for me to comment on the four oral presentations and the eight posters, dealing with access for total parenteral nutrition (TPN). The problem with administering TPN is the high osmolality of 1800 milliosmoles of the different feeding solutions. That is why it is so important to administer these hyperosmolar solutions not through a peripheral vein, but through a large-bore catheter with its tip in the superior vena cava.

However these centrally placed catheters are not, as mentioned by Brian Rowlands in his excellent review, without technical and long-term complications.

As the results presented in the posters and oral presentations are not comparable, I have divided them into three subjects: the technical aspects of catheter insertion, catheter-related sepsis and thrombosis of the central vein.

Concerning the technical aspects of catheter insertion, there is first the choice of which vein to use and how? Theoretically we can choose between the internal and external jugular vein, the subclavian vein and the saphenous and femoral veins. Both the jugular veins are popular with anaesthetists, because they are relatively easy to use during anaesthesia and extremely useful for rapid delivery of blood products and isotonic salt solutions during periods of shock. However the catheters are difficult to maintain for extended periods of time, as in TPN. Moreover they are difficult to fix to the skin of the neck and very uncomfortable for the patient, unless they are subcutaneously tunnelled to the chest as is demonstrated in the poster by Gouzi and co-workers from Toulouse, France. That is the only way in which the jugular vein can be used for administering TPN for a longer period of time. That the insertion technique is relatively easy is nicely demonstrated in the presentation of Casciani's group from Rome with 502 catheterizations of the internal jugular vein with only 0.8% technical insertion complications.

That is a lower complication rate than, for example, the subclavian route where an insertion complication rate of 4–12% is reported. However they do not mention their long-term complications such as catheter-related sepsis, to compare with the subclavian route.

The saphenous and femoral veins are not satisfactory access routes to the central system, except in dire emergencies, because of the high incidence of thrombophlebitis associated with venous catheters in lower extremities. Asepsis is extremely difficult, if not impossible, to maintain in these areas as evidenced by the high incidence of infection and septicaemia. That makes the subclavian vein the 'vein of choice' for insertion of central venous catheters for long-term TPN. Either through puncture or through a cut-down, insertion is relatively easy with a minimal number of complications in the hands of experienced operators. The position of the subclavian vein beneath the clavicle gives maximum stability for long-term use and minimizes the risk of catheter contamination.

Furthermore aseptic changing of the dressings is easily performed at this site and can even be done by the patients themselves during home TPN.

The question of 'to tunnel or not to tunnel' the catheter brings me to the most serious complication of centrally located catheters: catheter-related sepsis. Catheter sepsis can be defined as an episode of clinical sepsis for which no anatomical septic locus can be identified and which resolves upon removal of the centrally located catheter (with or without a positive blood culture). Besides meticulous aseptic care of the catheter during cannula insertion and dressing maintenance, from a theoretical point of view subcutaneous tunnelling of the catheter could lower the incidence of catheter-related sepsis.

This hypothesis is investigated by several groups and their results presented in four posters in this symposium. However, as was said several times before at this meeting, most of the investigations are not prospective randomized studies. For example, Smith and Lindop (Cambridge, England) tunnelled 120 silicone catheters with a sepsis rate of 8%, while Gouzi and his group (Toulouse, France) tunnelled 126 catheters with a sepsis rate of 10%. Schmidt *et al.* from Cologne (FRG) tunnelled 182 catheters as a pilot study for a randomized study currently being performed, and found a sepsis rate of 5%. Von Meyenfeldt (Maastricht, the Netherlands) reported the only randomized study in 150 patients and found no difference in incidence of catheter sepsis. So although it seems logical that a subcutaneous tunnel should diminish catheter sepsis, this could not be proven in a randomized prospective study, keeping the incidence of catheter sepsis around 6%.

A very interesting aspect of the study from Cologne (FRG) is the insertion of 89 Broviac catheters, using the peel-away introducer technique described by Hickman and mentioned by Rowlands. This will probably greatly facilitate the insertion of these very large-bore catheters.

The group of Bozzetti from Milan (Italy) had another very interesting and laborious idea to diminish catheter sepsis using a weekly exchange of the catheter over a wire guide, as well as in the presence of sepsis. Although they did not perform a prospective study, and compared their sepsis rate only retrospectively, the idea is intriguing; especially the fact that in seven septic patients the sepsis resolved spontaneously upon catheter exchange without stopping the TPN. However I cannot understand how, from a theoretical point of view, the infected sleeve or thrombus will stay *in situ* during this exchange?

The third subject is thrombosis of the subclavian and/or caval vein as diagnosed by phlebography, and I want to congratulate de Leeuw's group from Antwerp (Belgium) with a nice study in which in 35 consecutive patients with a central venous catheter a transcatheter phlebography was performed during removal of the catheter. They found in 29 of the 35 catheters, or 83%, a sleeve or thrombus in the subclavian vein. In this positive group they encountered three cases of pulmonary embolism and two clinical evident cases of thrombosis of the caval vein. I must agree that these last figures are disturbingly high, and this makes one once more aware of the morbidity of the procedure. Firstly it would be interesting to perform sequential phlebographies to see what happens to the sleeves, and secondly we should not worry too much as only the clinical cases are relevant.

Phlebography was also used by Lindberg *et al.* from Örebro, Sweden, to diagnose thrombosis of superior vena cava in 750 central venous catheters. These workers found an incidence of 1.2% in which most cases remained clinically unnoticed, and I agree with their conclusion that immediate thrombolytic treatment is recommended only when a clinical syndrome develops.

In studying the incidence of thrombosis during central venous catheterization it is important to mention what kind of catheters are used as it was already shown, by Welch[1] in 1974, that silicone catheters caused much less intimal reaction and thus less thrombosis than any other catheter. At the moment it seems that a tunnelled silicone catheter inserted via the subclavian route is the access of choice for TPN!

Reference

1 Welch, G. W., McKeel, D. W. Jr., Silverstein, P., *et al.* (1974). The role of catheter composition in the development of thrombophlebitis. *Surg. Gynecol. Obstet.*, **138**, 421

Section IX
Access for chemotherapy

45

Vascular access for chemotherapy: results of a simple procedure

TH. WOBBES, M. J. H. SLOOFF, D. TH. SLEYFER
AND N. H. MULDER

Vascular access in patients receiving cytostatics is often a serious and significant problem. In cases of long-standing chemotherapy especially, the superficial veins of the lower arm are often thrombosed due to the sclerosing effect of the drugs. It is likely that in future the oncologist in charge will be confronted more and more with this problem owing to the increased use of chemotherapeutic agents.

In 1975 we started creating arteriovenous (A-V) fistulas in patients who were already receiving, or about to be treated with, cytostatics (similar to the procedure in end-stage renal disease). The purpose of such a fistula is to increase the flow in the arterialized veins, so producing a rapid dilution and therefore reducing the damaging effect of the drug on the vessel wall. Moreover the vein is easier to cannulate, thus producing benefits for both the patient and the doctor. Several types of fistulas are mentioned in the literature. Some authors advocate the radiocephalic fistula as described by Brescia[1-4]; others use a PTFE graft in the thigh[5] or a bovine graft in the lower arm[6].

This chapter describes our experiences with the radiocephalic fistula between the radial artery and the cephalic vein as vascular access for chemotherapy.

MATERIALS AND METHODS

In the Groningen University Hospital we prefer to create an arteriovenous fistula in the lower arm as described by Brescia[1]. We use a variant of the originally described procedure by ligating the cephalic vein distally and making an end-vein-to-side-artery anastomosis. In this way arterialization of the vein distal to the anastomosis is prevented.

In the period April 1975 to December 1980, 115 radiocephalic A-V fistulas were created in 100 patients – 65 males and 35 females. The minimum follow-up was 6 months. The patients were treated for various types of malignancies: 47 malignant testicular tumours; 19 leukaemia; 13 Hodgkin-, non-Hodgkin's disease; seven malignant ovarian tumours; 12 sarcoma; two other malignancies. The operation was performed under local anaesthesia, on both an outpatient and an inpatient basis. From the day prior to the operation all patients received salicylates (500 mg daily) in order to prevent thrombosis, except in cases of severe thrombocytopenia.

RESULTS

In 66 of the 100 patients it was possible to create an A-V fistula, which functioned at least 4 weeks. The series included 12 patients who died with a functioning fistula. In 50 (77%) of the 65 males an effective fistula was performed and in 16 (44%) of the 35 females. In all cases the fistula was well tolerated. Figure 45.1 shows a survival curve of the 102 fistulas in 88 living patients. After 3 months 40–50% were still functioning. In 12 patients the fistula thrombosed within 3 to 10 months during a restaging laparotomy. In two cases the thrombosis was due to an anaphylactic reaction to cisplatinum. The thrombosis was the only complication encountered. There were no haemodynamic or infectious complications.

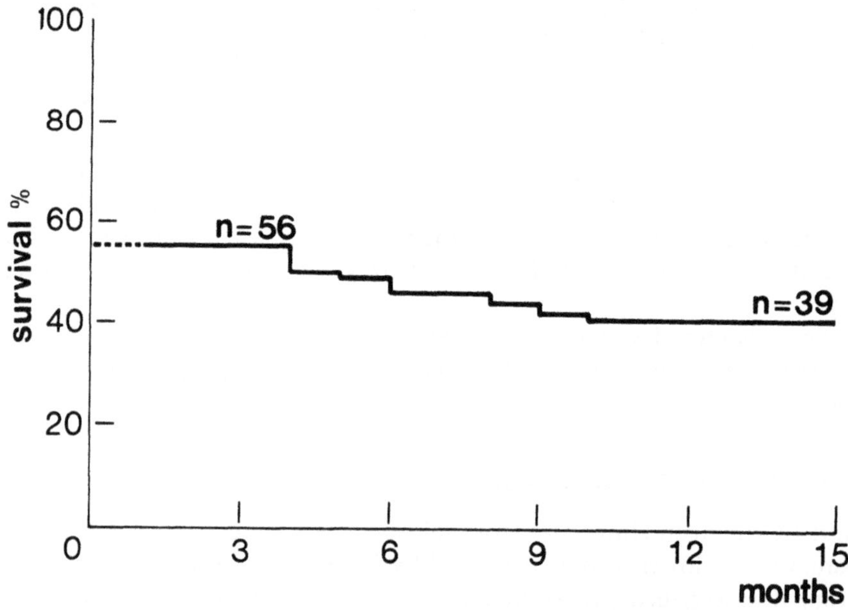

Figure 45.1　Survival curve of 102 fistulas in 88 living patients

Table 45.1 Relation between duration of preoperative chemotherapy and functioning of A-V fistula

Duration of preoperative chemotherapy	Proportion of functioning A-V fistulas
< 4 weeks	74% (60/81)
> 4 weeks	31% (6/19)
	66/100

In our series functioning of the fistula seemed dependent on the period of preceding chemotherapy. Either no chemotherapy, or treatment for less than 4 weeks, was received by 60–66 (91%) patients with a functioning fistula. In the 34 patients in whom the procedure failed 13 (38%) were treated for more than 4 weeks, and only in 31% in the 19 patients treated for longer than 4 weeks (Table 45.1).

DISCUSSION

Creating A-V fistulas in patients to be treated with chemotherapeutic agents is not yet a common procedure. Our results show that in a large number of patients convenient access can be performed. We have opted for a simple procedure, which can be performed under local anaesthesia even on outpatient basis. Most of the other access operations need general anaesthesia and hospitalization.

The most important reason for early failure of the operation was early thrombosis. This may be due to technical imperfections; most of the time, however, the reason is impairment of the outflow of the fistula caused by the sclerosing effect of the chemotherapeutic agents[2–4]. A remarkable difference in success rate was found between patients who received no chemotherapy and those who were treated for longer than 4 weeks preoperatively. It is therefore advisable to create an A-V fistula before the start of the chemotherapy, or as soon as the condition of the patients permits. Another reason for early failure of the procedure is the possible increased clotting tendency as a form of chronic intravascular coagulation[4]. This is in contrast to chronic haemodialysis patients, who have a decreased clotting tendency caused by the uraemic thrombopathy.

The cause of late thrombosis was nearly always identifiable as a decrease in blood pressure, either at operation or as a result of shock. Experience had taught us that a radiocephalic A-V fistula can function for a long time, while early thrombosis can be avoided. Thrombosis during an operation can effectively be prevented by a continuous infusion of saline solution in the fistula. If it is not possible to perform the radiocephalic fistula as a primary operation we have to resort to secondary access procedures in the elbow or the thigh. In that case the success rate of the operation will be much lower[4,7].

The conclusion is that the radiocephalic fistula can be a good solution as convenient access for chemotherapy, provided it is created before commencing chemotherapy.

References

1 Brescia, M. J., Cimino, J. E., Appel, K. and Hurwich, B. J., (1966). Chronic hemodialysis using venipuncture and a surgically created arteriovenous fistula. *N. Engl. J. Med.*, **275**, 1089

2 Bell, S. N., Sullivan, J. R., Hurley, T. H. and Marshall, V. C. (1977). The creation of artificial subcutaneous arteriovenous fistulas in patients with malignant haemotologic disease. *Aust. N.Z. J. Surg.*, **47**, 614

3 Steckler, R. M., Martin, R. G., Speer, J. F. and McCredie, K. B. (1974). Vascular access by means of surgically created arteriovenous fistulas in the chemotherapy of acute leukemia: a preliminary report. *South. Med. J.*, **67**, 821

4 Wobbes, Th., Slooff, M. J. H., Sleyfer, D. Th. and Mulder, N. H. (1982). Five years experience in access surgery for polychemotherapy. An analysis of results in 100 consecutive patients. *Cancer*. (In press)

5 Raaf, J. H. (1979). Vascular access grafts for chemotherapy. Use in forty patients at M. D. Anderson Hospital. *Ann. Surg.*, **190**, 614

6 Lempert, N., MacDowel, R. T., Karmody, A., Knight, E., Cunningham, T. J., Sponzo, R. W., Horton, J. and Ruckdeschel, J. (1975). Vascular access for cancer chemotherapy. *Cancer*, **43**, 1934

7 Slooff, M. J. H. (1981). Secondary access surgery for hemodialysis and chemotherapy. *Neth. J. Surg.*, **33**, (suppl.), 1

46

Indwelling right atrial venous access in the cancer patient

J. J. REILLY JR, D. L. STEED AND P. S. RITTER

INTRODUCTION

The cancer chemotherapy patient must undergo frequent venipuncture. Blood samples must be obtained to establish a diagnosis and to monitor therapy. Many chemotherapeutic agents and antibiotics administered intravenously produce chemical phlebitis. Plastic and metal disposable venipuncture needles must be changed every few days. In this setting, peripheral veins rapidly become inadequate as a route for reliable venous access.

Because of these problems we began evaluating surgically implanted venous access catheters in a series of acute leukaemia patients. The Hickman catheter (Evermed Corporation, Medina, Washington, USA), is a Silastic double-lumen catheter. The device is created by melding together two single-lumen catheters with outside diameters of 3.2 and 2.2 mm; it is 90 cm in length and is radiolucent. A Dacron cuff is incorporated onto the catheter to facilitate tissue ingrowth and minimize bacterial migration.

TECHNIQUE

The catheter is inserted in the operating room under local anaesthesia. A cephalic vein or external jugular vein cut-down is performed. After isolating the vein and ligating it distally, a long subcutaneous tunnel is created from a stab wound in the upper abdomen. The catheter is drawn through this tunnel and passed through a venotomy into a large-bore central vein within the mediastinum. The catheter is flushed with heparinized saline and its position confirmed by injecting water-soluble radiopaque contrast medium (Renografin) and obtaining a chest X-ray. The wound is closed with absorbable suture material.

The oncology nursing service performs initial catheter care. This regimen consists of an aseptic daily dressing change and flushing both limbs of the catheter with heparin solution after each use. Patients are taught both the dressing change and irrigation technique prior to discharge.

RESULTS

We have inserted 26 catheters in 25 acute leukaemia patients. Thrombocytopenic patients received a preoperative platelet transfusion. Prophylactic cefazolin was administered as a single dose immediately prior to surgery.

Table 46.1 Catheter survival (26 catheters)

In situ: 101 ±97.4 days (range: 11−331 days)	
Removed for complications	11
Inadvertent removal	1
Patient died − catheter functional	6
Patient alive − catheter functional	8

The 26 catheters remained *in situ* an average 101 ±97.4 days (range 11−331 days) (Table 46.1). Eleven catheters were removed for complications. A single catheter was dislodged inadvertently. Six patients have died of complications of acute leukaemia with functional catheters. There have been no catheter-related deaths. Eight outpatients are currently alive with functional catheters.

Each patient received on average 12 courses of combination drug chemotherapy (Table 46.2). Packed red blood cells (11.5 units/patient), fresh frozen plasma (4.2 units/patient), and platelets (48.0 units/patient) were readily administered via the Hickman catheter. All blood samples were also obtained through the catheter.

Despite this utility, the Hickman catheter is not without complications (Table 46.3). Our complications were of three types: (1) haemorrhage, (2) occlusion, and (3) infection, and are similar to those previously reported[1].

Table 46.2 Utility

Chemotherapy	12 courses/patient
PRBC	11.5 units/patient
FFP	4.2 units/patient
Platelets	48.0 units/patient

Table 46.3 Complications

Haemorrhage − 2 patients
1 re-exploration
Occlusion − 6 patients
5 catheters removed
Infection − 14 bacteraemias
8 resolved with antibiotics
6 catheters removed

Two patients suffered haemorrhagic complications in the immediate postoperative period. Re-exploration was undertaken in one patient. The catheter was bleeding around an inadequately tightened silk ligature. A second patient was treated conservatively.

Catheter occlusion occurred in six patients necessitating the removal of five catheters. In three patients catheter venography demonstrated an external fibrin sheath surrounding the intravascular portion of the catheter. Streptokinase infusion through the catheter successfully dissolved this sheath in two of these three patients. Reocclusion necessitated catheter removal in one streptokinase-treated patient.

The most serious complication of the Hickman catheter is bacteraemia[2]. There were 14 instances of this problem. All patients were febrile, but none suffered cardiovascular collapse. Bacteraemia invariably occurred in the setting of profound leukopenia after several courses of chemotherapy. The organisms cultured from the blood included 12 Gram-negative rods, one Gram-positive coccus, and one fungus. This bacteriology suggests a gastro-intestinal, pulmonary, or urinary source of the sepsis. Broad-spectrum antibiotics were begun in all such patients, with resolution of bacteraemia in eight of the 14 instances. In six, a persistently febrile course and/or bacteraemia led to catheter removal. Only one catheter grew an organism on direct culture.

CONCLUSION

Our overall experience with the Hickman catheter in the acute leukaemia patient has been satisfactory. The Hickman catheter provides a reliable means of venous access for obtaining blood samples and for administering a wide variety of drugs and blood products. Haemorrhagic complications occur in the immediate postoperative period and can be minimized by preoperative platelet transfusions in the thrombocytopenic patient and by meticulous attention to surgical technique. Catheter occlusion is commonly caused by extraluminal fibrin sheath formation, similar to that occurring in subclavian hyperalimentation catheters[3]. Such fibrin sheaths can be dissolved by streptokinase infusion, but may recur, necessitating catheter removal. Infection is the most serious complication. Bacteraemia should be treated with broad-spectrum antibiotics. If bacteraemia is persistent or recurs, the catheter should be removed.

References

1 Blacklock, H. A., Hill, R. S., Clarke, A. G., Pillai, M. V., Mathews, J. R. D. and Wade, J. F. (1980). Use of modified subcutaneous right-atrial catheter for venous access in leukaemic patients. *Lancet*, **1**, 993
2 Larson, E. B., Wooding, M. and Hickman, R. O. (1981). Infectious complications of right atrial catheters used for venous access in patients receiving intensive chemotherapy. *Surg. Gynecol. Obstet.*, **153**, 369
3 Hoshal, V. L., Ause, R. G. and Hoskins, P. A. (1971). Fibrin sleeve formation on indwelling subclavian central venous catheters. *Arch. Surg.*, **102**, 353

47

Seventy-five patient-years' experience with right atrial catheters for chemotherapy

W. P. REED, K. A. NEWMAN, C. A. De JONGH, S. C. SCHIMPFF AND P. H. WIERNIK

INTRODUCTION

Modern chemotherapeutic management of a number of malignancies depends upon repeated safe access to the venous system for the administration of drugs, fluids and blood products, and for the periodic assessment of cell counts and serum chemistries[1-3]. In the treatment of acute leukaemia we have found large-bore (Hickman) right atrial catheters to provide a more reliable means of access to the venous system than arteriovenous (A-V) fistulas[2]. We now document the long-term safety of these catheters when used for permanent venous access in patients with leukaemia and other malignancies.

METHODS

Patients with inadequate veins and acute leukaemia, or other malignancy requiring repeated courses of chemotherapy, were offered Hickman catheter insertion as a means of improving venous access. The features of this catheter have been previously described[1,2]. All catheters were inserted under local anaesthesia and aseptic conditions in an operating room equipped with fluoroscopy. The right external jugular vein was used whenever possible. If this vein proved to be inadequate, the internal jugular vein could be exposed and cannulated through the same incision. A subcutaneous tunnel was developed from the cervical incision to an exit site along the sternal border by means of a neurosurgical shunt passer[2,4]. The catheter was then threaded along the tunnel into the cervical incision through the lumen of the passer, and positioned with the Dacron cuff 6–8 cm deep to the exit site. Trimmed to proper length, the catheter was next directed into position near the junction of the superior vena cava and right atrium through a small venotomy in the exposed vessel. The catheter's capacity for withdrawal and infusion was tested before it was secured in place, and its position was confirmed by fluoroscopy. Catheters that extend too far into the atrium have a tendency to occlude during blood withdrawal. If hesitancy on withdrawal was noted, additional length was trimmed from the catheter until free flow was obtained. Once position and function were assured, the lumen was filled with 2 ml of heparin solution and occluded with a threaded cap. The wound was closed in two layers with absorbable sutures.

In October 1980 a double-lumen catheter, permitting simultaneous continuous infusion of incompatible chemotherapeutic agents, became available. This catheter consists of two single-lumen tubes attached together longitudinally. The resulting hybrid has the cross-sectional configuration of a figure '8'. The two grooves running along each side of this '8' have been plugged with cement over the length of catheter destined to lie in the venotomy site. Unless care is taken to position this contoured segment of the catheter within the venotomy, haemostatic closure of the vessel about the catheter will not be possible. With the exception of this placement detail, double-lumen catheters have been inserted in a manner identical to that used for the single-lumen ones.

Access to the catheter was not limited to any specific purpose, such as hyperalimentation or drug infusion, or to any specified number of daily uses. A heparin lock was left in all catheters not being used for infusion, and this lock was renewed daily. Patients and their families were carefully trained in catheter care so that catheters could be maintained during periods of out-patient care.

RESULTS

Patient characteristics

One hundred and seventy-two catheters have been employed in 159 patients over the 40-month period from November 1978 to March 1982. One hundred and thirty-one of these patients had acute leukaemia or chronic leukaemia in blast crisis (Table 47.1), and double-lumen catheters were used in 75 of these. One hundred and forty-seven patients received only one catheter, 12 required a second one, and one of these 12 patients needed a third catheter. All patients requiring more than one catheter were being treated for acute leukaemia. Ages ranged from 14 to 75 years (mean 43 years), and the male/female ratio was 67/92.

Table 47.1 Patient characteristics at catheter placement

	Patients ($n = 159$)	Insertions ($n = 172$)
Sex		
Male/female	67/92	71/101
Diagnosis		
Acute non-lymphocytic leukaemia	109	121
Acute lymphocytic leukaemia	17	18
Chronic myelogenous leukaemia	5	5
Lymphoma	11	11
Lung cancer	5	5
Breast cancer	5	5
Ovarian cancer	3	3
Other	4	4
Disease status		
Prior to initial therapy		34
First induction		29
Remission		15
Relapse		94
Platelet count/μl		
<50 000		74
50 000–100 000		41
>100 000		57
Granulocyte count/μl		
<100		48
100–499		27
500–999		16
≥1000		81

Catheters were placed prior to therapy in 34 patients, during induction in 29 patients, during relapse in 94 patients and during remission in 15. Partly as a result of disease status at placement, the preoperative haemograms (Table 47.1) showed a median platelet count of 48 000/μl, with 74 insertions taking place at counts less than 50 000/μl. The median granulocyte count at placement was 980/μl.

Catheter function

The mean longevity of function of these catheters was 167 days, with 48 catheters still functioning 3–873 days after placement. Catheters were in place and functioning at the time of patient death from the primary disease 1–491 days after placement in 102 patients. Eight catheters were lost for mechanical reasons from 7 to 358 days after insertion. Such loss was most often the result of a too superficially placed cuff working free. Four catheters were pulled because of tunnel infections. This complication usually occurred early after placement (6, 15 and 18 days) before the tunnel was well sealed. One patient developed a haematoma over the tunnel as a result of a seat-belt injury in an automobile accident. Secondary infection of this haematoma during a period of granulocytopenia necessitated catheter removal at 626 days. Six catheters were removed as suspected sources of systemic infection after 11–275 days. Only the catheter removed at 275 days had confirmed colonization at the time of removal.

Sixteen catheters have remained in place for more than 1 year, and 10 of these are still in place. Five catheters have remained in place for more than 2 years, and three of these are currently functioning.

Haemorrhage

Although the preoperative platelet counts were low there were only eight instances of postoperative haemorrhage requiring transfusion and only one of these was secondary to thrombocytopenia. Four episodes occurred in patients with active disseminated intravascular coagulopathy (DIC) at the time of operation. Haemorrhage was controlled in each instance by the application of pressure and by the administration of fresh frozen plasma and 1–8 units of red cells. DIC is now considered to be an absolute contra-indication to catheter insertion. Likewise, newly admitted patients with acute progranulocytic leukaemia (and hence a high propensity for DIC during initial therapy) are not now given catheters until coagulation parameters have had a chance to normalize after induction. One haemorrhage that required 5 units of transfusion and reoperation was attributed to the laceration of a small subcutaneous artery that had gone unrecognized at the time of the initial procedure. Two haemorrhages were secondary to capillary fragility induced by steroid administration and by leukaemic infiltration. The only patient to bleed as a result of thrombocytopenia was initially thought to have a platelet count of $100\,000/\mu l$ because of the presence of white cell fragments. Bleeding was arrested by the administration of platelets, once the problem was recognized after 9 units of blood were lost.

Infection

One hundred and nineteen episodes of bacteraemia have occurred during 28 675 days of catheter use in these patients, for a rate of 0.4 episodes per 100 catheter days. Most of these bacteraemias occurred at times of profound granulocytopenia or in association with terminal leukaemia (Table 47.2). Sources of sepsis remote from the catheters, such as pneumonias or perirectal abscesses, were generally present at the time that bacteraemias developed. Very few septic periods were noted during first induction chemotherapy and only 13 episodes were catheter-related (same organism in blood and at exit site, positive cultures only through catheter, or fever and positive blood cultures unassociated with a source other than the catheter). Unless the tunnel was inflamed or the patient was in the terminal stages of leukaemia, bacteraemias could be cleared by appropriate antibiotic therapy without removing the catheter. Catheters were removed from three early patients during antibiotic treatment. In retrospect, all had cleared their infections by the time of removal and the catheters were sterile in each instance. Two patients with terminal fungaemias had their catheters removed without apparent benefit. Both died within 24 h, their course further complicated by the loss of venous access. Only one patient had confirmed colonization of the catheter at removal. This patient had never fully co-operated with the daily flushing care of his catheter and had developed repeated episodes of poor withdrawal as a result. It is likely that a small fibrin plug had been present at the tip of his catheter for some time prior to the onset of his bacteraemic episodes.

Table 47.2 Bacteraemias in patients with right atrial catheters

	Leukaemia	*Other*	*Total*
Bacteraemias	114	5	119
Granulocytes <1000	98	3	101
Granulocytes <100	83	2	85
Terminal	25	3	28
First induction	6	0	6
Catheter-related	13	0	13

COMMENT

Management of patients acutely ill with leukaemia requires that reliable access to the venous system be maintained for the administration of chemotherapeutic agents, antimicrobials, blood components, fluids and occasional hyperalimentation[1-4]. Blood withdrawal capability is also necessary for the periodic sampling of blood indices and chemistries and for platelet phaeresis. The Hickman catheter has been shown to be well suited to provide such access, but experience with extended use of this device is still limited.

In many series[1,5-7] the catheters have been removed after completion of the planned course of therapy, usually within 100 days, although there are reports of catheters being left in place for more than 300 days[4,8].

The present report includes 16 patients who have kept their catheters for a year or more, including five patients with continuously functioning catheters for more than 2 years. The only serious complication to develop in any of these long-term patients was the result of an automobile accident producing tissue injury along the subcutaneous tunnel.

The rate of bacteraemias has not been increased from our previous report[2] by the inclusion of these long-term catheter placements, an observation which is consistent with our view that bacteraemias are usually secondary to disease status and only rarely to catheter-related factors. Only 13 bacteraemias were catheter-related, a rate of 0.045/100 catheter-days. Most were related to profound granulocytopenias, with infections at sites removed from the catheter, that were a direct result of leukaemia in relapse.

We conclude that the Hickman catheter offers an excellent choice for long-term venous access in cancer patients. The catheter is reliable and safe, even after prolonged periods of use extending beyond 1–2 years, and can be left in place permanently with little danger to the patient.

References

1 Hickman, R. O., Buckner, C. D., Clift, R. A., Sanders, J. E., Stewart, P. and Thomas, E. D. (1979). A modified right atrial catheter for access to the venous system in marrow transplant recipients. *Surg. Gynecol. Obstet.*, **148**, 871

2 Wade, J. C., Newman, K. A., Schimpff, S. C., Van Echo, D. A., Gelber, R. A., Reed, W. P. and Wiernik, P. H. (1981). Two methods for improved venous access in acute leukemia patients. *J. Am. Med. Assoc.*, **246**, 140

3 Copeland, E. M., Daly, J. M. and Dudrick, S. J. (1977). Nutrition as an adjunct to cancer treatment in the adult. *Cancer Res.*, **37**, 2451

4 Reed, W. P., Newman, K. A., de Jongh, C. A., Wade, J. C., Schimpff, S. C., Wiernik, P. H. and McLaughlin, J. S. (1982). Prolonged venous access for chemotherapy by means of the Hickman catheter. *Cancer* (In press)

5 Abrahm, J., Mullen, J. L., Jacobson, H. and Polomano, R. (1979). Continuous central venous access in patients with acute leukemia. *Cancer Treat. Rep.*, **63**, 209

6 Blacklock, H. A., Hill, R. S., Clarke, A. G., Pillai, M. V., Matthews, J. R. D. and Wade, J. F. (1980). Use of modified subcutaneous right-atrial catheter for venous access in leukemic patients. *Lancet*, **1**, 993

7 Thomas, M. (1979). The use of the Hickman catheter in the management of patients with leukemia and other malignancies. *Br. J. Surg.*, **66**, 673

8 Thomas, J. H., MacArthur, R. I., Pierce, G. E. and Hermreck, A. S. (1980). Hickman–Broviac catheters: indications and results. *Am. J. Surg.*, **140**, 791

48

The arteriovenous fistula and the Ommaya capsule – two accesses for long-term therapy

N. WALDSTEIN, K. RENDL AND K. PRENNER

The conditions for using the various forms of vascular catheters, such as subclavian catheters, are suitable veins, precise puncturing techniques and proper care of the catheter. However, such preconditions do not often exist, especially when long-term intravenous chemotherapy with almost thrombogenic agents is required.

In such cases we resort to the arteriovenous (A-V) fistula or the Ommaya capsule as alternative methods.

Provided there is adequate vascular expansion, the A-V fistula represents a good solution for long-term injection of drugs in larger quantities. We have experience in six cases. The A-V fistula is not always successful and despite corrective operations and the use of graft material the overall patency is so poor that an alternative method had to be adopted. We implanted eight Ommaya capsules.

MATERIALS AND METHODS

Six of our patients were provided with A-V fistulas for long-standing chemotherapy. Most patients had an inoperable malignancy. Those six patients represent 5.2% of the total fistulas constructed in our hospital between 1975 and 1981. The average age of these six patients was 56 years.

John H. Burrows of St John's Hospital, Detroit, Michigan, introduced the implantation of a subcutaneous reservoir for intravenous therapy[1]. This capsule, called after its inventor Ommaya, was first used in 1963 for injection of medicaments into the cerebral ventricle.

The capsule consists of a semispherical polyethylene container, 0.8 mm in diameter. A Silastic tube with a slit valve is connected with the Ommaya capsule. The operation is performed under local anaesthesia. On the right side of the neck the tube is inserted into the vena jugularis externa and introduced into the vena cava superior in front of the right atrium under X-ray control. The capsule is lodged subcutaneously in front of the sternum, which provides the necessary abutment. The tube is then connected with the capsule. Sclerosing therapeutic agents of this kind are a useful alternative when surface veins are not available or are introgenic. Strict observation and following of the rules for venipuncture are essential:

(1)   skin disinfection;
(2)   puncture of the capsule with thin sharp needle;
(3)   preliminary injection of approximately 5 ml of 0.9% NaCl;
(4)   injection of drug;
(5)   follow-up injection of NaCl;
(6)   1000 i.u. of heparin for irrigation;
(7)   withdraw needle from capsule during heparin instillation;
(8)   never aspirate blood.

The advantages and disadvantages of the Ommaya capsule and the A-V fistula can be seen from Table 48.1.

Table 48.1   Ommaya capsule and A-V fistula compared

	Ommaya capsule	*A-V fistula*
Operation technique	simple	tedious
Cost	high (about 1000 Austrian sch.)	low
Capacity	small quantities of drugs	larger quantities of drugs
Handling	experience required	relatively simple
Risk of infection	few long-term instances ($n = 0$)	low ($n = 0$)
Patency rate	not yet determinable	57% after 2 years ($n = 99$)
Contraindications	none	local: unsuitable veins and arteries; general: serious cardiac decompensation or coagulopathy

RESULTS

The survival time of the six A-V fistulas, and the patients, are seen in Figure 48.1. Inadequate outflow resulted, in two patients, in immediate occlusion of the fistula. Three A-V fistulas functioned well until the patients died of their malignancy. One patient, suffering from an acute allergic syndrome, had an A-V fistula for over 24 months.

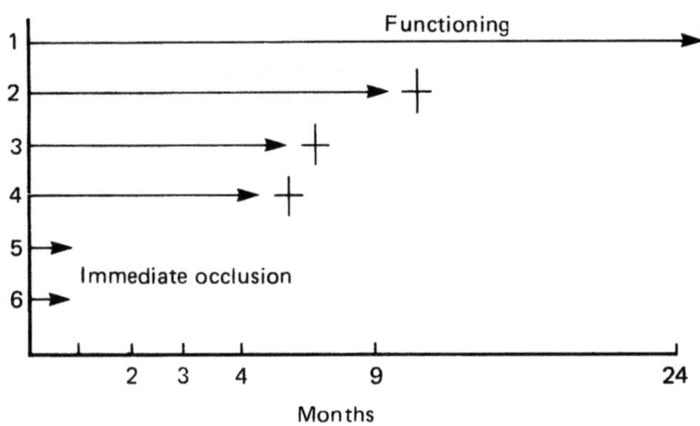

Figure 48.1 Function of A-V fistula for chemotherapy

In eight cases of intravenous treatment with the capsule, we saw no thrombosis of the vein. One of our patients used his capsule for more than 24 months. There was one case of dysfunction of the capsule, due to a riding accident involving this patient.

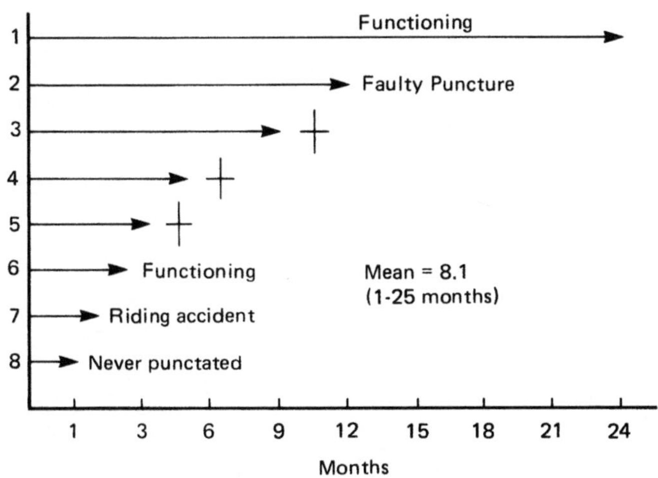

Figure 48.2 Function of Ommaya capsule for chemotherapy

CONCLUSION

Our experience with the Ommaya capsule is small, but we think that in the absence of suitable veins for chemotherapeutic agents, the implantation of a capsule like Ommaya's is a useful alternative for A-V fistulas or grafts. It is quite possible to lead a normal life with an Ommaya capsule.

References

1 Burrows, J. H., Yap, J., Coello, E., Casas, E. R. and Cera, D. (1977). Presentation at the American Society of Clinical Oncology meeting, Denver, Colorado, 17 May

49

Abstracts of posters in
Access for chemotherapy

Thirty-five direct and interposition arteriovenous fistulas for chemotherapy
L. LAMY and P. BOURQUELOT

Since September 1976, 35 angioaccesses for cancer chemotherapy have been constructed on 25 patients. The mean age was 45 years (19–73). Primary diseases were malignancies of breast (8), ovary (4), bronchus (3), testicle (3) or Hodgkin's disease (4). Chemotherapy had been initiated before surgical angioaccess in all but one case. Arteriovenous fistulas were: 12 direct (wrist: 6, elbow: 6), 23 graft fistulas (bovine: 16, PTFE: 6, saphenous vein: 1). Immediate complications are: 2 infections (PTFE), 6 thrombosis. Secondary complications and reoperations are detailed. Follow-up ranges from 1 to 43 months. Direct arteriovenous fistula should be settled at the beginning of cancer chemotherapy before exhaustion of superficial veins. Later on graft fistula is usually possible at the arm: operative infection and thrombosis due to secondary stenosis of the venous anastomosis have to be prevented.

Vascular access in bone marrow transplantation (BMT)
G. F. ADAMI, U. BONALUMI, U. BACIGALUPO and
F. GRIFFANTI-BARTOLI

A Hickman[1] right atrial catheter (HRAC) was placed in 60 patients with acute leukaemia (30) or aplastic anaemia (30) who were eligible for BMT. The HRAC was sterilized for 30 min at 131 °C, was inserted in the venous system via the cephalic vein (45 cases) dissected under local anaesthesia in the delto-pectoral groove, or via the internal jugular vein, under general anaesthesia: this was not tied and the anterior wall of the vein was fastened around the catheter by a silk purse-string suture. The tip of the HRAC was radiologically guided to the right atrium, the extravascular portion was placed in a subcutaneous channel on the chest wall. Blood was drawn daily for routine tests through the HRAC. Total parenteral nutrition compound, chemotherapy drugs, hydration solutions, antibiotics, blood products and the bone marrow graft were all administered through the HRAC. Between infusions, and twice daily, the HRAC was washed with miconazole 10 mg and heparin 100 i.u. in 20 ml saline, closed and taped to the chest wall. HRACs were in place for an average of 73 days (10–402). In 20% of cases there was local haematoma, in 25% (15/60 patients) infection developed. In seven patients causative agents were *Candida albicans*, in five, *Staphylococcus aureus* and in three, *Escherichia coli*. Only in 1/60 cases was the catheter removed for infection. Complications linked to percutaneous subclavian venipuncture (pneumothorax, haemothorax, brachial plexus and thoracic duct injuries) are avoided. In addition blood could be drawn easily and blood products infused without catheter clotting. The use of the HRAC, easily inserted, easily manageable and fairly safe from infections also in profound immunosuppression, is mandatory for patients undergoing BMT.

Reference

1 Hickman, R. O. *et al.* (1979). A modified right atrial catheter for access to the venous system in marrow transplant recipients. *Surg. Gynaecol. Obstet.*, **148**, 871

Secondary access surgery for chemotherapy; the elbow arteriovenous fistula
P. J. H. SMITS, D. T. SLEYFER, TH. WOBBES, N. H. MULDER AND M. J. H. SLOOFF

Secondary access surgery for chemotherapy is considered when the superficial lower arm veins are destroyed by the sclerosing effect of infused chemotherapeutics and when primary access surgery fails. Experience was gained with two types of elbow arteriovenous (A-V) fistula; the first type being the end-to-side brachiocephalic or brachiobasilic A-V fistula (E-S type) and the second type an end-to-side A-V fistula created between a perforating vein in the elbow and the brachial artery (Gracz type). Of the 31 E-S A-V fistulas 13 (42%) functioned compared to 16 (59%) out of the 27 Gracz A-V fistulas. Functioning of the A-V fistulas seemed dependent on the period of chemotherapy given before construction of the A-V fistulas. Of the 58 elbow A-V fistulas 22 were created in patients with no previous chemotherapy courses; 16/22 (73%) of these A-V fistulas functioned compared to 13/36 (36%) A-V fistulas created in patients which had undergone multiple courses of chemotherapy before construction of the fistula ($p = 0.016$). Mean survival time of both types of A-V fistula was 12 months. No major complications were encountered.

When secondary access surgery is considered the elbow A-V fistulas are serious alternatives to other secondary access methods like the bovine graft or PTFE graft or the autologous saphenous vein. The elbow A-V fistulas are constructed with autologous material. The operation is minor and is performed under local anaesthesia, on an outpatient basis. The Gracz type of A-V fistula showed the best results. This fistula has the additional advantage that when chemotherapy is ended, the fistula is easily abolished with a ligature around the perforating vein.

By doing this the continuity of the superficial and deep brachial veins is left intact, and normal anatomy is restored. Construction of the A-V fistulas should be attempted before the start of the chemotherapy.

Long-term discontinuous vascular access using silicon rubber catheters
J. F. GILLETTE, J. SUSINI and J. F. BERNARD

Long-term discontinuous vascular access is often a problem, either for total parenteral nutrition or chemotherapy. Silicon rubber catheters, properly inserted and managed, offer a simple solution. Silicon is a safe material, perfectly tolerated by the vein. Insertion can be percutaneous (subclavian) or through a cut-down of the deep humeral vein. The access is always done using the Seldinger method. A subcutaneous tunnel is always made.

Discontinuous use and discharge of patients between chemotherapies is possible: the catheter is rinsed with heparin and locked; the tip is covered by an occlusive bandage. The patency can be kept for 3–4 weeks without reinjection.

Since January 1981, nine subclavian and seven humeral catheters have been used discontinuously from 50 to 178 days. Out of 12 cultures on removal none was positive. Only one catheter had to be removed, because of clotting, at 155 days.

Vascular access for recurring life-threatening ketoacidosis
M. G. WALKER, R. NEWTON and B. LANE

A type 1 insulin-dependent diabetic, now aged 21, first required subcutaneous insulin at 12 years of age. Control was satisfactory until at the age of 16 her requirements rose progressively to more than 1500 i.u. insulin daily and she became exceptionally ketosis-prone. The artificial pancreas showed that her i.v. insulin requirements were approximately 90 i.u. daily, supporting subcutaneous insulin degradation. Treatment of recurring ketoacidosis with i.v. infusions caused progressive loss of venous access and four arteriovenous shunts at conventional sites failed. A PTFE femorosaphenous shunt also rapidly occluded. Control (poor) at this time was by combined maintenance continuous s.c. insulin infusion and supplementary i.m. insulin. An intra-deltoid cannula had to be discontinued because of haematoma formation following dipyridamole and anticoagulant therapy for shunt maintenance. A left femoral artery to popliteal vein shunt using a Dardik® (human umbilical vein) graft fashioned in January 1981 lasted until October 1981, having been used for most of its life for continuous maintenance and intermittent acute access – an average of two punctures per week. A second Dardik graft shunt, right femoropopliteal, has been in use since October 1981 with the exception of 2 months during which central venous catheters were used. Three of these failed due to sepsis and two Hickman catheters were factitiously damaged by the patient. In this patient the Dardik shunts have been free of infection and aneurysmal dilatation and have been longer-lasting than other arteriovenous shunts. This technique has allowed vascular access for continuous i.v. infusion of insulin but more importantly for fluid replacement and resuscitation during multiple spectacular episodes of diabetic ketoacidosis.

An intracaval shunt for the isolated perfusion of the pig liver
B. J. L. KOTHUIS, C. J. H. VAN DE VELDE, H. W. M. BARENBRUG and A. ZWAVELING

The median survival time after diagnosis of hepatic metastases is 75 days, and few effective modalities exist for prolonging this period of time. The best responses are obtained at present with hepatic artery perfusion, and remission induction has been shown to be dose-dependent limited by systemic toxicity.

An experimental study was undertaken in the pig, to develop an intracaval shunt allowing the delivery of high concentrations of cytotoxic agents to the hepatic parenchyma without loss to the systemic circulation (Figure 50.1).

Dosages up to 80 mg/kg body weight (maximum systemic dosage) were given to the isolated circuit. Concentrations of drugs measured by chromatography showed an average leakage of the isolated liver circuit to the systemic circulation of less than 1% ($n=25$).

Technical problems due to temporary portal hypertension, measured preoperatively, showed to be lethal if uncorrected in the pig. Systemic toxicity was minimal and liver function was restored within 2 weeks postoperatively after initial deterioration.

50

Invited comment on papers and posters in Vascular access for chemotherapy

R. MARGREITER

Patients requiring prolonged chemotherapy for malignancy, such as those receiving haemodialysis, often experience long-term problems with vascular access. Administration of antitumour drugs over long periods of months or years requires multiple venipunctures with progressive thrombosis, sclerosis and obstruction of all available surface vessels due to the irritating effect of these agents when in contact with veins. Moreover, chemotherapy is often combined with parenteral nutrition and in patients undergoing bone marrow transplantation is combined with supportive care, including antibiotics and platelet and granulocyte transfusions. The search for a suitable vein can then become a painful ordeal for the patient and a frustrating experience for the nurse or physician, and thus becomes a serious and challenging problem.

The results of four oral and six poster presentations on various modalities of vascular access for chemotherapy will be summarized and discussed in the following report.

Th. Wobbes *et al.* reported on 88 radiocephalic arteriovenous (A-V) fistulas which they created in 76 patients with various malignancies, though mainly solid tumours, with a 50% overall functioning rate at 3 months and a maturation time of 10–14 days, which is very short. It seems to be of great importance that 50% of their patients with no functioning fistula had had previous chemotherapy for more than 4 weeks, while 90% of the patients with patent fistulas had had no chemotherapy, or for less than 4 weeks, preoperatively.

J. J. Reilly *et al.* demonstrated their results with 26 indwelling double-lumen right atrial (Hickman) catheters in 25 patients suffering from acute leukaemia. Two cases of haemorrhage were seen, which was suggested to be due to the '8'-shaped cross-section of the catheter. In 14 cases of bacteraemia six catheters were removed for presumed haematogenous seeding. In 12 of these 14 patients Gram-negative bacteria were cultured, suggesting a gastrointestinal, urinary or pulmonary source, thus being a systemic rather than a local problem. Five other catheters had to be removed because of occlusion. Furthermore, it seems worthy of note that infectious complications were seen exclusively in granulocytopenic and immunosuppressed patients.

W. Reed *et al.* gave a survey of their wide experience with 167 Hickman catheters, inserted in patients with leukaemia and solid tumours. Bleeding and infectious complications were very much the same as in Reilly's group. They calculated 0.04 bacteraemic episodes per 100 catheter-days, which is quite low. They also emphasized that the majority of their infectious complications were related to granulocytopenia.

The number of A-V fistulas, on which N. Waldenstein *et al.* report, is too small (six) to draw any conclusions from their data. On the other hand they gave an account of the use of the Ommaya capsule; this is an implantable device, which has been used in the past for the instillation of chemotherapeutic agents intraventricularly for various cerebral disorders. The capsule is connected with a silicon rubber tube, which is inserted into the cava via the jugular vein. Although this is a very interesting approach, further experience has to be gained. However, three of their seven capsules were still functioning after 8–24 months.

L. Lamy and P. Bourquelot performed 35 A-V and graft fistulas for chemotherapy in 25 tumour patients suffering mainly from cancer. Twelve were A-V fistulas (wrist, ten; elbow, six) and 23 graft fistulas (bovine, 16; PTFE, six; saphenous vein, one). In all but one patient chemotherapy had been initiated before surgical angioaccess. Five A-V and one graft fistula occluded immediately after surgery, while seven further fistulas thrombosed after 5–19 months. In PTFE grafts two infections and three stenoses were reported. Their results are distinctly better than those of other groups reported at this meeting.

G. F. Adami *et al.* presented a poster on 'Vascular access in bone marrow transplantation'. They inserted 60 Hickman catheters in 30 patients with acute leukaemia and 30 others suffering from aplastic anaemia undergoing marrow transplantation. Their reported haemorrhage and infection rate of 20% and 25%, respectively, is slightly higher than that of Reilly and Reed. Interestingly, they had to remove only one catheter for these reasons.

P. J. Smits *et al.* exhibited an interesting poster on 'Secondary access surgery for chemotherapy; the elbow arteriovenous fistula'. They differentiate between two types of fistulas: Type I, which is a brachiocephalic fistula, and Type II, where they anastomosed a perforated vein with the brachial artery; 31 and 27 fistulas, respectively, were created. Considering the fact that in all these patients primary access surgery had failed, the patency rates of 42% and 59% are excellent and, interestingly, better for Type II than for Type I fistulas. Furthermore, the results were very much dependent on previous chemotherapy.

The poster 'Long-term discontinuous vascular access using silicon rubber catheters' by J. F. Gillette *et al.* presents the results with 16 of the above-mentioned catheters inserted via the subclavian or brachial vein, using the cut-down technique for the latter. Only one catheter had to be removed for thrombosis and no infection occurred. This is unusual and does not correlate with the general experience but may be due to their accurate technique and mode of dressing.

M. G. Walker *et al.*'s poster on 'Vascular access for recurring life-threatening ketoacidosis' gives the case report of an insulin-dependent diabetic patient requiring up to 1500 i.u. insulin daily and i.v. infusions for recurring ketoacidosis. After having created four A-V fistulas, which all occluded, and after inserting five right atrial catheters, they put in a Dardik graft (human umbilical vein) between the left femoral artery and the popliteal vein, which functioned for 10 months. Since a second Dardik graft on the right thigh is still patent after 6 months they suggest that human umbilical veins can be an alternative in such desperate cases.

The last poster from B. J. L. Kothuis *et al.* on 'An intracaval shunt for the isolated perfusion of the pig liver' shows exciting experimental results with an implantable device for the isolated liver perfusion (Figure 50.1). Less than 1% of the cytotoxic agent has been lost to the systemic circulation. Since some of these drugs are excreted by the bile, the systemic effect of these cytotoxic agents absorbed by the gut will have to be evaluated to prove its clinical value.

Apart from the Ommaya capsule and the relatively small number of simple silicon rubber catheters, two major possibilities for vascular access for chemotherapy were offered: The shunt procedures, either as A-V fistula or graft fistula using different materials, and the right atrial catheter.

Altogether 187 A-V and graft fistulas were reported in this session. The patency rate for more than 4 weeks was 57%, the mean survival time 12 months. Thrombosis turned out to be the main cause of failure, whereas hardly any other complications were observed. The success rate was very much dependent on the fact of whether the patient had had previous chemotherapy or not.

On the other hand, 253 Hickman catheters, mainly inserted in patients suffering from acute leukaemia or aplastic anaemia, were reported. The patency rate was about 100%, the longest survival time 34.8 months. The main causes of failure were infection (5%) and thrombosis (2.7%), dislocation being another complication.

The A-V and graft fistula offers the advantage of being a minor operation, which can be carried out under local anaesthesia on an outpatient basis, of no septic problems and fairly good long-term results. Definite disadvantages of this method are the high clotting rate, the maturation time and the discomfort associated with its use. Advantages of the Hickman catheter are the high patency rate, the possibility of immediate use and the comfort for the patient

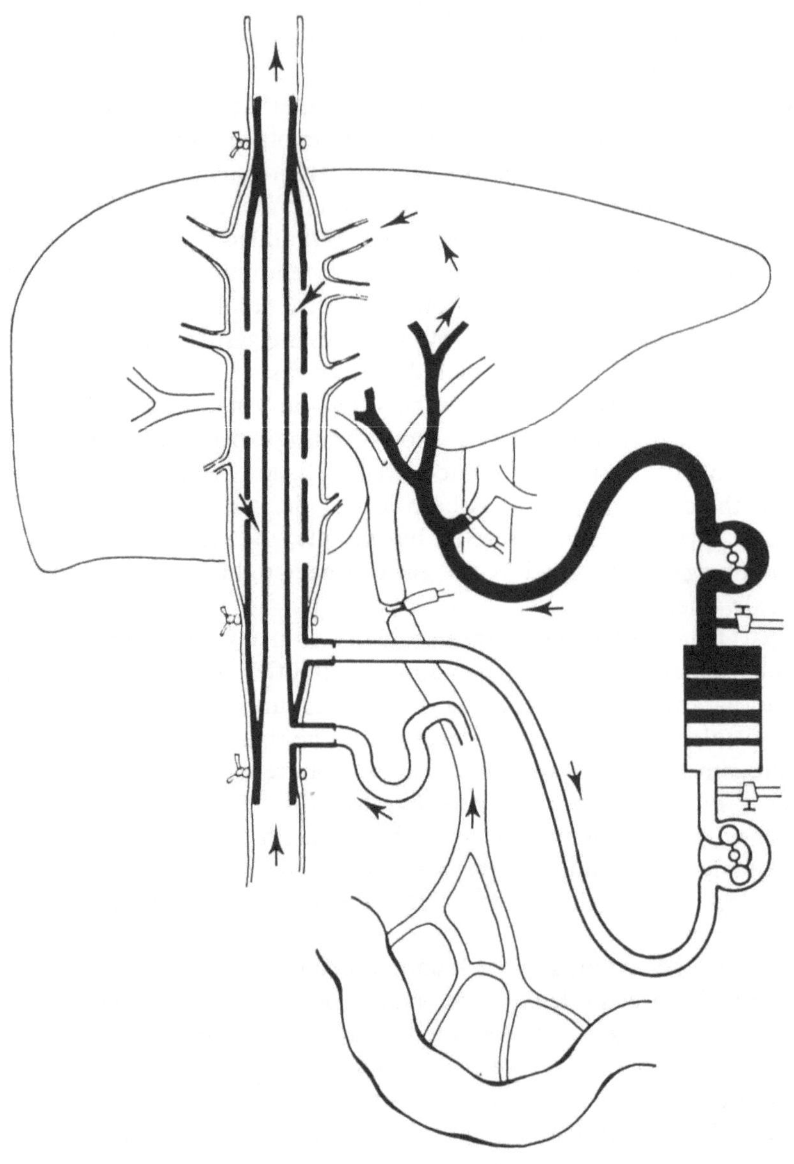

Figure 50.1 Isolated liver perfusion (animal model) (Kothuis)

as well as for the nursing staff. Infectious complications and the necessity for meticulous care of the catheter are probable disadvantages. It should be possible to avoid haemorrhage by altering the cross-section of the catheter.

Therefore my recommendations for vascular access for chemotherapy would be: fistulas for outpatients with solid tumours and good prognosis receiving chemotherapy at greater intervals and with insufficient superficial arm veins. The fistula should be created before the onset of chemotherapy.

Right atrial catheter (Hickman) for patients with acute leukaemia or aplastic anaemia requiring (immediate) chemotherapy, blood products and/or parenteral nutrition or undergoing bone marrow transplantation.

Section X
Unusual procedures and desperate cases

51

Multicentre clinical experience with the Hemasite blood access device

A. J. COLLINS, F. L. SHAPIRO, P. KESHAVIAH, K. ILSTRUP,
R. ANDERSEN, T. O'BRIEN AND L. C. COSENTINO

INTRODUCTION

The Hemasite® blood access device was first introduced into clinical evaluation in July 1980. Early results with thigh implants showed good device survival but infection was a concern[1,2]. In March 1981 the device was modified to improve septum life. This report summarizes the multicentre clinical experience with the modified blood access device between March 1981 and March 1982.

PATIENTS AND METHODS

Patient and dialysis centre characteristics

Twenty-three chronic haemodialysis centres throughout the United States participated in the evaluation. All dialysis patients being considered for bovine or polytetrafluoroethylene (PTFE) grafts were considered as potential candidates for a Hemasite vascular access shunt. Patients with existing fistulas, bovine, or PTFE grafts who strongly objected to needle punctures were also considered candidates. The Hemasite (Renal Systems, Inc., Mpls., Mn.) blood access was provided as a carbon-coated device body with or without 6 mm arterial and venous PTFE grafts (Gore-tex®). Figure 51.1 is a schematic representation of the device, and Figure 51.2 shows the device 4 weeks after implantation. The grafted device was placed either in the proximal anterior thigh or the upper arm, or spliced into an existing upper arm PTFE graft. The graftless device was placed into the venous side of a simple forearm or upper arm fistula or an existing forearm bovine graft.

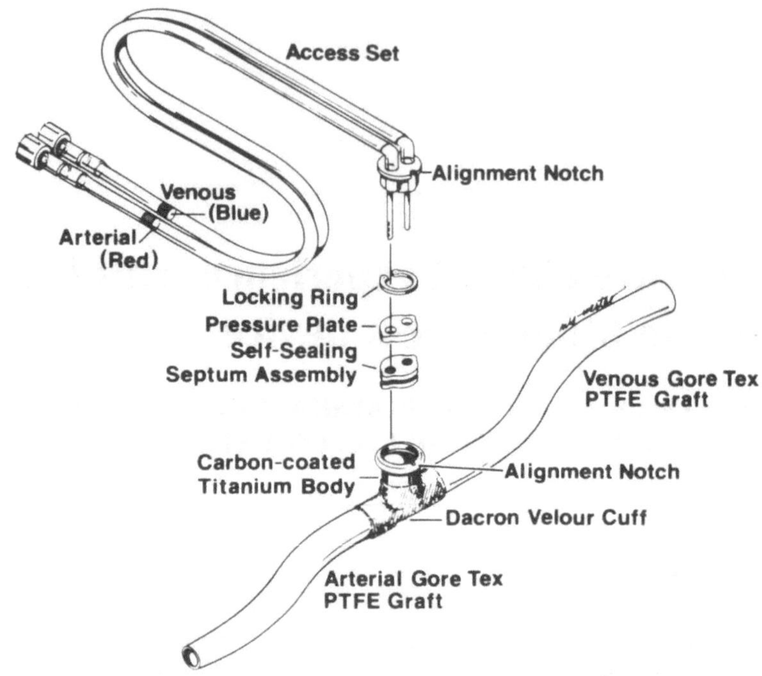

Figure 51.1   Schematic diagram showing the device and internal septum assembly

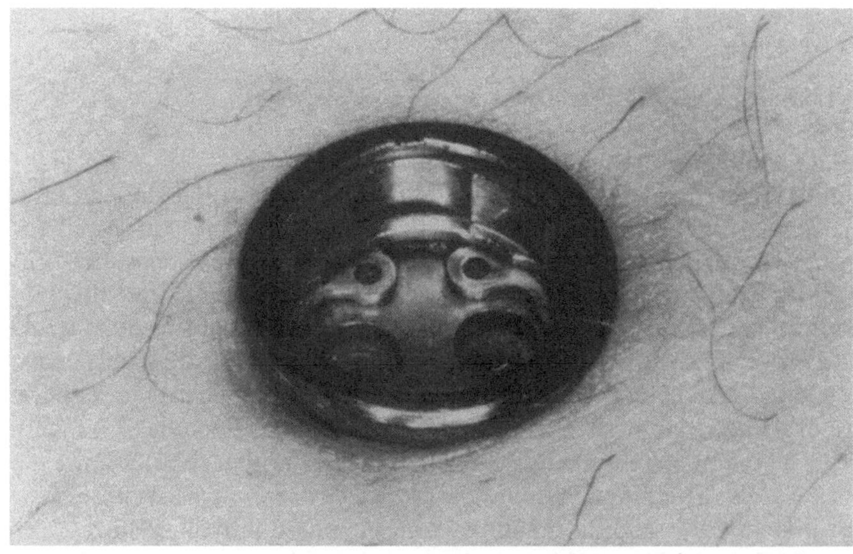

Figure 51.2   Blood access 4 weeks after placement

Blood access survival data were calculated using cumulative life-table analysis[3]. The participating haemodialysis centres reported the following: type of device and site of placement, incidence of thrombosis, declotting procedures, infection, steal syndrome, congestive heart failure, seroma, reasons for device removal, cause of death, and reasons for patient removal from the study. Secondary surgical procedures to treat device-related complications were also reported.

RESULTS

The overall multicentre experience included 124 patients receiving 129 devices. The mean follow-up was 3.2 patient-months with the median 3.7 patient-months. Figure 51.3 compares the overall cumulative survival for the blood access device to the cumulative survival of standard PTFE grafts from a multicentre study in southeastern Michigan[4]. Cumulative survival of the Hemasite calculated with patient deaths as withdrawals from the study, shows a 90.25% survival at 11 months.

Eighteen of the 129 implants were considered non-functional. Nine devices were removed; four for thrombosis, two for infection, two for seroma and one because of renal transplantation. Nine patients died with functioning accesses, six because of cardiac disease, one from vasculitis, one from uraemia and the last being secondary to pneumonia. There were no device-related deaths.

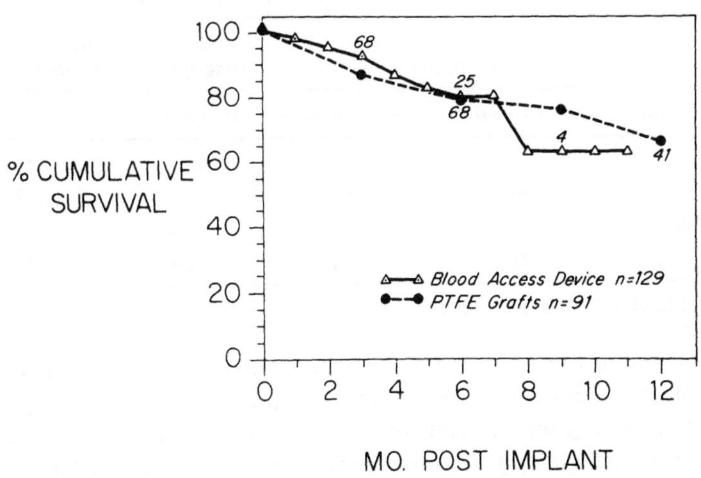

Figure 51.3 The blood access device showing comparison of survival with PTFE grafts

Table 51.1 Device-related complications; multicentre experience

	Thigh	Arm–graft	Arm–graftless
No. of implants	23	89	17
Infection	4	12	2
Thrombosis	4	24	4
Stenosis	4	11	3
Seroma	2	2	—
Steal syndrome	—	3	1
Jump graft	1	3	1
Congestive heart failure	1	2	1
Contact dermatitis	1	6	1
Device below skin	2	5	0

Data from March 1981 to March 1982

The device-related complications are summarized in Table 51.1. The grafted arm device shows a 27% incidence of thrombotic complications and 14% incidence of infectious complications. Further analysis of the infectious complications in the first month post-implant show three devices with incisional infections, three with exit-site infections, one with a graft infection and two with combinations of the exit-site, well and device graft infections. These last two implants were removed for infectious complications. Nine devices had infectious complications after the first month. There were no devices removed during this period for infection.

Table 51.2 summarizes the incidence of the initial thrombotic episodes. In the first month the arm implants had a higher incidence of thrombosis compared to the thigh, the incidence decreasing thereafter.

Table 51.2 Multicentre incidence of initial thrombosis in the blood access device

Implant site	No. of implants		Incidence of initial thrombosis (one episode per patient-month)	
	0–1 month	2–12 months	0–1 month	2–12 months
Thigh	2	2	10.8	21.0
Arm–graft	16	8	4.8	17.1
Arm–graftless	3	1	4.2	31.0
TOTAL	21	11	5.4	19.1

Data from March 1981 to March 1982

Surgical and technical problems with the blood access device are related to placement of the device and replacement of the septum, pressure plate and locking ring during septum change procedures. A large exit site incision in combination with a deep graft tunnel in an obese patient resulted in retraction of the device below the skin in seven patients. Three devices had improper placement of the locking ring after a septum change procedure. On removing the needle set, the septum, pressure plate and locking ring were pulled free. A plug was placed in the device and the septum change procedures were repeated.

DISCUSSION

The 1980 results with the prototype device in the first five patients with leg implants had significant complications related to the high graft flows with high-output heart failure and a 56% incidence of infectious complications[1,2]. The overall device survival was good with a median of 19 months. The incidence of infectious complications was greatly reduced with the modified device, with only one implant having a device-related bacteraemic episode.

The cumulative survival of the modified Hemasite blood access device appears to be comparable to plain PTFE grafts as reported in a multicentre study on access morbidity[4]. With survival of the Hemasite being comparable to an existing PTFE graft, the other benefits of the device appear to offer distinct advantages. Declotting procedures are primarily done through the device which may reduce hospitalizations. Easy monitoring of blood flow through the device has been used to diagnose access problems. Patient acceptance has been extremely high because of elimination of skin needle punctures. Staff acceptance has been high related to easy and rapid 'on and off' procedures with minimal blood loss. The newest application, of placing a graftless device into the venous side of a fistula or bovine graft, will need further follow-up to evaluate longer-term survival and complications.

Acknowledgements

The authors wish to extend their appreciation for the co-operation given by the nephrologists and surgeons at each centre, the technical support for data analysis given by Ginger Hansen, Carol Miles and LeRoy Fishbach, and the manuscript preparation by Bridget Stellmacher.

References

1 Shapiro, F. L., Keshaviah, P. R., Carlson, L. D., Illstrup, K. M., Collins, A. J., Andersen, R. C., O'Brien, T. J., Fishbach, L. J., Martinus, S. J., Amiott, D. T., Cracauer, R. F. and Cosintino, L. C. (1982). Blood access without percutaneous punctures. *Proc. Clin. Dial. Transplant* (In press)

2 Collins, A. J., Shapiro, F. L., Keshaviah, P. R., Illstrup, K. M., Andersen, R. C., O'Brien, T. J., Martinus, F. J. and Cosintino, L. J. (1981). Blood access without skin puncture. *Trans. Am. Soc. Artif. Intern. Organs*, **27**, 308

3 Peto, R., Pike, M. C., Armitage, P., Brezlow, N. E., Cox, D. R., Howard, S. Z., Mantell, N., McPherson, K., Peto, J. and Smith, P. G. (1976, 1977). Design and analysis of randomized clinical trials requiring prolonged observation of each patient. *Br. J. Cancer*, **34**, 585, Part 1; **35**, 1, Part 2

4 Aman, L. C., Levin, N. W. and Smith, D. W. (1980). Hemodialysis access site morbidity. *Proc. Clin. Dial. Transplant Forum* (In press)

52

Popliteal region – a new site for vascular graft implantation

K. OTA, K. TAKAHASHI, R. ARA AND T. AGISHI

INTRODUCTION

It cannot be overemphasized that blood access holds a key for long-term haemodialysis. Vascular grafts have been used to create arteriovenous (A-V) fistulas for cases in which native blood vessels of their extremities have been damaged. The fore and upper arm and the thigh have been proved to be suitable sites for vascular graft implantation in such patients. There are, however, a group of patients who have had their blood vessels damaged so extensively that no suitable blood vessels remain patent in such ordinary sites.

For these patients it is necessary to look for other blood vessels available for anastomosis. In this report the popliteal region is evaluated as a site for vascular graft implantation.

MATERIALS AND METHODS

Case records
Vascular grafts were implanted four times to three patients in the popliteal site.

Case 1
A 19-year-old boy had been operated 11 times including six external shunts, two fistula creations, and four graft implantations prior to admission to our hospital. His low blood pressure (100/69 mmHg) and susceptibility to infection were considered to be the causative factors of his repeated access failure. An expanded polytetrafluoroethylene (ePTFE) graft of 35 cm in length and 0.6 cm in internal diameter was anastomosed to the popliteal vessels using the method described hereafter.

Case 2

A 64-year-old male dialysis patient with polycystic kidney disease was admitted to our hospital because of repeated blood access trouble. He had undergone access operations including one external shunt, four fistula creations and five graft implantations prior to admission. His low blood pressure (90/60 mmHg) in addition to high haematocrit (43%) and fibrinogen (600 mg/dl) levels were considered to be the main causes of repeated access failures. Implantation of vascular graft at the popliteal region was performed twice in this case. The first operation was done using a PTFE graft which occluded 37 months after implantation. Umbilical cord vein graft was used for the second operation.

Case 3

A 49-year-old male patient had undergone vascular access surgery up to 75 times including approximately 60 external shunts, two fistula creations and 13 graft implantations. His original disease was chronic glomerulonephritis. He had his extremities severely damaged as shown in Figure 52.1. The popliteal artery and vein were the only vessels untouched at the time of admission. A PTFE graft was implanted in the popliteal region similar to the other cases.

Operative procedure

Operation is performed in a prone position under epidural anaesthesia. A transverse incision of 4–5 cm is placed 2–3 cm distal to the popliteal joint. The popliteal artery and vein are exposed and isolated approximately 3 cm from adjacent tissues. Small arterial and venous branches are ligated and severed.

Anastomosis starts at the venous side. After application of vascular clamps, a longitudinal incision of approximately 2 cm is made on the venous wall. After irrigating the vessel lumen, vascular graft which is severed obliquely to fit the anastomotic ostium is sutured carefully using 7–O or 6–O nylon monofilament. After completion of the venous anastomosis, the opposite side of the graft is brought to the anastomotic site of the artery through a U-shaped tunnel extending subcutaneously to the sural region. Arterial anastomosis is performed similar to the venous anastomosis (Figure 52.2).

RESULTS

Operation was done successfully without any difficulties. No complication was observed except for local oedema caused by filtrate from the ePTFE grafts. Puncture started approximately 2 weeks after operation without any difficulties. The prone position was preferable at the time of puncture (Figure 52.3). During the course of dialysis, however, the patients could change their

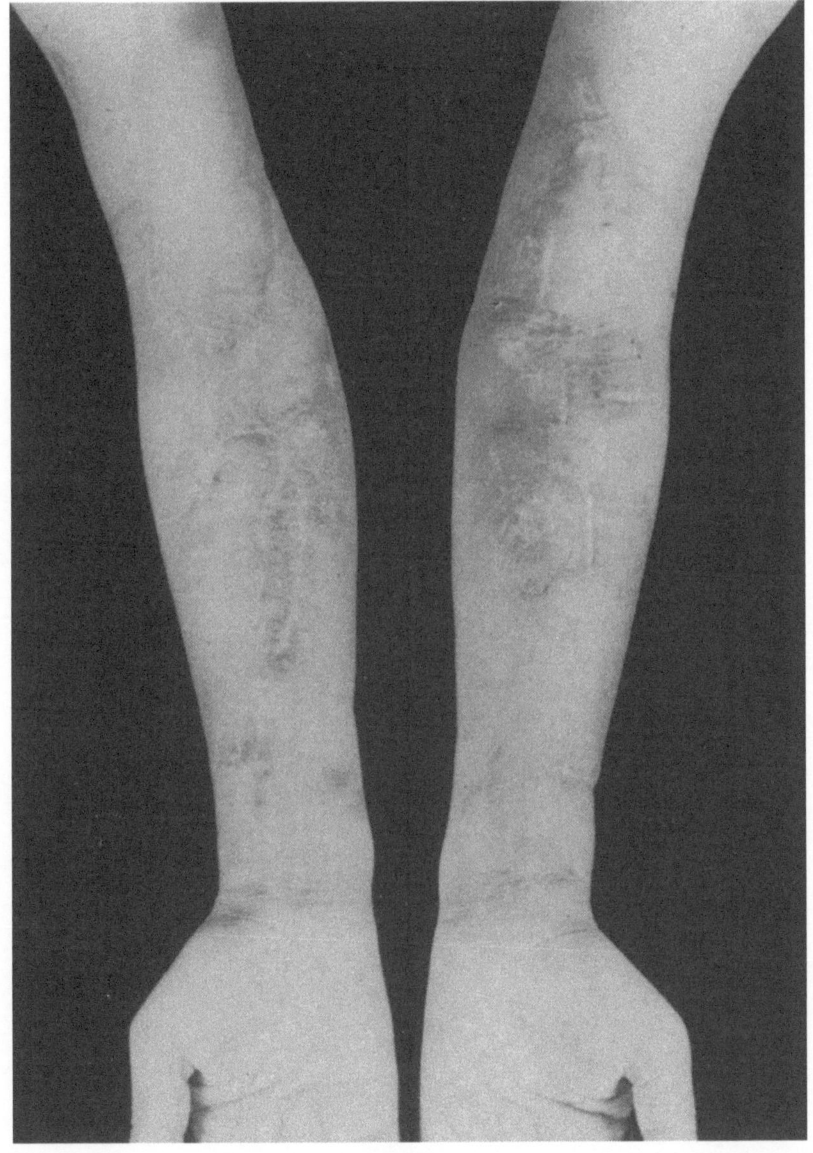

Figure 52.1   Severely damaged upper extremities (case 3)

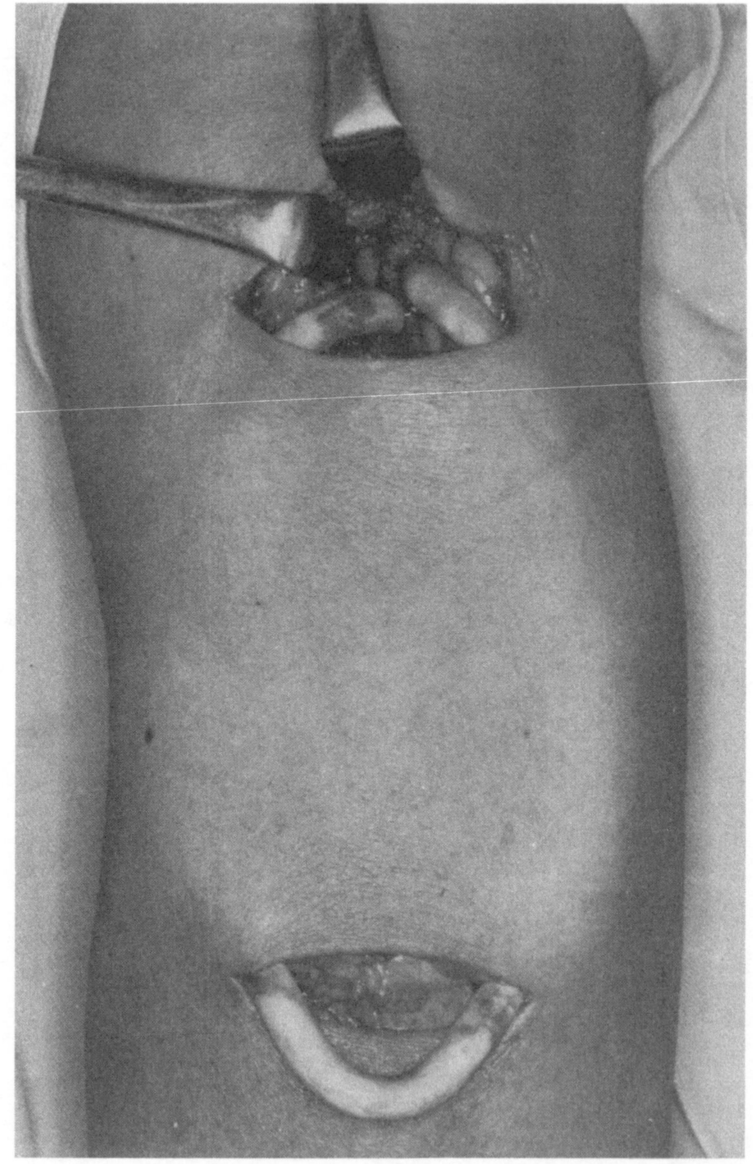

Figure 52.2   ePTFE graft just after implantation (case 3)

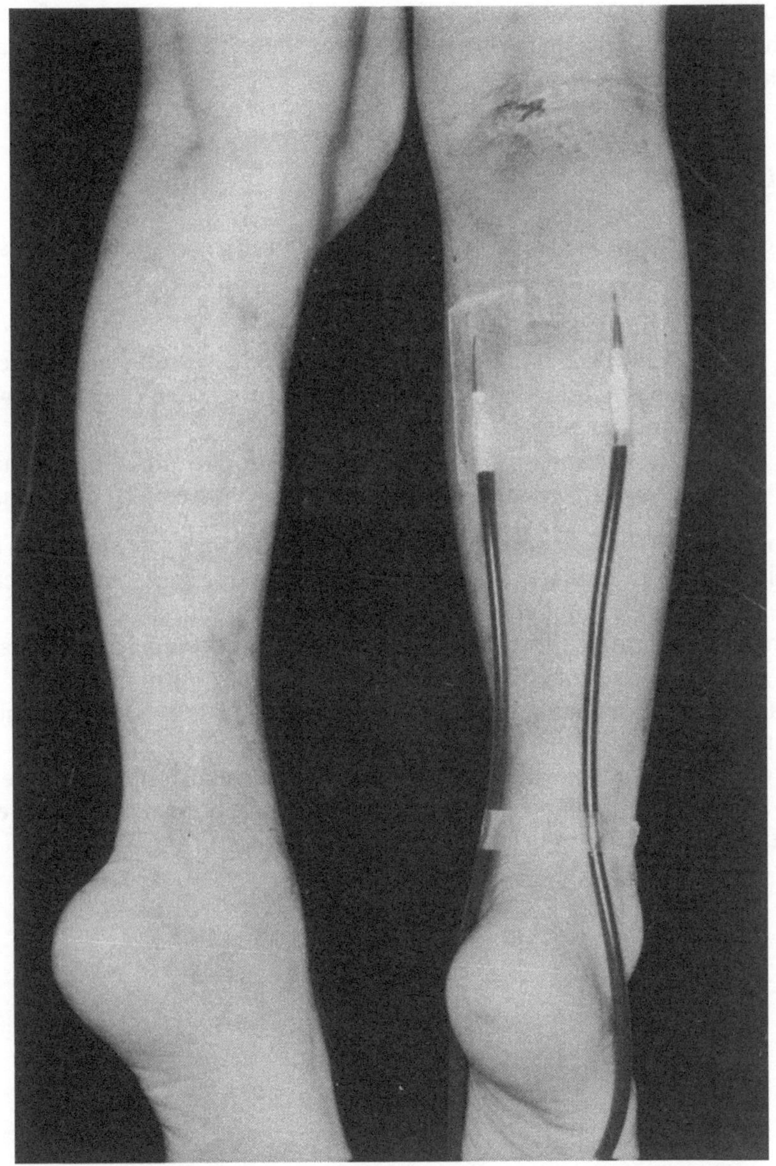

Figure 52.3 Puncture is carried out in prone position (case 3)

posture according to their choice. Function of the grafts was excellent in all cases without any side-effects such as steal syndrome or venous congestion. Haemostasis was completed usually within 15 min. No high-output cardiac failure was observed in any of the cases.

Survival of the graft was terminated with occlusion of the venous side at 30 months in case 1, 37 and 5 months in case 2. In case 3, however, the function of the graft was terminated by the death of the patient at 16 months after implantation.

DISCUSSION

Basic requirements for blood vessels available to create arteriovenous fistula using vascular grafts are as follows:

(1)   diameter of the vessels should be more than 3 mm;
(2)   artery and vein should be located in the same extremity, with space for graft implantation and, if possible, no joint should exist between arterial and venous sides;
(3)   steal syndrome and local congestion should not be caused by the shunt;
(4)   no serious complication should develop at occlusion of the vessels.

With respect to these requirements, the popliteal region is considered to be a qualified site for vascular graft implantation. It is a quite acceptable selection since the site is the 'cubital fossa' of the lower extremities.

The average graft survival was shortened by the unexpected death of case 3 and an early occlusion of the umbilical cord vein graft in case 2. The remaining two cases maintained their functioning grafts as long as 30 and 37 months respectively.

From these results it is concluded that the popliteal region is a suitable site for vascular graft implantation in patients who have presented difficulties in creating blood access in ordinary sites.

53

Subclavian catheter as a vascular access for single-needle haemodialysis

R. VANHOLDER, M. De CLIPPELE, A. De CUBBER AND
S. RINGOIR

INTRODUCTION

Sporadic reports on subclavian haemodialysis in small groups of patients
have appeared during the last few years in the literature[1-5]. As far as we
know, overall experience in larger groups with this technique has not yet been
published. For a period of more than 5 years, over 300 patients have been
treated in our haemodialysis unit by this approach, making use of a
pressure–pressure monitored single-needle technique. The advantages and
possible risks have been studied on a prospective basis.

Subclavian puncture is easy to realize and has been in use for years as a
vascular access for fluid administration and in chronic intravenous hyperalimentation[6]. The use of the subclavian vein technique in chronic haemodialysis seemed equally suitable, especially in ambulatory patients.

In the present article the eventual pitfalls of the subclavian technique are
studied. It is concluded that when an internal vascular access is not immediately available, subclavian vein haemodialysis appears to be a valuable alternative approach.

PATIENTS AND METHODS

Two different catheter types were used. During the first 4 years of our
experience a non-radiopaque modified Shaldon dialysis catheter (Femoral
catheter, Extracorporeal, Medical Specialties, King of Prussia, Pennsylvania,
USA), was introduced over a Seldinger guidewire, slipped through a first-
introduced opaque non-dialysis catheter. Later, a radiopaque Uldall catheter

(Vas-cath® , Missironga, Ontario, Canada) was used. Both catheter types were introduced using the infraclavicular Aubaniac pathway[7].

Haemodialysis was performed using a single-needle procedure with a pressure monitored double-headed pump system (Bellco, BL 760). If a regular infusion was unnecessary, the catheter was flushed with 5 ml of saline and then filled with 1 ml of pure heparin (5000 i.u./ml). The catheters were not further manipulated during the period separating the haemodialysis sessions. Air-occlusive dressings were changed every 48 h under sterile conditions, after checking of the catheter's integrity.

Between January 1976 and March 1982, 3525 subclavian vein haemodialyses were performed in 307 patients of whom 112 presented acute renal failure and 173 chronic renal failure. Furthermore, the subclavian access method was used for haemoperfusion in 15 patients and for pure ultrafiltration in seven patients. By means of 367 subclavian punctures, a total of 466 catheters were inserted in these 307 patients.

Occurring complications and reasons for stopping subclavian haemodialysis were studied in a prospective way.

RESULTS

Acute patients
The technique was used in 134 acute patients, necessitating 154 subclavian punctures. In 24 patients a new catheter was introduced over a Seldinger guidewire. A single catheter remained in place over a range of 1–28 days. Catheter dialysis was performed over a range of 1–41 days per patient. As a whole, a total of 35 complications occurred. They are listed in Table 53.1. No complications had lethal implications.

Table 53.1 Complications of subclavian haemodialysis in 134 acute patients

Inadequate flow	27
Malposition	2
Infection	1
Disconnection	2
Haemothorax	1
Pneumothorax	1
Kinking	1

Chronic patients
The technique was performed in 173 chronic renal failure patients, using 213 subclavian punctures and 288 catheters. The absence of an adequate vascular access was the main indication (170 of 173 patients).

As a whole 2671 haemodialysis sessions were performed (average duration of catheter haemodialysis period ranging from 1 to 202 days).

Table 53.2 Complications of subclavian haemodialysis in 173 chronic patients

Inadequate flow	48
Inadvertent withdrawal	28
Kinking	19
Catheter sepsis	9
Bleeding	6
Malposition	4
Haemothorax	2
Thrombosis of the superior vena cava	2
Tear in catheter wall	2
Disconnection	2
Pneumothorax	1
Pulmonary embolism	1

A total number of 124 complications were observed. They were most often mechanical and could be corrected by replacement of the catheter by Seldinger technique. The complications are represented in Table 53.2. The most impressive complication was superior vena cava obstruction. Clinical arguments in favour of such a diagnosis were only present in two patients. Slight oedema of one upper limb persisted in both patients. It should be stressed that subclinical vena cava thrombosis might further be present in some more patients, as phlebographic studies demonstrated thromboses without clinical implications in several randomly designed patients treated with subclavian catheter haemodialysis[8].

Eighty-three patients were instructed to flush the catheter with heparin in a sterile way and were subsequently dialysed on an ambulatory basis. This method became progressively more popular in our subclavian patient population with chronic renal failure (13.6% were treated this way in 1977, 45.7% in 1978, 55.6% in 1979, 60% in 1980 and 64% in 1981).

DISCUSSION

Subclavian catheterization recently became progressively more popular as a method for vascular access in haemodialysis, especially in the absence of other accesses. Studies of the possible complications are scarce and of limited extent[1-5].

In the present study, essentially two types of complications are seen. First, early problems, due to or arising shortly after the catheter insertion, are similar to the complications seen with subclavian catheterization for other indications. Late problems, however, are mostly due to the prolonged intraluminal presence of the catheter and arise within a certain interval after the insertion. These complications are more specifically correlated to the haemodialysis technique.

There is a high incidence of mechanical problems in the present series. This might be due to the often prolonged use of these catheters. Another possible reason is that the catheters are submitted to strong mechanical forces.

The most alarming complication of subclavian haemodialysis in our series appears to be thrombosis of the superior vena cava. Clinically manifest venous thrombosis, however, only occurred in two of 307 patients, corresponding to a rate of 0.65%, which is comparable to the average values observed in other series[3,9].

In conclusion, our experience with the use of subclavian catheters as vascular access for haemodialysis is presented in this chapter. The complication rate was low. Moreover, most complications appeared to be relatively mild. Subclavian catheter haemodialysis is a valuable access method, in those situations where other vascular accesses are lacking.

References

1 De Cubber, A., De Wolf, C., Lameire, N., Schurgers, M. and Ringoir, S. (1978). Single needle hemodialysis with the double headpump via the subclavian vein. *Dial. Transplant.*, **12**, 1261
2 Uldall, P. R., Woods, F., Bird, M. and Dyck, R. (1978). Subclavian cannula for temporary hemodialysis. Abstract, *8th Ann. Clin. Dialysis Transplantation Forum* (1978), p. 40. New Orleans, Louisiana, USA
3 Schwarzbeck, A., Brittinger, W. D., Henning, G. E. and Strauch, M. (1978). Cannulation of subclavian vein for hemodialysis using Seldinger's technique. *Trans. Am. Soc. Artif. Intern. Organs*, **24**, 27
4 Vaz, A. J. (1980). Subclavian vein single needle dialysis in acute renal failure following vascular surgery. *Nephron*, **25**, 102
5 Uldall, R. and Williams, P. (1981). The subclavian cannula: temporary vascular access for hemodialysis when longterm peritoneal dialysis has to be interrupted. *Perit. Dial. Bull.*, **1**, 97
6 Linos, D. A., Mucha, P. and Van Heerden, J. (1980). Subclavian vein. A golden route. *Mayo Clin. Proc.*, **55**, 315
7 Aubaniac, R. (1952). L'injection intraveineuse sous-claviculaire: avantages et technique. *Presse Méd.*, **60**, 1456
8 Vanholder, R., Lameire, N., Verbanck, J., Van Rattinghe,'R., Kunnen, M. and Ringoir, S. (1982). Complications of subclavian hemodialysis. A 5 year prospective study in 257 consecutive patients. (Submitted for publication)
9 Ryan, J. A., Abel, R. M., Abbott, W. M., Hopkins, C. C., Chesney, T. C., Colley, R., Phillips, K. and Fischer, J. E. (1974). Catheter complications in total parenteral nutrition. *N. Engl. J. Med.*, **290**, 757

54

Antecubital arteriovenous fistulas with reverse flow

Z. SHAPIRA, D. SHMUELI, A. YUSSIM AND C. SERVADIO

A Brescia–Cimino[1] type of arteriovenous (A-V) fistula is still regarded as the preferred initial angioaccess operation for patients who require chronic haemodialysis[2-4]. It can provide the patients with an arterialized network of superficial veins at the forearm which permits easy and repeated cannulation to be effected by the staff and even by the patient himself. However, only about 62% of these fistulas are patent after 36 months[5]. The major second choice for creation of angioaccess is utilization of the blood vessels at the antecubital level for performing either direct A-V fistulas or for A-V inter-positioning of autologous or synthetic grafts[6-10]. By either method there is no deliberate attempt to arterialize or to rearterialize solely the superficial forearm vein by complete reversal of the blood flow in the distal direction.

Adar *et al.*[4] in 1975 and Geis *et al.*[3] in 1977 described their satisfactory experience with reverse A-V fistulas at the antecubital level in shunt-exhausted patients but this alternative procedure did not seem to gain popularity. We decided to utilize the antecubital reverse A-V fistula in two different indications:

(a) as the preferred alternative after failure of Brescia–Cimino fistulas via both wrists;
(b) as the preferred initial angioaccess procedure in children weighing 12 kg or less.

We describe in this chapter our experience with this type of fistula in 32 uraemic patients.

MATERIALS AND METHODS

From January 1980 to December 1981, 32 A-V fistulas with reverse-directed flow were performed at the antecubital level in 32 uraemic patients. The majority of the patients were referred to our centre from nephrology departments of other medical institutions. Twenty-six were adults, with age range of 32–58 years (average 47 years). They had all previously undergone two or more angioaccess operations at the wrist level of both hands. There were also six children, ages ranging from 4 to 5½ years (average age 4.8 years). Their body weight at time of presentation was between 11 and 12 kg. None of them had any previous angioaccess operation.

We employed a surgical technique similar to that described by Geis *et al.*[3], with some modifications (Figure 54.1). The skin is incised above and parallel to the antecubital crease. The distal brachial artery as well as the basilic vein are isolated and approximated. Care must be taken not to disrupt perforating veins. A side-to-side anastomosis of 8–10 mm length is preferred. Thereafter, a thrill is usually palpable at the vein proximal and distal to the anastomosis site. The proximal arm of the basilic vein is now clamped. If, following the clamping, the thrill in the distal vein arm exists then the proximal vein arm is double-ligated and separated close to the anastomosis. Thus the side-to-side A-V fistula is converted to end (vein)-to-side (artery) with reverse pulsatile flow. Should the thrill in the distal vein weaken significantly or disappear after clamping of the proximal vein, the use of aFogarty catheter in the distal vein may result in reappearance of thrill. Otherwise the anastomosis may be left as a side-to-side fistula.

RESULTS

In 20 adults and five children the reverse A-V fistulas at the antecubital level have been functioning from 2 to 24 months (average 6.5±3 months). The 24-month cumulative patency rate for the initial fistulas in the children's group was 83% and for the adult group 77% (Table 54.1).

Table 54.1 Cumulative patency rate of the antecubital reverse A-V fistula at 24 months

Age group	No. of patients	Patency rate (%)
Adults	26	77
Children	6	83
TOTAL	32	78

In three adult patients a marked forearm oedema developed 2–8 weeks after the operation: in two of them the oedema subsided gradually. In the third, profound progressive swelling necessitated operative suppression of the fistula 6 months after its construction.

In the adult group cannulation of the forearm veins for haemodialysis could be started after 10–12 days. The maturity period in the children's group extended from 6 to 8 weeks.

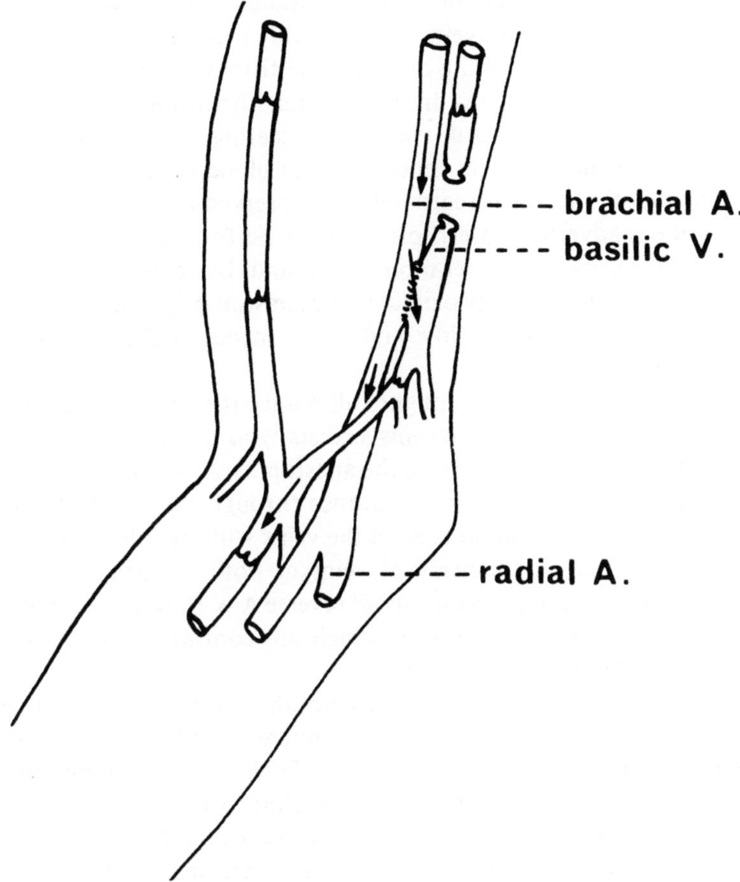

Figure 54.1   Basilic vein to brachial artery, end-to-side fistula with reverse flow

DISCUSSION

The infrequent utilization of reverse fistula for arterialization of the forearm veins is due probably to the following assumptions:

(a)   that the vein valves might slow down the reverse-flowing blood, resulting in stasis and thrombosis;

(b)   that the same unsuitable condition in the veins which might have caused failure of the initial wrist fistula would also endanger the reverse fistula;

(c)   that the massive retrograde arterialization would result in severe progressive oedema.

Adar and his colleagues[4] showed that the reverse pulsatile pressure in the vein is capable of dilating the veins and rendering the valves incompetent. On the other hand, many of the patients who are candidates for creation of reverse fistula have dilated forearm veins and probably incompetent valves, due to previous temporary functioning of antegrade fistulas at the wrist.

The excess of the blood flow drains itself readily through the deep venous system of the arm and forearm via communicating veins[3]. Thus the intact communicating venous system should prevent blood stasis and thrombosis. We assume that the severe forearm oedema observed in three patients is due in part to the inadvertent interruption of the perforated veins at the antecubital fossa during the operation. Geis and his colleagues[3] advocate narrowing of the basilic vein proximal to the anastomosis by plication to such a grade that enough reverse flow and simultaneous cephalad drainage of excess blood will occur.

We think that such plication might still reduce the necessary reverse flow velocity which should dilate the veins as distally as possible.

Clamping of the vein proximal to the anastomosis should serve to indicate whether there is sufficient blood clearance through the perforate veins to permit direct retrograde blood flow in the veins with its full velocity.

Extensive occlusion of superficial veins at both forearms is a serious obstacle; thus performing an antecubital reverse A-V flow in these patients is undesirable. However, vein injuries which are confined to the wrist level leave enough potential accessibility areas.

The 77% cumulative patency rate at 24 months of the reverse A-V fistula in the adults is higher than the 24-month cumulative patency rate of several salvage procedures of the wrist A-V fistula (Table 54.2). Although only salvage by interposition of expanded polytetrafluoroethylene grafts shows a higher survival rate[5], they are, however, expensive and their interposition is more time-consuming. They can still be used in case of failure of the reverse A-V fistula.

Table 54.2 Cumulative patency rate of different salvage procedures of wrist A-V fistulas compared to antecubital reverse A-V fistula at 24 months*

Type of salvage procedure	No. of patients	Patency rate (%)
Patch angioplasty	25	68*
Direct repair	21	52*
Declotting	41	33*
New A-V fistula	62	30*
Reverse A-V fistula	26	77
Interposition of PTFE grafts	19	88*

*From Ref. 5

The use of the antecubital reverse A-V fistula as the initial angioaccess in uraemic children weighing 12 kg or less may solve one of the major problems in their treatment. The lumen size of their antecubital vessels is large enough to allow conventional surgery. The maturation period is shorter than that of a wrist fistula created with the aid of microsurgery[11,12]. It has satisfactory patency rate at 24 months and we did not notice any growth difference between the two arms.

To perform a sufficient angioaccess in uraemic patients is a formidable surgical challenge, especially in patients with previous failure of A-V fistula or in small children. The reverse antecubital A-V fistula might serve in selected patients as an additional simple and easy-to-perform alternative without eliminating the possibility of reverting to other alternatives.

References

1 Brescia, M. J., Cimino, J. E., Appel, K. and Hurwich, B. J. (1966). Chronic hemodialysis using venipuncture and a surgically created arteriovenous fistula. *N. Engl. J. Med.*, **275**, 1089

2 Gracz, K. C., Ing, T. S., Soung, L. S., Armbruster, K. F. W., Seim, S. K. and Merkel, F. K. (1977). Proximal forearm fistula for maintenance hemodialysis. *Kidney Int.*, **11**, 71

3 Geis, W. P., Giacchino, J. L., Iwatsuki, S., Vaz, A. J., Hano, J. E. and Ing, T. S. (1977). The reverse fistula for vascular access. *Surg. Gynecol. Obstet.*, **145**, 901

4 Adar, R., Antebi, E., Iaina, A. and Mozes, M. (1975). Retrograde arteriovenous fistula for chronic hemodialysis. *Vasc. Surg.*, **9**, 160

5 Silcott, G. R., Vannix, R. S. and DePalma J. R. (1980). Repair versus new arteriovenous fistulae. *Trans. Am. Soc. Artif. Intern. Organs*, **26**, 99

6 Beven, E. and Hertzer, N. (1975). Construction of arteriovenous fistulas for hemodialysis. *Surg. Clin. N. Am.*, **55**, 1125

7 Dagher, F., Gelber, R., Ramos, E. and Sadler, J. (1976). The use of basilic vein and brachial artery as an A-V fistula for long term hemodialysis. *J. Surg. Res.*, **20**, 373

8 Adar, R., Siegal, A., Bogokowsky, H. and Mozes, M. (1973). The use of arteriovenous autograph and allograph fistulas for chronic hemodialysis. *Surg. Gynecol. Obstet.*, **136**, 941

9 Toledo-Pereyra, L. H., Kyriakides, G. K., Ma, K. W. and Miller, J. (1977). Proximal radial artery−cephalic vein fistula hemodialysis. *Arch. Surg.*, **113**, 226

10 Anderson, C. B., Etheredge, E. E. and Sicard, G. A. (1980). One hundred polytetrafluoroethylene vascular access grafts. *Dial. Transplant*, **9**, 237

11 Hardy, M. A., Schneider, K. M. and Levitt, S. B. (1974). An improved technique for the construction of internal arteriovenous fistulas in uremic children. *J. Ped. Surg.*, **9**, 465

12 Robinson, H. B., Wenzl, J. E. and Williams, G. R. (1979). Internal vascular access for hemodialysis in children weighing less than fifteen kilograms. *Surgery*, **85**, 525

55

Abstracts of posters in
Unusual procedures and desperate cases

Straight thigh fistulas in chronic haemodialysis – a 9-year follow-up report
E. M. GORDON

A straight subcutaneous fistula between the saphenous vein and popliteal artery was developed in 1974. Since 1980 velour Dacron has been used when the vein was unsuitable, or an earlier fistula had failed, and may be sited parallel to a thrombosed fistula, allowing maximum preservation of the patient's own vessels. Thirty-one fistulas have been made, 18 venous and 13 Dacron. There has been one immediate failure, and one was ligated within 24 h on account of ischaemia of the lower limb. The remaining fistulas have been usable for up to 375 weeks, with a mean of 57 weeks.

Use of large-bore catheters in the internal jugular vein as an access for acute haemodialysis
R. BAMBAUER

For almost two decades the chosen method for haemodialysis has been the transcutaneous Seldinger technique, using large-bore catheters. Tradition-ally, the femoral or subclavian veins have been used. We report our experience on introducing the catheter (Shaldon catheter) into the internal jugular vein in 350 cases in 287 patients. The percutaneous insertion was necessary for acute haemodialysis, haemofiltration, haemoperfusion, or for temporary vascular access. This method was also used for plasmapheresis. Major complications did not occur, which is in agreement with other authors, whereby the frequency of complications relating to the catheter itself has been lower using this approach.

It thus seems that the cannulation of the superior vena cava through the internal jugular vein is a suitable means of obtaining fast vascular access for the purposes of haemodialysis, haemofiltration, haemoperfusion or plasmapheresis.

Femoral vein catheterization (FC) for chronic haemodialysis (RDT)
L. CATIZONE, A. SANTORO, E. DEGLI ESPOSTI and P. ZUCCHELLI

The present study reports our experience with FC in patients on RDT. We used the technique described by Seldinger and modified by Shaldon in 5704 FC for the last 12 years, for patients waiting for available vascular prothesis, with temporary unavailability of their own angioaccess, with acute renal failure or unable or unwilling to use peritoneal dialysis. Usually we employ two catheters (and occasionally only one with a double-headpump system), which were always removed at the end of every dialysis session. A lot of patients have dialysed for long continuous periods with FC, some for more than a year. The complications have been an insignificant haematoma (4.7% of all FC), more severe haematomas (0.17%), severe fibrosis of the groins (0.09%) and four cases (0.07%) of important retroperitoneal bleeding, three of which required surgical intervention. The patients have always tolerated FC very well and they have been able to go home 40–60 min after dialysis. Haemodialysis efficiency is good and no patient has had signs of insufficient treatment. In conclusion, this technique permits an effective treatment for several months for patients without an efficient blood access or unable to use peritoneal dialysis. The complications are usually insignificant.

The straight upper arm bovine graft in chronic haemodialysis
K. H. ONG, T. I. YO and R. A. F. v.d. NESTE

The usefulness of the bovine graft in access surgery for chronic intermittent haemodialysis has been in doubt. We present the results of our experience in 20 patients in the period from 1975 till 1982. The series consists of patients with terminal uraemia, in whom previous arteriovenous fistulas in both upper extremities had failed. In most cases the implantation of a bovine graft was considered a last resort. A total of 24 grafts were implanted in 17 females and three males; on 20 occasions the location was the upper arm. The inguinal regions have been used twice. In two instances grafts were implanted in the axillo-axillary position. The mean age was 52 years. We stress the importance of implantation in a straight position, preferably in the upper arm; also the use of single-needle haemodialysis may add to graft patency. The shortest patency was 2 weeks; the longest 62 months; mean patency was 14 months. Complications consist of aneurysm formation, postoperative bleeding, and graft disintegration due to sepsis.

Right atrial catheters as access for haemodialysis

W. P. REED, P. D. LIGHT and J. A. SADLER

Broviac and Hickman right atrial catheters have permitted up to 960 days safe continuous access for hyperalimentation and up to 1044 days for chemotherapy. Similar catheters should offer an attractive means of alternate access in patients requiring repeated dialysis for end-stage renal disease provided sufficient flow be available. A modification of the standard Hickman catheter with an internal diameter of 2.6 mm, instead of 1.6 mm, and length of 26 cm, instead of 90 cm, was used to provide repeated access for haemodialysis in two patients with no available standard access sites. Insertion was easily accomplished by cut-down of the external jugular vein. Dialysis was carried out through a Y adapter by single-needle technique on the Gambro AK-10 machine, with a peak flow setting of 300–350 cc/min producing flows of 150–180 cc/min. Removal of up to 8 kg of fluid was possible in 6 h of dialysis. Pre- and post-dialysis chemistries were similar to those obtained during standard two-needle technique. Between runs the catheters were flushed daily with saline and heparin and recapped. One patient needed alternate access when she developed candida peritonitis after 3 years of chronic ambulatory peritoneal dialysis necessitated by prior ablation of the last of her peripheral veins. Although she ultimately succumbed to her abdominal sepsis, the right atrial catheter permitted haemodialysis to continue over a 2½-month period and in support of three abdominal explorations. A second patient was known to have extensive intra-abdominal adhesions from a recent vascular reconstruction. When her only arteriovenous (A-V) fistula irreversibly thrombosed, a right atrial catheter provided access during the 1½ months required for a new A-V fistula to mature.

Long-term vascular access for haemodialysis using a peritoneal dialysis catheter in the superior vena cava

D. M. A. FRANCIS, M. K. WARD, G. PROUD and R. M. R. TAYLOR

While most chronic renal failure (CRF) patients successfully undergo haemodialysis (HD) by conventional methods of vascular access, a small number have major difficulties because of severe atherosclerosis, arterial and venous thrombosis and infection. Four patients are described in whom conventional HD, as well as peritoneal dialysis and renal transplantation, repeatedly failed, but in whom long-term vascular access and subsequent successful HD was achieved by surgical implantation of a Tenhkhoff peritoneal dialysis catheter (Quinton, Seattle, Washington) into the superior vena cava (SVC). Patients were female, aged 44–64 years and had end-stage CRF for 15 months to 8 years. A total of 21 separate vascular access procedures had been undertaken previously, including arteriovenous fistulas, shunts and autogenous vein and PTFE grafts; all had failed, 67% before dialysis could be commenced. In each patient a Tenckhoff peritoneal catheter (internal diameter 2.6 mm) was inserted into the SVC via an external jugular vein using a simple surgical technique. A 'single-needle' technique is used for HD and blood flow rates of 130–190 ml/min are achieved. Catheters have remained *in situ* for 5–82 weeks and have been used for a total of 375 haemodialyses. In contrast to previous attempts at vascular access this technique was easy to perform, has allowed adequate HD and has been free of major complications. While not recommended for routine long-term vascular access this procedure has proved to be life-saving in patients in whom conventional access methods failed.

Needleless dialysis using the Biocarbon device
J. J. JAKIMOWICZ, T. S. KWAN, F. DIDERICH, J. H. M. TORDOIR and A. L. GOLDING

A new Biocarbon (Bentley Laboratories) transcutanous haemodialysis access device (CTAD), which eliminates needle puncture, is described. The device is made from vitreous carbon and is mounted on a PTFE vascular prosthesis. By means of disposable connectors the patient can be dialysed without puncture of the implant.

Indications for the use of CTAD are as follows: failure of multiple previous access procedures; hypercoagulable patients; patients with scleroderma and other skin complaints and patients with needle phobia.

From April 1979 until December 1981, 69 CTAD were implanted in 60 patients. Eighteen patients died of reasons not related to the implant; one patient was transplanted; 32 CTAD are still patent. 18 were removed; six due to thrombosis and 12 due to infection, 12 successful thrombectomies were performed.

CTAD offers the following advantages: it eliminates the use of needles; it can be used directly after implantation; it can be implanted at different sites; home dialysis is possible and use of long-term anticoagulant therapy is possible. Our conclusion is that CTAD is a welcome contribution to the tertiary blood access procedures. Improvement of the connector systems would further lessen the infection rate and in future make the device acceptable as secondary access procedure.

Temporary subclavian catheter in 62 haemodialysed patients
F. KHAZINE, O. SIMONS, J.-L. COY, J. BECART, J. VILLEBOEUF, T. HAAS and G. DONGRADI

From 1977 to 1982, 62 patients underwent the temporary use of a subclavian catheter for failure of the permanent blood access or terminal renal failure.

The catheters were left in place for 1–247 days permitting 1–82 dialysis sessions. We observed one pneumothorax, two local infections, two subclavian vein stenosis and two septicaemias. This technique seems to be safe and efficient respecting patients' vascular system and patients' comfort, and permitting ambulatory dialysis. This method is the ideal temporary vascular access.

Vascular access strategy when CAPD has to be interrupted: a dilemma!
M. BITKER, J. ROTTEMBOURG, J. L. POIGNET and J. L. GALLEGO

Long-term continuous ambulatory peritoneal dialysis (CAPD) has been over the last years a definitive mode of therapy for a regularly increasing number of patients with end-stage renal failure. Between August 1978 and December 1981 83 patients (48 men, 35 females; mean age 67.4±8.6 years) chose CAPD as first mode of therapy for renal failure. Seventeen patients required, after a mean period of 14±4.2 months, a permanent transfer to haemodialysis for various reasons (recurrent peritonitis eight cases, cachexia six cases, abdominal pain two cases, poor ultrafiltration one case). None of these patients had a previous constructed vascular access. At that time clinical and biological status of the patient were very poor: mean arterial blood pressure 82±16 mmHg, protein level 52±6 g/l, albumin level 21±4 g/l. In seven cases direct creation of an arteriovenous (A-V) fistula failed. Because of poor vascular conditions in seven cases a Buselmeier shunt was implanted near the wrist and transformed successfully in five cases after a delay of 53±12 days in an A-V fistula using the same vessels. In five cases a subclavian catheter was inserted and used during 30–360 days before a permanent vascular access was created. In only five cases was immediate creation of an A-V fistula possible. Strategy for creation of permanent vascular access when CAPD has to be interrupted is debated. Should all the patients entering a CAPD programme have an A-V fistula previously created? When permanent transfer from CAPD to haemodialysis is required, direct creation of an A-V fistula is difficult. Subclavian catheter insertion or Buselmeier shunt implantation offer a temporary vascular access for haemodialysis before creation or transformation in A-V fistula becomes possible when clinical and vascular conditions are improved.

Well-maintained external blood access for chronic haemodialysis using expanded polytetrafluoroethylene (ePTFE) graft
H. NISHI and K. OTA

There are many access troubles for the long-term haemodialysis patient. Therefore bovine or swine xenograft, synthetic graft, saphenous vein autograft and Dardik Biograft are currently in use. Such grafts are used as internal access. But their maintenance is very difficult, because of infection, pseudoaneurysm, haematoma, obstruction and many problems arising through puncture. Therefore, we tried to change to the external access using expanded polytetrafluoroethylene (ePTFE) graft. The change resulted in a significant decrease in complications.

Among 875 cases which were operated in the last 3 years, 26 cases of the long-term haemodialysis patients (14 persons) had external access constructed using ePTFE grafts. They were six males and eight females. Mean of age was 48 years. Mean of haemodialysis period was 7.4 years.

Thirteen patients were maintained without complications. But one case needed re-operation eight times because of frequent obstruction and infection. Therefore he is now changed to continuous ambulatory peritoneal dialysis (CAPD).

Internal access is usually the first choice to maintain haemodialysis, but external access should be constructed in the patient whose internal access using synthetic graft repeatedly gives many complications. External accesses using ePTFE graft are easily maintained even in complicated long-term haemodialysis patients.

56

Invited comments on papers and posters in Unusual procedures, desperate cases

F. O. BELZER

To summarize the need for access surgery, this can be divided into three groups: (1) haemodialysis, (2) hyperalimentation, and (3) chemotherapy. Under haemodialysis we would include indications other than renal failure, such as plasmapheresis, dialysis for drug overdose, etc. I will briefly summarize these three areas and try to make some predictions about future innovations and methods.

Table 56.1 Vascular access problems

Thrombosis	Embolization
Stenosis	High output failure
Infection	Venous hypertension
Aneurysm formation	Absence of access sites
Ischaemia	

During this First International Congress on Access Surgery the majority of papers addressed the problems of vascular access for haemodialysis. These problems can be summarized in Table 56.1. *Thrombosis* continues to plague the vascular access surgeon and is usually due to one of three causes, namely: (1) technical errors at the time of surgery; (2) anatomical problems, such as inadequate arterial inflow or inadequate venous outflow; (3) the requirement for repeated puncture of the graft which may lead to the development of an intimal flap or haematoma leading to compression of the graft; and (4) hypercoagulability. Two papers were presented in this session attempting to eliminate the need for repeated puncture by the use of a transcutaneous haemodialysis port. Collins *et al.* from Minneapolis described their clinical experience with the Hemasite blood access device and Jakimowicz *et al.* in a

325

poster session presented their experience with needleless dialysis using the Biocarbon device. These new procedures are at present undergoing clinical evaluation. The early experience suggests that thrombosis and infection are two of the main problems.

Stenosis usually occurs at the puncture sites but in autogenous veins or at the venous anastomosis when artificial grafts are used. This is in all probability due to the different compliance of the thin-walled distensible vein and the much stiffer prosthetic material. Future research and the development of more expansile compliant vascular prosthesis might decrease the development of distal stenosis.

Infection is almost always associated with the use of an artificial graft such as the expanded polytetrafluoroethylene graft, the bovine graft or the umbilical vein graft. In my opinion the vascular surgeon should make every attempt to use autogenous tissue and use of the saphenous vein either placed subcutaneously in the thigh or transposed to the forearm is probably not utilized as often as could be done. It is of interest that the vascular surgeons in Sydney, Australia (J. M. Day, personal communication), rarely use artificial grafts for venous access but rely heavily on the use of the saphenous vein. Aneurysm formation either of the true or false type is a direct result of repeated percutaneous puncture required for haemodialysis. Fortunately the aneurysm can usually be excised without losing the vascular access site.

Distal ischaemia secondary to a steal phenomenon almost exclusively occurs in the upper arm fistulas and usually in patients with arterial obliterative disease, such as diabetics. Occasionally it is seen in Cimino fistulas of the wrist when a steal occurs through the palmar arch. Careful examination of the patient prior to surgery and preoperative arteriography in selected cases should make this a rare complication.

Embolization is a rare but occasionally catastrophic complication which can be eliminated by not utilizing a side-to-side arterial venous anastomosis. However, the side-to-side anastomosis has multiple advantages and at least this author has not given up the use of side-to-side anastomosis because of embolization.

High-output failure, in my opinion, will never occur if the fistula or the feeding arterial vessel does not exceed 6 mm. Although it occasionally can occur in bilateral Cimino fistulas in the wrist, it usually is found in fistulas where the brachial or femoral artery is used. If a large artery is to be used in the creation of an arteriovenous (A-V) fistula, the surgeon should make every attempt to make a permanent fistula which is less than 6 mm wide. A tapered Gore-tex® graft is now available which measures 4 mm on one side and 6 mm on the distal side; these should be used preferentially if a large artery is to be used.

Finally, and probably one of the most frequent problems in the past, is the absence of vascular access sites because of previous failed grafts. This problem should be less frequent in the future, as emergency vascular access should rarely require the utilization and perhaps sacrifice of a peripheral artery. Seven of the papers, both in the presentation as well as in the poster session, showed that both short-term and even long-term haemodialysis access can be performed using a venous site only. Vanholder *et al.* from Belgium showed that a subclavian catheter was quite satisfactory as a vascular access for single-needle haemodialysis. Bambauer from Germany showed that the use of large-bore catheters in the internal jugular vein were quite satisfactory as an access for acute haemodialysis. Catizone *et al.* from Italy showed that the femoral vein could be used repeatedly for chronic haemodialysis, as did several of the other authors. The needless sacrifice of a distal artery by the insertion of a Scribner shunt should rarely or never be used in the 1980s. In the past the absence of additional access sites was a major problem and was only overcome by the ingenuity of access surgeons. Dr Russ Lawton (personal communication) many years ago successfully used Scribner shunt modification using the femoral artery alone. He also suggested placing the femoral artery subcutaneously in the thigh, thus allowing percutaneous puncture of the artery for dialysis. In desperate cases axilloaxillary grafts have been placed and Lawton even suggested the creation of an axillofemoral graft. These ingenious but rather extensive procedures are now rarely needed, and time for maturation of fistula can now be obtained by the use of venous access or peritoneal dialysis.

Although in general during this congress not too many papers addressed the problems of hyperalimentation and chemotherapy, this also is an extremely important topic. Both entities often require prolonged infusion of often highly sclerosing solutions, making the use of peripheral veins impossible. Both hyperalimentation and chemotherapy can be divided in short-term and long-term therapy, and chemotherapy may have to be given either intravenously or interarterially. The use of the central venous catheter by the subclavian or jugular route is extremely satisfactory for short-term hyperalimentation or chemotherapy and will not be further discussed. Long-term hyperalimentation or chemotherapy can be done by utilizing A-V fistula or a permanent central venous catheter. The use of A-V fistula for hyperalimentation was first suggested by Conolly *et al.*[1]. in 1968 and has been used by many authors including Scribner for both chemotherapy and hyperalimentation. This author had the pleasure of seeing a patient of Dr W. Altmeier of Cincinnati who required total intravenous nutrition because of extensive scleroderma of the gastrointestinal tract. This patient was maintained quite well on total intravenous feeding by utilizing an arm A-V fistula as an outpatient for a period of 5 years, at which time she succumbed because of complications of her underlying disease. A-V fistulas, however, in the non-uraemic patient who have normal haematocrits and normal clotting factors, may have a high tendency for thrombosis. The central venous catheters such as the Broviac or Hickman catheter have been utilized successfully for long periods of time but have the disadvantage of being external catheters which may produce aesthetic as well as infectious disadvantages. The use of totally implantable venous access systems to replacement external catheters is a recent development. Such an injection port system is currently manufactured by the Infusate Corporation of Sharon, Massachusetts. Dr Niederhuber and his colleagues from Ann Arbor, Michigan, recently presented their experience with this device in 30 cancer patients receiving chemotherapy for their underlying disease[2]. Their total time on arterial access ranged from 70 to 370 days. All devices were inserted under local anaesthesia and can be used immediately. In their series they had no documented incidents of catheter sepsis with this total implantable system. The development of a catheter with a one-way valve should further decrease the incidence of catheter occlusion. The use of these implantable devices in the 1980s will probably replace that of A-V fistulas. Finally, the development of total implantable pumps as pioneered by Dr Henry Bookwald from Minnesota, USA, and others may allow constant infusion over long periods of time of chemotherapeutic agents. At present, most of these implantable pumps are developed for the infusion of insulin and thus are designed for infusion of low volumes only. However, modification of these pumps to include a reservoir which can be filled percutaneously will be an obvious modification in the future. A combination of the components of the inflatable penile prosthesis which include a reservoir and pump with an implantable delivery system could be a readily available system. As most of chemotherapy is still palliative, every effort to allow these patients to receive their chemotherapy at home would obviously be of great value.

The title of this last section of this congress on desperate cases obviously suggests that prevention is better than cure. I have tried to outline some of the pitfalls of vascular access, but it is more important to suggest new approaches so that in the future desperate cases hopefully will be a rarity.

References

1 Conolly, W. B., Murphy, J. B. and Belzer, F. O. (1968). Intravenous feeding by an arterio-venous shunt. *Surg. Forum*, **19**, 383
2 Niederhuber, J. A., Ensinger, W. *et al.* (1982). Totally implanted venous and arterial access systems to replace external catheters in cancer treatment. *Surgery* (In press)

Index

FSC
www.fsc.org
MIX
Papier aus verantwortungsvollen Quellen
Paper from responsible sources
FSC® C105338